Power Plants

POWER PLANTS

New Evidence That
Nature's "Phyto-Fighters"
Are Your Best Medicine

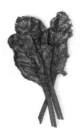 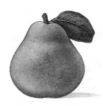 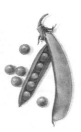

Kim O'Neill, Ph.D. & Byron Murray, Ph.D.

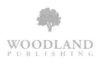

WOODLAND
PUBLISHING

For ordering and information, contact:
Woodland Publishing, P.O. Box 160, Pleasant Grove, UT 84062
(800) 777-2665

A CIP record for this book is available from the Library of Congress.

Note: The information in this book is for education purposes only and is not recommended as a means of diagnosing or treating an illness. All matters concerning physical and mental health should be supervised by a health practitioner knowledgeable in treating that particular condition. Neither the publisher nor author directly or indirectly dispenses medical advice, nor do they prescribe any remedies or assume any responsibility for those who choose to treat themselves.

ISBN 1-58054-351-0

Printed in the United States of America

Please visit our website:
www.woodlandpublishing.com

Contents

Acknowledgments

Our book is not the sole effort of the two individuals whose names appear on the cover. There are many that helped in different ways to bring about this work—from moral support and encouragement to lending expertise in various fields. We have hopefully produced a book that will allow everyone, young and old, to walk away with a greater respect for the health-related benefits of a plant-based diet. We appreciate the support of many colleagues in the field whose research efforts have made invaluable contributions to this book. We have diligently attempted to recognize them in the reference section and throughout the book. For any that we may have inadvertently omitted we apologize in advance.

We would also like to recognize those who assisted us in our library research. These include but are certainly not limited to the following: Lana Fort, Troy Russon, Jina Shin, Hyram La Turner, Stephen Standage, and Travis Torngren. We also appreciate the forbearance and encouragement of our friends, colleagues, and students. We specifically would like to recognize the critical evaluation by Dr. Ron Watson. His expert review and suggestions were greatly appreciated.

It also goes without saying that this book could not have been written without the strong support of our families, especially our wives Allison and Ilene and our children who sacrificed valuable hours in order to let us focus on writing this book.

We are also indebted to the understanding staff at Woodland publishing: Ted Hartman, Calvin "The Undertaker" Harper, Allison Yrungaray, Cord Udall and all others that have helped to bring this book to the public eye. Finally, we would like to thank you, the reader, hoping this book will be a useful tool that you can easily apply in your daily life.

In addition, this book is dedicated to our children; Anu, Shannon, Connor; Ryan, Blake, Dawn, Randall, Brooke, and Dana.

Introduction

I
t may seem unusual for two scientists involved in cancer research
to write a book on phytonutrition. After all, a book on the
healthy benefits of plants would seem a more appropriate topic
for a nutritional biologist or botanist. However, in our combined fifty-
three years in biological research, it has become obvious that the
answer to many of the human diseases has been staring us in the face
for thousands of years—a diet based on fruits and vegetables is one
way to prevent many of the lifestyle and chronic diseases, including
cardiovascular disease, stroke, diabetes, osteoporosis, many forms of
cancer, arthritis and afflictions associated with aging. We both have
vast experience with cancer and diabetes, on both a personal and
clinical level. As have many, we have experienced the loss of a loved
one and the frustration of realizing we can only stand helplessly by
and watch someone we love suffer. These experiences, more than any
others, have been the driving force behind our research.

A Cure for Cancer?

Since much of our research has focused on studying cancer, we
intend to use it as a model for the prevention of other lifestyle and
chronic diseases. However, as our knowledge of molecular biology,

cell biology and immunology increases, it is becoming clear that cancer and other debilitating diseases may never be totally cured; still, we hope that they can be controlled or prevented.

Cancer is a name given to many different diseases, each having its own unique properties and genes involved in the general cancer process. Though we now have a greater understanding of the actual mechanisms behind the production and establishment of a cancer cell, the overall goal of total eradication of cancer cannot and will not take place with the limited knowledge of molecular biology currently available. Our understanding of cancer must increase dramatically before we will be able to conquer it.

This seems well beyond our scope at the present time. Recent scientific findings certainly have enlarged our understanding of the genes involved in the cancer process. Science has discovered and labeled genes involved in cancer as "tumor-suppressor genes" and "oncogenes." Many hoped "gene therapy" (manipulating and correcting defective genes to affect a cure) would already be possible. In order to do this, scientists need to be able to go into each individual cancer cell and alter specific, mutated genes. There have been some successes against cancer, and in certain cases, gene therapy may prove very useful and is showing great promise. But overall, it is quite clear that the war against cancer will not be won only by molecular biology techniques in the near future.

Prevention Is the Only Cure

As we have studied the mechanisms of cancer, we have also watched and read with interest the many different reports on prevention. For many years in the Western world, it has been thought that the best medicine was the one that cured the disease. However when you think about it, it is better to never contract the disease in the first place. For years people have known that cigarette smoking causes many forms of cancer. The American Cancer Society estimates that if everyone stopped smoking, deaths from cancer in the U.S. would drop over 30 percent. One would think this knowledge would make it hard to find a smoker. Sadly, this is not true. There are still many people unable to kick the habit, and still others who do not care to quit. We feel most for those who begin smoking during the "young, invincible years" and find themselves held captive by a weed that will eventually rob them of their most precious possession.

The American Cancer Society also states "about 33 percent of all U.S. cancer deaths can be attributed to the adult diet." In addition, some estimate that if people quit smoking and ate a proper diet based on fruits and vegetables, the cancer incidence would drop by more than 60 percent. That is an impressive statement— *60 percent of cancers are preventable.*

As the evidence mounted on the major role of fruits and vegetables in the prevention of disease, we started to investigate what it is in fruits and vegetables that gives us this protection. That investigation is the basis of this book.

You Can Prevent Cancer

It is very easy for some authors to print testimonies of individuals who experience miraculous cures while on certain regimes of chemicals obtained from fruits and vegetables. However, that is not the aim of this book. While anecdotal evidence and testimonials certainly have their place in society, this book focuses on the science behind the claim that chronic and lifestyle diseases may be prevented by a diet rich in fruits and vegetables. Fruits and vegetables are rich in vitamins, minerals and phytochemicals that enhance your body's defense systems such as the antioxidant mechanism, mitochondrial protection, DNA repair mechanisms, apoptotic systems, metabolic physiology systems and the immune system, enabling you to fight disease-causing agents more efficiently.

Contained within your body are many powerful defense mechanisms that continually function to prevent disease. Many of these systems work together to enhance the body's overall ability to deal with serious assaults from such things as free radicals (discussed in detail later). Science is now beginning to understand the role of phytonutrition and how phytochemicals (the chemicals from plants) function to prevent many diseases. The body has many antioxidant protection mechanisms that are enhanced by phytochemicals. These systems protect proteins, membranes, mitochondria (organelles in your cells that provide energy) and DNA from being damaged by oxidants or free radicals. Much of this protection comes from phytochemicals and allows our biological systems to function correctly to prevent lifestyle diseases such as cancer, heart disease, strokes, etc.

Science is now discovering the important role that phytochemicals play in helping our many defense systems to function and provide protection. This book details many of these mechanisms and provides the scientific research that has helped in their discovery.

For example, the human immune system is one of several protection systems. The immune system functions through interactive cells and bioactive compounds. If our immune system's are weak, then our bodies are more open to disease-causing agents. Our immune system can be affected by stress, aging, nutritional deficiencies, and the environment, to name a few. Fruits and vegetables have been known to enhance the immune system in humans. Fruits and vegetables have been shown to affect many aspects of the immune system.

Two studies were recently conducted that indicated that fruits and vegetables stimulate the immune system. The participants of the study who had their diet enhanced with fruits and vegetables, showed an increase of antibody response and natural killer cell activity. In comparison to the group that ate less fruits and vegetables, the subjects who consumed more fruits and vegetables were less likely to suffer from illness due to infection during that same year.

Foods rich in flavonoids and carotenoids have also been shown to enhance your immune system. These phytochemicals are found in rich abundance in fruits and vegetables. There are many herbal products known to enhance the immune system as well. A few of these include garlic, echinacea, licorice, and cat's claw. Recent studies indicate that garlic can improve the immune system in AIDS patients.

Another study indicates that the consumption of garlic on a regular basis can dramatically reduce the incidence of prostate cancer. Echinacea was initially used for its anti-inflammatory and immunostimulatory activity, but it also promotes the activity of lymphocytes and increases phagocytosis (a process used by immune cells to attack invading bacteria and viruses). Studies have demonstrated that taking echinacea can reduce the severity and duration of flu symptoms. In a recent study, researchers gave HIV patients 200 mg of licorice root. The results indicated the licorice root increased their count of immune helper T-cells and also improved liver function within two months. By making your immune system strong, you are able to decrease your risk of many chronic degenerative diseases.

Other Valuable Resources

This book does not set out to be a comprehensive review of everything written on phytonutrition. In fact, there are many areas we feel we have not covered in appropriate depth. There are many excellent books from established authors we wish to call attention to. Those of you wishing to expand your knowledge beyond this book may look to the following list for interesting and credible information on phytonutrition. We will not provide a complete list, and we apologize in advance to the authors we have not mentioned. Many of these books have served as excellent resources for various chapters in this book. (Many of the authors have several books on the subject. For convenience we only list one but recommend the reader look for other books by the same author.)

Natural Health, Natural Medicine, by Andrew Weil.
The Johns Hopkins Complete Guide to Preventing and Reversing Heart Disease, by Peter Kwiterovich, Jr.
The Vitamin E Factor, by Andreas Papas.
Stopping Cancer Before it Starts, by The American Institute for Cancer Research's Program for Cancer Prevention.
The Importance of Good Nutrition, Herbs and Phytochemicals, by Getty T. Ambau.
The Nutraceutical Revolution, by Richard Firshein.
Antioxidants and Disease Prevention, edited by Harinder S. Garewal.
The Homocysteine Revolution, by Kilmer S. McCully.
Miracle Cures, by Jean Carper.
Reversing Memory Loss, by Vernon H. Mark and Jeffery P. Mark.
Gary Null's Ultimate Anti-Aging Program, by Gary Null.
The Power of Superfoods, by Sam Graci and Harvey Diamond.
The Antioxidant Miracle, by Lester Packer and Carol Colman.
Power Foods, by Stephanie Beling.

The difference between our book and many of these lies in the approach and content. We explain what phytonutrition is and the role of fruits and vegetables in health. Our goals are to first, identify the mechanisms of disease prevention and educate the public to these mechanisms; second, enhance the body's own systems for fighting disease; and third, aid in the early detection of disease.

Preventing Other Major Diseases

The more we study cancer, it is becoming more and more obvious that fruits and vegetables also play a major role in the prevention of all major lifestyle diseases, such as cardiovascular disease, strokes, diabetes, Alzheimer's, arthritis, aging and many others. Our original intent was to write a book on phytonutrition and cancer, but as we began collecting information it became obvious that there are many lifestyle diseases affected by the consumption of fruits and vegetables.

This book also explains the importance of antioxidants, vitamins, and several well-established alternative medicine treatments. For your benefit, we have included a large appendix and glossary to be used as a reference.

Our diets have changed as we have put this book together. The knowledge we have gained while researching this book has changed our outlook on health and nutrition. We hope *Power Plants* will help you change your lifestyle and eating habits, too.

In the end, we hope to present you with basic principles, together with the promise of increased physical, emotional, intellectual and spiritual health. Eating a healthy diet of fruits and vegetables is the single greatest thing you can do to prevent disease and increase the quality of your life. Although no one can be assured they will never contract one of these lifestyle diseases, taking precautions as early as possible in your life and changing your diet can significantly decrease the risks.

Although we focus heavily on the benefits of fruits and vegetables, we are not advocating a strict vegetarian diet. In fact, we feel some red meat in your diet can be healthy. However, we hope this book will make you more prone to order extra fruits and vegetables the next time you sit down to eat in a restaurant.

CHAPTER 1

Promoting Optimal Health Through Phytonutrition

I t has never been easier to eat fruits and vegetables. Our grocery stores and supermarkets are stocked year round with "seasonal" citrus, and the vegetable aisle has everything from avocado to zucchini. And yet, recent surveys and studies indicate that the average American still does not eat enough fruits and vegetables. It seems that we have yet to understand how important they are for healthy living. For example, the average American consumes only one serving of vegetables and one serving of fruit each day. According to a recent survey, two out of three feel two or fewer servings of fruits and vegetables are sufficient for good health. Only one in five children eats the recommended servings of fruits and vegetables. However, even this may be misleading, because nearly one-fourth of all the "vegetables" these children consume are French fries. One researcher found that one in every nine ate no fruits or vegetables on the day they were interviewed.

When it comes to disease of any kind, prevention is always preferable to treatment. As the old adage goes: an ounce of prevention is worth a pound of cure. The dominant trend in conventional science has been to find solutions for problems, rather than to find ways to prevent problems in the first place. However, the trend seems to be changing, and more time, energy and money are now spent on preventive science than ever before.

Emerging Scientific Proof

Numerous studies continue to demonstrate the power of various fruits and vegetables in fighting cancers. The American Cancer Society recently stated that one-third of cancer deaths in the United States could be attributed to diet in adulthood. Many cancers should not be viewed as unpreventable tragedies—the real tragedy is that many deaths caused by cancer could be avoided with a balanced diet.

The Journal of the National Cancer Institute recently reported that men eating three servings of vegetables per day cut their chances of prostate cancer nearly in half. The report claims that cruciferous vegetables (broccoli, cabbage, cauliflower, Brussels sprouts and mustard) seem to be the most potent in combating cancer. A research team at Nagoya City University Medical School and Kyoto University in Japan reports that prostate cancer is directly related to low levels of beta-carotene (found in dark vegetables and fruits).

Another study conducted at the Johns Hopkins School of Hygiene and Public Health found a strong correlation between beta-carotene and decreased risks of lung cancer, melanoma and bladder cancer. A British study found that men who eat garlic at least twice a week have a 50 percent lower risk of prostate cancer than men who never eat garlic.

It seems like every day someone publishes a new study that links diet with cancer prevention. But the benefits of eating fruits and vegetables do not end with cancer.

A balanced diet of fruits and vegetables can also help prevent heart disease, atherosclerosis, Alzheimer's disease, premature aging, memory loss, cardiovascular disease and obesity. In addition, it can also contribute to immune system response, healthy pregnancy, virility, proper growth and emotional health.

Dr. C. Stoney of Ohio University recently reported, "People who have deficiencies in folic acid and the B vitamins are at increased risk for cardiovascular disease." Another study found that high quantities of lutein (found in tomatoes and other vegetables) have been implicated in the prevention of lesions of the heart.

A recent survey from researchers at Cambridge suggests that a healthy diet of seasonal fruits and vegetables dramatically decreases the risk of cardiovascular disease. Swedish researchers conducted a long-term study of middle-aged men and found a strong correlation between daily fruit intake and longer life. A study analyzing the diets of people in Austria, Hungary and Switzerland found a high correlation between the consumption of fruits and vegetables and the length of life: those eating fruits and vegetables live longer.

A high fruit and vegetable diet has recently been linked to reductions in risk for atherosclerosis, angina, diabetes, stroke and loss of sight. Dietary fiber (available in most fruits and vegetables) has been demonstrated to decrease the risk of coronary heart disease in women. A recent study in Poland credits changes in diet (specifically the increase in available fruits and vegetables) to a sharp decrease in deaths caused by heart disease. A study conducted in 1999 indicates that a diet providing eight to ten fruits and two to three low-fat dairy products per day significantly reduces blood pressure.

There are literally hundreds of similar studies indicating that an increased consumption of the right fruits and vegetables profoundly decreases blood pressure.

Which Foods Are the Best Foods?

In choosing which foods to eat it is important to keep several factors in mind. A good diet is a balanced diet—adequate, varied, moderated, dense in nutrients, and not too high or too low in calories. Nutritional needs change according to age, gender, stage of life (pregnancy, development) and weight. Therefore it is important to keep in mind that an appropriate diet for one person may not meet the nutritional needs of others. However, recommendations on diet seem to come back to a few basic principles dealing with the most important aspects of health:

- Don't smoke.
- Maintain appropriate body weight.
- Make sure your energy intake is equal to or less than your energy output.
- Eat a wide variety of foods.
- Consume complex carbohydrates.
- Reduce fat (mainly saturated fats) in the diet.
- Eat more fiber, fruits and vegetables.
- Eat less cholesterol.
- Eat less sodium.
- Abstain from alcohol or drink it only in moderation.

As the American public becomes more conscious of health and image, many different diets have become wildly popular. On one hand, these include low-carbohydrate/high-protein diets, and on the other hand there are low-protein/high-carbohydrate diets. There are also many kinds of vegetarian diets, liquid diets, combination food diets, timed diets—the list goes on and on. All of these diets promise, and often result in, great weight loss in the beginning; however, they often sacrifice proper nutrition, which is much more important than simply looking good and losing weight.

Often, the lack of complete nutrition from these diets stresses your body more than the extra weight you just lost. Do not rely on a crash diet cycle to stay thin; rather, make your diet a part of your lifestyle. That is, when you take a look at the foods you eat, you need to make decisions based on long-term health goals. A successful diet must be comfortable for you for the rest of your life. We suggest that you ensure your diet follows the basic guidelines provided by the United States Department of Agriculture's (USDA) Food Guide Pyramid. The Food Guide Pyramid not only serves as a guideline for what kinds and amounts of food to eat, but it also encourages you to eat a variety of foods within each food group. It is not enough to simply eat five apples to meet your body's nutrient needs from the fruit and vegetable group. It is important to eat a few different types of fruit to meet your body's needs.

Principles of Nutrition

Before actually getting into the ways that fruits and vegetables prevent disease, we need to take a look at general principles of nutri-

High Green Vegetable Intake Reduces Cancer Risk

In a study of 367 males and 240 females published in the May 2001 issue of the *British Journal of Cancer*, scientists concluded, "Decreased odds ratios for squamous cell and small cell carcinomas were observed in males with frequent consumption of raw and green vegetables, fruit and milk." This study also suggests cooked/raw fish consumption lowers the risk of adenocarcinoma of the lung in Japanese subjects.

tion. Nutrients are elements that regulate body processes, and provide energy and building materials. Nutrients can be organized into six groups: carbohydrates, fats (lipids), proteins, water, vitamins and minerals. These nutrients are further broken down into two categories depending on how we obtain them. Nutrients the body must obtain from food are known as essential nutrients. Nutrients the body makes itself are known as nonessential nutrients.

In order to operate at optimal health and performance levels, we require roughly forty to fifty nutrients from all the six groups. These nutrients give energy to the body and work together to extract more nutrients from food. All must be present for healthy living. The body can derive all the energy, structural materials and regulating agents it needs from the food we eat, as long as our diet provides enough of them.

However, if you fail to eat foods rich in a variety of nutrients, you force your body to operate without important elements. Continual nutritional deficiency leads to disease; on the other hand, a healthy diet rich in various nutrients prevents disease and maintains health.

A variety of foods are essential to ensure that you are getting all of the required nutrients to maintain health. No single food has the right amount or kinds of nutrients to sustain life. Nutrients will often interact with each other to perform important functions; so when there is a deficiency in one necessary nutrient, many processes may suffer. For example, vitamin D, calcium and phosphorus are required for bone formation. A lack of any one of these nutrients will inhibit the formation, growth or repair of bones.

Still, we have a long way to go in understanding how the interaction of various nutrients promotes good health. We agree with the statement, "To extract one particular component of a healthy diet and think people can replicate the benefits by taking a pill is usually a fallacy. Instead of an exclusive focus on individual nutrients, I like the idea of looking at the whole diet."

History Will Repeat Itself

As we see in history, even the smallest changes in diet have played a great part in preventing disease. The eradication of scurvy was the result of a small change in diet—sailors started eating citrus fruits, and the rest is history. We honestly foresee similar progress in the war with cancer, cardiovascular disease and other destructive illnesses. The idea here is that eating a healthy and balanced diet will prevent many diseases before they get started. Again, prevention is preferable to treatment.

In order to better understand how nutrients function, we need to look more closely at macronutrients, micronutrients and non-nutrients. There are fruits and vegetables that provide the macronutrients, micronutrients, water and non-nutrients necessary to maintain a healthy life.

Macronutrients

Macronutrients are nutrients that are needed in large amounts. They produce energy (measured in calories) for physical activities and assist in the chemical reactions that occur in living cells, and provide building blocks for tissues. Macronutrients are divided into three categories: carbohydrates, lipids and proteins. (See Appendix A for more information on macronutrients.)

CARBOHYDRATES

Carbohydrates keep our digestive systems fit, feed our brains and nervous systems, and keep our bodies lean (within correct calorie limits). There are two types of carbohydrates, simple and complex. Simple carbohydrates are sugars; i.e., relatively small compounds of carbon, hydrogen and oxygen that form the basic source of fuel for our bodies. Sugar molecules are frequently referred to as carbohydrates because of their carbon and hydrogen components. Simple carbohydrates are readily absorbed in the body, meaning that enzymes found on the tongue digest them. In times of need, the body can use other molecules as its fuel source, but it prefers sugars when they are available.

If carbohydrates were necessary solely as an energy source there would be no reason to prefer fruits, vegetables and whole grains to candy. When it comes right down to it, the body will utilize the concentrated sugars in candy as an energy source as readily as the sugar in fruits, vegetables and whole grains. However, there are many compelling reasons to prefer fruits, vegetables and whole grains. Not only are they sources of carbohydrates, but they are excellent sources of vitamins, proteins, minerals and many other health-promoting chemicals.

Though the sugar in candy is able to fuel the body and provides necessary calories, it is unable to provide the body with fiber as efficiently as fruits, vegetables and whole grains. Fiber is a complex carbohydrate that is indigestible. There are many problems associated with eating foods dense in calories but deficient in fiber. First, foods lacking fiber will not provide satiety as well as foods high in fiber. In other words, you can eat a lot more candy before feeling full than you can fruits, vegetables and whole grains. If you eat more sugar than your body will use for fuel then the excess sugar is converted to fat, leading to unhealthy weight gain and eventually obesity—a serious health condition.

On the other hand, a diet with adequate fiber intake can foster weight control, lower blood cholesterol, help prevent colon cancer, diabetes, appendicitis and diverticulosis (the formation of small pockets in the intestines) and can alleviate hemorrhoids. Though a diet low in fiber is not healthy, a diet too high in fiber is unhealthy as well. It is important to eat a balanced diet to ensure that the proper amounts of nutrients are available, avoiding extremes in deficiency or excess. Too much fiber in a diet can interfere with mineral absorption and energy production. It is essential that your diet include a variety of foods rich in fiber because there are two different types of fiber.

FAT

Another important macronutrient is fat. Fats, or lipids, are absolutely necessary for good health. Fat is the primary form of energy storage; it acts as a shock absorber for vital organs; it maintains skin and hair; it stores and transports fat-soluble vitamins; it protects cell walls; and it keeps our bodies warm.

There are two basic kinds of fats: saturated and unsaturated. Saturated fats have all the hydrogen atoms they can hold. They are appropriately named because they are saturated with hydrogen. Thus, they are highly efficient for storing energy because they utilize more bonds. Unsaturated fats do not have all of the hydrogen atoms they are capable of holding. So, unsaturated fats are not as efficient for storing energy as saturated fats. However, the key here is not efficiency as much as it is balance. Though saturated fats are more efficient in storing energy, they are very unhealthy.

Saturated fats are among the most prevalent fats in our diet. They are found in animal foods like meat, poultry, dairy products, and even in tropical oils like palm and coconut. Unsaturated fats

are found in vegetable oils (olive, canola, peanut, safflower, sunflower and soybean), nuts and in fatty fish.

You have probably heard of many different words relating to
fat: monounsaturated, polyunsaturated, triglycerides, lipids, fatty
acids, LDL, HDL and cholesterol. When talking of unsaturated fat,
it is helpful to keep in mind that there are only two kinds of unsaturated fats: monounsaturated fats are unsaturated fats with one
double bond, while polyunsaturated fats are unsaturated fats with
two or more double bonds. Unsaturated fats are further divided
into monounsaturated fatty acids and polyunsaturated fatty acids.
Monounsaturated fatty acids are mostly found in vegetable oils
(olive, canola, and peanut). Polyunsaturated fatty acids are found
in nuts and other vegetable oils (safflower, sunflower, and soybean)
and in fatty fish.

Occasionally there is a study or discussion revolving around
alpha-linolenic and linoleic acids. Both alpha-linolenic acid and
linoleic acid are polyunsaturated fats, coming from two entirely different families of polyunsaturated fatty acids. Alpha-linolenic acid
is part of the omega-3 family and linoleic acid is part of the omega-
6 family. These two essential fatty acids supply the basic components, or precursors, to other crucial polyunsaturated fatty acids.

Even though it is important to decrease saturated fat intake, it's
also important to keep fat intake in perspective. Do not consume
either an excessive or deficient amount of fat. We will discuss fats
in greater detail in chapter 4.

PROTEIN

Proteins are made up of long strings of smaller molecules
called amino acids. Our bodies use twenty basic amino acids to
form proteins. These chains of amino acids fold and twist into special shapes that allow the proteins they comprise to perform
important structural and mechanical duties. Many proteins are
made of long chains of amino acids, often 200 in length. Different
proteins are made up of different sequences of amino acids.

COMPLETE PROTEINS

Proteins that utilize all twenty amino acids in various sequences
are known as *complete*. They can be found in meat, fish, poultry,
eggs, milks and soy products. These proteins have all of the essential amino acids needed for the body.

INCOMPLETE PROTEINS

On the other hand, proteins that are lacking in one or more amino acid are known as *incomplete*. Incomplete proteins are found in foods from plants. Eating a variety of fruits, vegetables, nuts, grains and beans makes a full compliment of amino acids as each plant food supplies the missing amino acid that others lack.

There are two basic divisions of proteins based on their activities. *Working proteins* include enzymes, antibodies, transport vehicles, hormones, cellular "pumps," and oxygen carriers. In essence, these proteins perform all the hard chemical labor that keeps us alive.

STRUCTURAL PROTEINS

Structural proteins include ligaments, bone and teeth cores, scars, filaments of hair, materials of toenails and fingernails, and more. Keratin, for example, is a fibrous protein that contributes to the structure of our hair, nails and skin. Hemoglobin is a protein in the blood with a special shape allowing it to carry oxygen from the lungs to the outer parts of the body.

Proteins are very versatile and are important because growth and maintenance are dependent on them. Proteins regulate the fluid and mineral composition of body fluids and act as buffers to maintain an appropriate acid-base balance. Proteins provide some fuel for the body's energy needs and help transport needed substances in the body (lipids, minerals and oxygen).

It is important to make sure that your diet supplies you with an adequate amount of protein. The best way to get enough protein is eating a variety of fruits, vegetables, nuts, grains, beans, meats, poultry and eggs.

WATER

Next to oxygen, water is the most essential element to life. The average individual can go without food for eight weeks, but can only last a few days without water. Sixty percent of an average adult's body weight is made up of water. The ratio is even higher for infants and children. Water mass generally decreases with age. Some of the most important functions of water are not involved in either the creation of energy or the construction or repair of body tissue directly. However, water is indirectly involved in almost everything that happens within the body. Water transports nutrients, removes waste, regulates body temperature, lubricates the eye, cushions tissues and sets the stage for vital chemical reactions. Because water is involved in all of these various processes, you need to make sure that you maintain a suitable water balance. Water balance occurs when you have enough water in your body to do all the various things that require water.

Without drinking 8 to 12 cups of water per day, your body would not have enough water to perform basic tasks. If you fail to drink enough water you risk dehydration and kidney damage. When dehydrated, your body does not have enough water to dilute the waste products in urine, causing the kidneys to work with waste build-up. Water acts to transport nutrients because it is a good solvent. In other words, nutrients dissolve into the water in the blood and are then carried throughout the body in order to be used by cells.

The quantity of minerals consumed in a diet has a direct bearing on the amount of water that must be ingested. Blood itself is about 85 to 90 percent water. When nutrients are absorbed into the blood supply, they are then transported throughout the body. Blood also moves nutrients to the cells of the body tissues and removes metabolic waste products from cells.

The water in the blood collects waste product from cells as it circulates and brings them to the kidneys. The kidneys work as the trash can for the body, filtering wastes and concentrating them. Water serves two important purposes in the removal of waste from the body. First it transports waste to the kidneys, and second it helps the kidneys dilute wastes, keeping them from becoming toxic.

Water also helps regulate body temperature through perspiration. It rests on your skin and lowers the temperature of the body through evaporation. It works much like a swamp cooler. The energy of heat is converted into motion in water molecules, which then carry off the heat with them when they are blown around. Water's main function is to act as a medium for cellular biochemical and physical reactions. Water is essential for body tissues and acts as a regulator—aiding in multiple metabolic functions. Water is an integral part of the structure of the soft tissues of the body.

Drinking water may contain both beneficial and harmful compounds. The beneficial ones include trace minerals such as calcium, magnesium, etc. Chlorine is beneficial as a treatment to kill harmful organisms, but it also may have long-term side effects that are unknown at this time. The best source of drinking water is filtered or spring water.

Also, there is considerable controversy regarding the use of fluoride in drinking water due to the possible harmful health effects of toxic fluoride compounds. Other known harmful compounds include heavy metals (lead and mercury), nitrates and organic chemicals (pesticides). Since vegetables and fruits are 60 to 98 percent water, they serve as a good source of dietary fluids.

Micronutrients

The next group of nutrients, micronutrients, is composed of vitamins and minerals. They do not provide energy or build tissue, but they are needed to get energy from macronutrients and are necessary for numerous cellular biochemical reactions. Micronutrients are called such because they are needed in smaller quantities than macronutrients.

VITAMINS

Vitamins are organic compounds required for body functions. They are needed in very small amounts. Like water, vitamins are not broken down to produce energy. Vitamins help our bodies perform a number of different functions. It is necessary to eat foods rich in vitamins because there is no other way to get them in sufficient quantities to promote and maintain life. If you do not get enough of a specific vitamin, you will begin to show signs of deficiency.

Vitamins	
Fat Soluble	**Water Soluble**
vitamin A	vitamin C
vitamin D	thiamin (B1)
7-Dehydrocholesterol	riboflavin (B2)
vitamin D2	niacin
vitamin D3	vitamin B6
vitamin E	folic acid
vitamin K	cobalamin (B12)
phylloquinone (K1)	pantothenic acid
menaquinone-n (K2)	biotin
menadione (K3)	pyridoxine

The degree and seriousness of vitamin deficiencies depend upon the extent of the deficiency and the vitamin you are missing in your diet. However, symptoms of deficiency can be relieved when the vitamin is included in the diet.

In the early 1900s, it became quite popular in the East to eat polished rice—rice without the shell. Unfortunately, as this practice became more and more popular, there was a marked increase in a disease known as beriberi. The symptoms associated with beriberi are loss of feeling and stiffness in the limbs, paralysis, muscular weakness and abnormal heart movements. Scientists hunted for a cause for beriberi for years—assuming it was a disease caused by nondietary factors. However, they finally traced the increase in beriberi to the change in rice. They discovered that a nutrient, thiamine (B vitamin), found in the shell of rice was necessary to maintain health. In 1912, a biochemist named Casimir Funk was studying this anti-beriberi micronutrient and realized this nutrient had a particular chemical structure known as an amine. He decided to call it a "vital-amine" because it was necessary for life. "Vital" is Latin for "life." In time, the name for this and similar nutrients was shortened to *vitamin.*

Our body needs thirteen different kinds of vitamins to work properly, each vitamin performing its own specific function. They are vitamin A, C, D, E, K and eight B-complex vitamins: B12, folate, B6, biotin, riboflavin, pantothenic acid, niacin and thiamin. Vitamins are complex and sensitive organic molecules. They can

Minerals

Macrominerals	Microminerals
calcium	iron
phosphorus	zinc
magnesium	iodine
sulfur	selenium
sodium	fluoride
potassium	copper
chloride	cobalt
	chromium
	manganese
	molybdenum

be damaged and even destroyed by heat, light and chemical agents. Vitamins can only function when they are intact. Almost every action in the body requires the assistance of vitamins. The vitamins' roles in supporting optimal health in the body extend far beyond preventing deficiency diseases. Almost all vitamins must be obtained from food because the body cannot manufacture them. Chapters 6 and 7 will address the importance of the two kinds of vitamins: fat soluble and water soluble.

MINERALS

Minerals are also extremely important in the maintenance of health. Like water and vitamins, minerals do not provide energy or building materials to your body. Minerals are inorganic (without carbon) compounds needed only in small amounts. At least sixteen minerals are essential to human nutrition. They are divided into two types of minerals: macrominerals and trace minerals.

Macrominerals are essential nutrients found in the body in amounts larger than five grams. The macrominerals are calcium, chloride, magnesium, phosphorus, potassium, sodium and sulfur. On the other hand, trace minerals are essential nutrients found in the body in amounts less than 5 grams. The trace minerals are chromium, copper, iron, fluoride, iodine, manganese, molybdenum, selenium and zinc. Although minerals are chemically indestructible, they can be lost if you don't take care in preparing foods. They also can be bound to substances that make absorption difficult. Each mineral works both individually and with other minerals. In other words, these minerals each have unique functions but also work together to do important things for the body.

Minerals fulfill several important missions in the human body. They preserve the body's structural skeleton, control the water balance in the body and regulate the acid-base balance of body fluids. Minerals also act as a catalyst in body reactions, facilitate nerve impulses and muscular contractions, and act as a component of hormones, vitamins, enzymes and other chemical compounds of the body. No one food contains all the minerals needed. Thus, a varied diet is necessary to provide an adequate mineral selection for good health.

PHYTOCHEMICALS

Phytochemicals are essential, non-nutrient plant chemicals found in plant foods. There are thousands of phytochemicals.

They are named based on their varying structures, though this area of science is so new that it has yet to have an established naming system. We will discuss the following phytochemicals in detail in subsequent chapters: alkaloids, carotenoids, flavonoids, indoles, organosulfurs, phenolics, phytosterols, saponins, tannins and terpenoids. Like vitamins and minerals, there is no single plant that is a source for all the necessary phytochemicals. This is why we recommend a diet rich in a variety of plants and vegetables. Different plants produce and utilize different kinds and quantities of phytochemicals.

Phytochemicals serve many different functions: some are antioxidants, helping to prevent disease, slow aging, and combat cancer and other diseases. Some help decrease cholesterol levels, prevent cancer cells from multiplying, and prevent cell damage. In fact, the most important thing to remember about phytochemicals is that they work to prevent disease and damage to your body. The real benefit to eating a diet rich in phytochemicals is that your body will be more capable of maintaining good health. In addition to increasing your ability to prevent disease, eating a healthy diet rich in phytochemicals will actually help you overcome diseases you may already have.

The Best Foods to Eat

So just what should you be eating? It may be helpful to clarify a few terms that have been circulating in the health-food industry: fortification, supplementation, and functional foods. Fortification is the addition of nutrients to a food product. The U.S. government is requiring an increasing number of foods to be fortified as we gain understanding of the body's needs. Supplements are sources of nutrients separate from food products either synthesized artificially or extracted from natural sources. A functional food is any food with a health benefit.

Nutritional supplementation is one of today's more popular health trends. However, it's important to distinguish between supplementation designed to ensure adequate nutrition and supplementation touting miraculous gains. A casual perusal of the "health food" section of any grocery store or any of the growing number of "health food" stores across the country will demonstrate the overwhelming variety and quantity of supplements available today. Many claim almost unbelievable benefits from a few pills or a tasty shake. Although these supplements are often useful or even necessary tools, a balanced diet based on whole foods is still the best way to adequate nutrition.

Too Much of a Good Thing?

First, it is possible to eat too much of a good thing. Megadosing, the process of taking extremely high concentrations of vitamins or minerals, is a dangerous practice. It can place unnatural stress on various organs and may cause serious illness and even death. Often people will take megadoses in order to protect against deficiency. However, overdoses can be just as dangerous as deficiencies. For example, megadoses of vitamins C and A have been shown to have harmful effects on the body. Megadosing on vitamin C can lead to lung cancer, and megadosing on vitamin A can cause blindness. Use caution in using supplements proclaiming their value with terms like "natural" and "phytochemical."

The word "natural" in supplementation often implies that a product is harmless. This could be very deceptive. In addition to finding healthy and beneficial nutrients in "natural" states, it is also possible to get potent narcotics and deadly poisons in "natural" forms. Cocaine is a "natural" chemical found in the coca leaf of South and Central America. Plants can be both nutritious and poisonous. To say that a particular supplement is "natural" says little about its fitness for consumption.

Many supplements now tout the value of "phytochemicals." Much like the use of the term "natural," "phytochemical" is often used to imply value, healthiness and safety. However, strictly speaking, to call something a *phytochemical* says almost nothing about its value to you as a health food. It merely says that something is a chemical produced by a plant. In this sense, it is not wholly inaccurate to say that opium is a phytochemical. But in science, *phytochemical* is usually used to denote only certain plant chemicals that studies have shown to have preventative and/or therapeutic potential. Others use *phytochemical* to refer to plant chemicals from fruits and vegetables only (excluding herbs, grains, nuts and beans), and still others use it to denote chemicals that have anticancer potential.

Often claims made by supplement producers are based on

"ancient" practices of various cultures and peoples. We are not claiming that the practices and understanding of herbs and curative medicinal therapies of folk traditions are invalid. In fact, much of what we now know about the various benefits of herbs, plants and vegetables as curatives comes from folk remedies and traditional practices. However, there are many claims and traditions that boast therapeutic effects, but hold no scientific value.

Recent turns toward preventive research in the sciences have focused attention on the various benefits of eating well. Hopefully, this book will help you become a more knowledgeable consumer, make you more capable of understanding the claims circulating in the health-food industry, and help you to choose components of a balanced diet that will meet your body's needs.

References

American Cancer Society Dietary Guidelines May 8 1997. Cancer—Eating To Beat The Odds.

Carolyn Katzin. Cancer and Nutrition: What is the Connection? 1997–99. Copyright © 1998, 1999 [foodandlife.com].

Eleanor Noss Whitney, Sharon Rady Rolfes. Understanding Nutrition. West Publishing Company, New York 1996.

Fances Sizer , MS, RD, FADA and Eleanor Whitney, PhD. Nutrition Concepts and Controversies. West/ Wadsworth: An International Thomson Publishing Company, Washington 1997.

Getty T. Ambau. The Importance of Good Nutrition, Herbs, and Phytochemicals for Your Health, Good Looks, and Longevity. Falcon Press International. CA, 1997.

Hegarty, Vincent Ph.D. Nutrition, Food, and the Environment. Minnesota: Eagan Press, 1993.

J. A. Milner. Functional Foods and Health Promotion. Nutrition Department and Graduate Program in Nutrition, The Pennsylvania State University, University Park, PA 16802.

Katherine Mitchell, BA. And Margaret Cowden Bernard BS. Food in Health and Disease. FA Davis Company, Philadelphia 1995.

LE Lloyd, BE McDonald, EW Crampton. Fundamentals in Nutrition. WH Freeman and Company, San Francisco 1978.

Martha Davis Dunn MS Public Health Nutrition, MPA. Fundamentals in Nutrition. CBI Publishing Company, INC. Mass 1983.

Martin Eastwood Principles of Human Nutrition: University of Edinburgh, Western General Hospital, Edinburgh, UK. Chapman and Hall, UK 1997.

Maurice E Shils, James A. Olson, Moshe Shike, A. Catherine Ross. Modern Nutrition in Health and Diseases. Maryland: Williams and Wilkins, 1999.

Richard A. Knox. New Research Backs A Balanced Diet. Source: NY Times Syndicate Wednesday, April 26, 2000.

Ronald M Deutsch and Judi S Morrill, Ph.D. Realities of Nutrition. Bull publishing Company, California 1993.

Rosemary C. Fisher. Some Recent Research About Foods and Cancer.

Sam Graci and Harvey Diamond. The Power of Superfood. Prentice Hall Canada Inc. Ontario 1999.

Stephanie Beling, MD. Power Foods. Harper Perennial. New York 1998.

The American Dietetic Association. Excerpts from The American Dietetic Association's Complete Food & Nutrition Guide.OSU

CHAPTER 2

Choosing the Right Phytonutrition Plan

Plants contain thousands of phytochemicals, and scientists are discovering more each year. It sounds like a lot to include in your diet, but there can be over 100 different kinds of phytochemicals in just one serving of vegetables. They include: carotenoids, capsaicin, flavonoids, indoles, isoflavones and protease inhibitors. Different plants supply different kinds and amounts of phytochemicals.

Certain phytochemicals are known for their aid in protection against cancers, heart disease and other chronic health conditions. A diet of a variety of fruits, vegetables, legumes and grains is the best way to get these phytochemicals. In general, the darker the leaf or the brighter the fruit or vegetable, the richer it is in phytochemicals. The carotenoids, for example, are responsible for the red, orange and yellow plant pigments that give fruits and vegetables their vivid colors. They are also found in dark-green leafy vegetables (such as spinach, collards, kale, mustard greens, and turnip greens), broccoli, carrots, pumpkins and calabasa, red peppers, sweet potatoes and tomatoes. Fruits like mangos, papayas and cantaloupes are also rich in carotenoids. In plants, carotenoids function as storage sites for solar energy to support photosynthesis, the process used by plants to make energy. In humans, carotenoids play a key role in immune system support and enhancement.

Plant-Based Diets Reduce Risk of Heart Disease

A recent study published in the December 2000 issue of the *Journal of the American Dietetic Association* states, "Epidemiologic evidence of a protective role for fruits and vegetables in cancer prevention is substantial. Current scientific evidence also suggests a protective role for fruits and vegetables in prevention of coronary heart disease, and evidence is accumulating for a protective role in stroke.

"In addition, a new scientific base is emerging to support a protective role for fruits and vegetables in prevention of cataract formation, chronic obstructive pulmonary disease, diverticulosis, and possibly, hypertension. Continued attention to increasing fruit and vegetable consumption is a practical and important way to optimize nutrition to reduce disease risk and maximize good health."

It is best to obtain these nutrients from whole foods rather than supplements. Many studies suggest that foods, not supplements, should be our main source of phytochemicals and other nutrient compounds. A variety of foods are important in obtaining all the essential nutrients necessary to maintain proper health.

Scientists are identifying the nutrients or phytochemicals found in fruits, grains, and vegetables that protect us from diseases. If all of the protective agents found in fruit were isolated, it would be possible to make a pill and take it as a supplement. However, science is far from determining how fruits and vegetables act in protecting us from many disabling diseases. Part of the problem is that fruits and vegetables contain literally thousands of chemicals. An apple, for example, contains thousands of different phytochemicals, each interacting with one another, making isolation very difficult.

While some think we could just take pills with manufactured or synthetic phytochemicals, it is very likely that the chemicals in plants are healthier than synthesized compounds. Recent studies indicate that many phytochemicals found in fruits and vegetables act together to protect the human body from the formation of cancers and heart disease. It is important to note that science has begun to understand that fruits and vegetables are instrumental in protecting you from disease, but science has yet to know all of the reasons why, or what it is in fruits and vegetables that is protective.

For this reason, it is important to eat a balanced and varied diet of whole foods, rather than relying solely on supplements.

Six Variables of a Healthy Diet

A healthy diet will have six different variables: adequacy, balance, calorie control, nutrient density, moderation, and variety. By adequacy we mean a diet must provide sufficient energy and nutrients to meet the needs of the body. By balance we mean a diet must provide a variety of foods in order to be adequate. To control your calorie intake, you need to pick foods that are nutrient dense and balance the amount of calories in the foods and drinks you consume with the amount of calories the body uses. Nutrient density is closely related to calorie control. Fruits and vegetables are denser in nutrients than candy bars or meat products. It also happens that fruits and vegetables are less dense in calories. Not only does eating fruits and vegetables ensure you receive adequacy, but it also prevents you from having an imbalance in caloric intake/expenditure. By moderation we simply encourage you to eat sweets and fatty foods sparingly. Finally, a healthy diet must include variety. Different foods contain different nutrients. Healthy diets contain the amounts of essential nutrients and calories needed to prevent nutritional deficiencies and excesses. They also provide the right balance of carbohydrates, fats and proteins.

The Right Diet for You

It is important to select an appropriate diet. You have to recognize that you are different from other people and may thus require a unique diet to ensure adequate health. There are outside factors that have a direct impact on what and how you eat. This can range from food availability and socioeconomic conditions to culture. In the end, you alone can decide what kind of diet you will be able to stick with. We would encourage you to think of your diet as a lifelong commitment. It is not a matter of losing 5 pounds, or even 40 pounds, to be able to wear your swimsuit. It is a matter of living a healthy lifestyle.

The Standards of Health

An adequate and balanced diet meets all your nutritional needs for maintenance, repair, life, growth and development. You should acquire all your energy and nutrient needs through food and supplementation following the Food Guide Pyramid. The Food Guide Pyramid is a guidance system created by the U.S. Department of Agriculture (USDA) in 1992 and is supported by the Department of Health and Human Services (HHS). This pyramid was based on research conducted by the USDA on foods Americans consume, nutrients supplied in these foods, and how we can choose the best foods for a healthy diet. The Food Guide Pyramid recommends food intakes our bodies need for optimal performance. The U.S. Food Guide Pyramid is designed to decrease the amount of fat in a diet. It is thus a response to a common problem: high-fat diets.

Obesity is becoming more and more common, and the pyramid guides us to consume fewer fats: mainly saturated fats, alcohol, sodium, sugar and cholesterol.

The Food Guide Pyramid works well in conjunction with nutrition labels found on food products marketed and sold in the United States. These labels make it easier to follow basic recommendations made by the Federal Nutrition Board.

Dietary Reference Intakes (DRI)

In 1941, the Federal Nutrition Board (FNB) established the Recommended Dietary Allowances (RDA), which serves as a goal for individuals planning a diet, not as a benchmark of adequacy of diets for a population. The RDAs were revised in 1989. In 1993, the FNB introduced the Dietary Reference Intakes (DRI), which consists of four different types of nutrient recommendations for healthy people. These DRIs provide helpful information for people trying to plan a healthy diet. Taken together they indicate a range of nutritional needs from a bare minimum to the maximum amount of a nutrient short of overdose. The four categories are based on the specificity and reliability of the information they provide. The four DRIs are: Adequate Intake (AI), Estimated Average Requirement (EAR), Recommended Dietary Allowances (RDA), and the Tolerable Upper Intake Level (UL).

ADEQUATE INTAKE (AI)

The Adequate Intake (AI) indicates the bare minimum amount of a nutrient necessary for basic health. The Adequate Intake is based on experiments and observations that lack rigorous scientific specificity. They are thus less accurate than the other measures, but nonetheless stand as a reliable guide for dietary planning when there is no EAR, UL or RDA available.

ESTIMATED AVERAGE REQUIREMENT (EAR)

The Estimated Average Requirement (EAR) indicates the average amount of a nutrient necessary for healthy individuals. This measure is set based on a functional or clinical assessment made with specific controls. The EAR is most appropriately used to assess whether a population as a whole is getting an appropriate amount of a particular nutrient and is less helpful for planning an individual diet.

UPPER INTAKE LEVEL (UL)

The Tolerable Upper Intake Level (UL) indicates the maximum amount of a nutrient a person can eat while still avoiding/reducing the risk of toxicity. It is important to take the UL into account when planning your diet to ensure that you do not overdose on a particular nutrient.

RECOMMENDED DIETARY ALLOWANCE (RDA)

The Recommended Dietary Allowance indicates the optimal amount of nutrients necessary for health based on a diet of 1,500 to 2,000 calories. RDAs are often split into two separate categories for men and women. This is because the nutrient needs of men and women are different in important ways. In fact, nutrient needs differ in people according to age, gender, stage of life (pregnancy, lactation) and weight. This is one reason that the RDAs are based on a standard calorie level, though it is important to recognize that every person may need to adjust the RDA to appropriately meet their own personal nutrient needs.

The Food Guide Pyramid

In addition to these Dietary Reference Intakes, the government has other resources available for planning a healthy diet. The Food Guide Pyramid, for example, is broken up into five major cate-

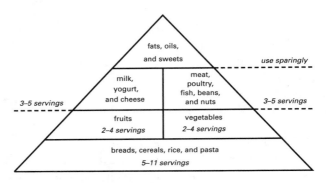

Figure 2.1 The Food Guide Pyramid

gories according to basic kinds of food groups. Each group provides important nutrients, though no individual food group provides all the nutrients needed to promote and maintain a healthy lifestyle. Food in one layer of the Food Guide Pyramid cannot replace another layer.

LAYER 1

At the base of the pyramid are breads, cereals, rice and pasta. The average adult should consume six to eleven servings of these foods per day. Breads, cereals, rice, and pasta are important in a healthy diet because they provide energy through complex carbohydrates, which provide fiber, minerals and vitamins. Generally, these foods themselves are not as fattening as many people believe. However, they are often prepared in ways that lead to a high fat content. The addition of butter, meats and cheese make these dishes high in fat. If you want to prevent the high-fat that often accompanies them, choose to prepare these foods with low-fat alternatives to high-fat additions: use lean meats, butter substitutes or unsaturated fatty oils, and go easy on the cheese.

In general, a serving size of breads, cereals, grains, etc., is the following:

- 1 slice of bread
- 1 ounce of cereal
- 1/2 cup cooked rice or pasta

LAYER 2

The next layer is divided into two separate categories: fruits and vegetables. Three to five servings of vegetables are recommended per day, while two to four servings of fruits are recommended.

Fruits are important in a healthy diet because they provide the necessary vitamins, minerals, phytochemicals and fiber.. Frozen, canned, or fresh, fruits are rich in vitamins A and C, and in the mineral potassium and are excellent sources of vitamins and minerals.

In a study conducted by the University of Illinois, the nutrient values of frozen, fresh, and canned vegetables and fruits were compared using both the USDA's nutrient database and nutrition label claims. The results of this study indicate that canned vegetables and fruits have equivalent nutritional values in most cases. However, the biggest difference between canned and fresh fruit is in the fiber content. Most of the fiber in fruit is found in the skin— a part of the fruit usually left out in the canning process. Whole, fresh fruits are therefore recommended over canned fruits, because of the differences between them in fiber content.

In general, a serving size of fruit is as follows:

- 1 medium sized fruit (apple, banana, or orange)
- 1/2 cup chopped, cooked or canned fruit
- 3/4 cup of 100 percent fruit juice

Vegetables are also rich in vitamins, minerals, phytochemicals and fiber. They also contain some proteins and are naturally low in fat and sodium. It is better to consume dark-green or deep orange and yellow vegetables because they are rich in nutrients.

There is growing evidence that vegetables are essential to preventing disease and maintaining health. In particular, broccoli, Brussels sprouts, carrots, garlic, peas, red peppers, spinach, squash and sweet potatoes seem to have power to guard against lifestyle diseases. Vegetables contain phytochemicals that are valuable antioxidants. Antioxidants are known for their ability to control free-radical damage. Free radicals are highly reactive compounds produced by the body through normal metabolism, pollution, cigarette smoke, radiation, UV light, alcohol, and pesticides that can damage cells, often causing cancer, eye damage and heart disease.

Vegetables are rich in vitamins and minerals. Vitamins A, C, folate (folic acid and folacin), B1 (thiamin), B2 (riboflavin), B5 (pantothenic acid), B6 (pyridoxine) and small amounts of vitamin E are all found in vegetables. Vegetables are also rich in minerals, iron being the only mineral not concentrated in vegetables. Vegetables can be a good source of calcium. For example, green beans contain about 36 milligrams for every 100 grams eaten. Vegetables are an important source of beta-carotene (vitamin A).

In general, a serving size of vegetables is as follows:

- 1 cup raw, leafy vegetable
- 1/2 cup chopped or cooked vegetable
- 3/4 cup vegetable juice

LAYER 3

The next layer consists of the animal foods: dairy and meats. These foods can provide needed protein, calcium, iron and zinc for the body. We wish to note that there is growing controversy over the necessity of animal products in a healthy diet. We will talk about these issues in greater length when we present alternative food guide pyramids. The dairy and meat layer includes milk, yogurt, cheese, poultry, fish, beans, eggs and nuts. Not all of these foods come from animals. However, they provide similar nutrients and are therefore classed together. These foods are needed in smaller amounts in comparison to plant-based foods. Plant-based foods also contain the important vitamins and minerals found in these groups, but in smaller quantities.

Meats, poultry, fish, dry beans, eggs and nuts can provide essential nutrients like protein, vitamin B (B12), iron and zinc. Meats, poultry and fish are generally richer in fats than plant foods because they come from animals. These foods contain more cholesterol. Consuming lean meats is more beneficial than regular meats. Beans, eggs and nuts also provide needed protein, vitamins and minerals for the body. However, egg yolks are high in cholesterol. In order to avoid the cholesterol-dense portion of the egg, try consuming egg whites rather than the entire egg.

Dairy products can also provide essential nutrients. Dairy products include milk, cheese, yogurt and ice cream. They provide protein, vitamins and minerals (most notably calcium). Often dairy products are fortified with other vitamins like vitamin D. Dairy products are also high in fat content, though there are often many low-fat alternatives still capable of meeting nutritional needs. Try consuming low-fat dairy products.

In general a serving size of dairy products is as follows:

- 1 cup milk or yogurt
- 1 ounce natural cheese
- 2 ounces processed cheese

LAYER 4

The last layer of the Food Guide Pyramid contains fats, oils, and sweets. These foods should be consumed sparingly, as they do not provide nutrients in important quantities. By sparingly, we mean once a week to once a month.

Servings are based on the number of calories an individual needs. In fact, there are separate Food Guide Pyramids for different age groups. There are three U.S. pyramids altogether: a pyramid for ages two to six, seven to fifty, and fifty and above.

A balanced diet will incorporate all the basic food groups. Try to consume a healthy portion of the recommended servings every day. However, keep in mind that these recommendations need to be flexible according to individual caloric intakes. Try to decrease the amount of fat in your diet and consume more fruits, vegetables and grains. Within each food group, try to maintain variety because no single food can provide all the minerals, vitamins, proteins, carbohydrates and fats needed for optimal performance.

Global Diet Pyramids

The Harvard School of Public Health, Oldways Preservation and Exchange Trust (a nonprofit organization) and other institutions introduced four new food guide pyramids in the United States. These four new "healthy eating pyramids" are dietary guidelines that are based on traditional diets of Asians, Latinos, Mediterraneans and Vegetarians.

Unlike the USDA Food Guide Pyramid, these pyramids represent traditional diets from cultures around the world. These pyramids have also been scientifically proven to enhance overall health if followed over a long period of time. The USDA Food Guide Pyramid is in the process of re-evaluation and will probably look more like these four new pyramids. They differ from the USDA pyramid primarily in the role of meat. As we have indicated, the role of meat in a healthy diet is under considerable debate.

Research indicates that over-consumption of red meat may be harmful. Eating less than the average American's diet of red meat has proven health benefits. The USDA pyramid currently recommends daily consumption of meat, and it clumps beans, poultry, fish and nuts in the same food group. Critics argue this implies that plant and animal proteins are the same, but in reality, they are not. In these new pyramids, nuts, beans and legumes are in a separate category and are recommended daily with fruits and vegetables. The Asian, Mediterranean and Latin pyramids recommend fish and poultry once or twice a week and red meat only monthly, in small quantities, while the Vegetarian pyramid cuts out red meats altogether and, in most cases, cuts out poultry.

Aside from differing from the U.S. Food Guide Pyramid, these pyramids also distinguish between animal and plant oils. Vegetable and plant oils (sesame, soy, olive and peanut oil) are rich in unsaturated fats, which are healthy for you, while animal fat is full of saturated fats that cause chronic diseases. Daily wine consumption and regular exercise are incorporated in these food guide pyramids, unlike the USDA pyramid where they have been omitted. See Figures D.2 through D.4 in Appendix D on pages 370 and 371 for graphic representations of the Global Diet Pyramids.

The Asian Diet

The Asian Diet Pyramid is based on the traditional plant-based rural diet of people in China, Japan, Korea and other Asian countries. Consuming adequate amounts of the traditional foods of these regions will allow you to obtain all the nutrients needed to maintain optimal health. The Asian diet is rich in fiber, vitamins, minerals and antioxidants and is extremely low in saturated fats.

Though this diet is low in meats and dairy foods, protein and iron are obtained from nuts, seeds and legumes. Dark leafy vegetables, nuts and soy products are rich sources of iron and calcium, traditionally obtained in the West from animal products. The Asian diet appears to be instrumental in lowering the risk of certain cancers, heart disease, obesity, osteoporosis and other chronic degenerative diseases found predominately in the United States.

The Asian diet is strong in plant-based foods, which range from vegetables to fruits, nuts and seeds. Animal products are incorporated in the Asian diet pyramid, but their importance is not emphasized. Current research supports the Asian diet's emphasis on fish. Weekly consumption of small to moderate servings of fish has a direct correlation with a healthy lifestyle. When making this diet a part of your lifestyle, you must remember to consume a wide variety of plant-based foods to receive the sufficient amounts of nutrients required for health (See Figure D.2, page 371).

At the base of the pyramid are rice products, noodles, breads and grains. This diet emphasizes whole grains and a minimal consumption of processed foods. It also places a deeper importance on fruits, vegetables, legumes, nuts and seeds in comparison to the USDA Pyramid. Daily physical exercise is incorporated in the Food Guide Pyramid, as well as a little consumption of plant-based beverages like tea (black and green), sake, beer and wine. Low-fat dairy products are preferred over other dairy sources while fish is a daily option. Sweets, eggs and poultry are recommended on a weekly basis, while red meat is recommended only monthly.

Saturated fat and total fat is very low in Asian diets. Many studies compare the Asian diet to the Mediterranean diet (which will be discussed later on), because both diets are effective in lowering the risk of chronic diseases. They are often used as models for healthy eating. While both diets are low in saturated fats, the Asian diet is lower in total fats.

Many people believe the obvious absence of dairy products in the Asian diet would lead to osteoporosis, but in reality populations traditionally following the Asian diet pyramid actually have lower risks of osteoporosis in comparison to those following a more Western diet. It appears that diets in which the major source of calcium is obtained from animal products show a greater risk of developing osteoporosis.

In recent years, the traditional Asian diet has been the center of a great deal of scientific attention. Chronic diseases such as certain cancers, diabetes and heart disease are not as common in Asia as in the United States and other Western countries. Researchers believe the Asian diet may protect you from these diseases.

The Mediterranean Diet

The Mediterranean diet, rich in fruits, vegetables, grains, omega-3 fatty acids and low in saturated fats, can reduce the risk of heart disease and cancer. A four-year study indicated that those consuming a Mediterranean diet were 60 percent less likely to develop cancer than others following the American Heart Association's "Step 1" diet for reducing high cholesterol. Six hundred men and women surviving a heart attack participated in the study. Seventeen people who followed the AHA diet developed cancer, while only seven developed cancer when incorporating the Mediterranean diet in their lifestyle.

This diet provides vitamins, minerals, fiber and antioxidants. Though rich in fat, the fats in the Mediterranean diet are primarily healthy monounsaturated fatty acids. The Mediterranean diet is grounded in plants: whole grains, fresh fruits and vegetables. Nuts, seeds, and dairy products are also staples in this diet, while fish and poultry are consumed occasionally. Red meat and eggs are eaten rarely. Moderate amounts of diluted wine and grape juices are also consumed.

The people of the Mediterranean region consume large quantities of complex carbohydrates in foods like pasta, beans, fruits, vegetables, rice and other grains. Protein is eaten in moderate amounts and olive oil is almost the exclusive source of fats, which is naturally cholesterol free. Regular physical activity is recommended for healthy weight and fitness (see Figure D.3 on page 371).

The Latin Diet

The Latin Food Guide Pyramid is based on two distinct time periods: the dietary traditions of the Incas, Mayas and the Aztecs; and the dietary patterns that emerged after the arrival of Christopher Columbus in the 1500s to the present.

A traditional Latin American Diet is associated with lower rates of chronic diseases and a high adult life expectancy. The Latin diet is high in plant-based foods, ranging from maize, potatoes, fruits, vegetables, tortillas, beans, nuts, corn and breads, to rice. The Latin diet is also dependent on chili peppers. Consumption of chili peppers daily contributes to a healthy lifestyle. Poultry (turkey) and fish are consumed weekly, and red meat is eaten sparingly. Since there is a limited availability of edible oils, the largest source of fats comes from nuts and vegetables (avocados). Fresh fruits and vegetables are consumed daily as well as chocolates. Moderated consumption of alcohol and daily physical exercise is also incorporated in this diet.

The Vegetarian Diet

The Vegetarian Food Guide Pyramid is the fourth of the series made by Harvard School of Public Health and Oldways Preservation & Exchange Trust. This pyramid is based on data from vegetarians across the world. Vegetarians have the lowest recorded rates of chronic diseases and the highest adult life expectancy of any population. (See Figure D.1 on page 370.)

The Vegetarian Food Guide Pyramid recommends eating multiple daily servings of fruits and vegetables, whole grains and legumes. The vegetarian pyramid also emphasizes the importance of eating nuts, seeds, plant oils, egg whites, soy milks and/or dairy products daily. This is to ensure adequate amounts of protein and minerals not found in large quantities in fruits and vegetables alone. As with the other pyramids, sweets and eggs should be eaten in small quantities on an occasional basis. The vegetarian food pyramid also indicates the importance of water, variety and exercise. Vegetarians ought to rely heavily on whole foods rather than processed foods and supplements. Finally, vegetarians should consider supplements as necessary according to various lifestyle factors. Those avoiding all animal products should consider supplementing their diet with vitamins B12 and D.

Many people believe vegetarians do not consume enough protein, but this is not so. Though meat provides the nine essential amino acids, plants are also a good source for them. A combination and variety of grains and vegetables can provide the nine essential amino acids needed to maintain proper health. *The Journal of Clinical Nutrition* indicates that plant foods contribute approximately 65 percent of the per capita supply of protein on a worldwide basis.

The term *vegetarian* is vague in the United States because the term has been used to describe a variety of lifestyles. There are a number of kinds of vegetarians including vegans, fruitarians, macrobiotics, lacto-vegetarians, ovo-lacto-vegetarians, pollo-vegetarians and pesca-vegetarians. These types of vegetarians are distinguished by the kinds of foods restricted from the diet. Here is a basic definition of the various types of vegetarian diets:

Vegan: a diet where only plant-based foods are consumed. A vegan diet excludes all animal products including honey. Some vegans even exclude yeast.

Fruitarian: a diet that is probably the closest to fitting the term "vegetarian." This diet consists of only raw fruits, nuts and berries. A fruitarian diet does not contain all the nutrients necessary for long-term sustenance and should therefore be followed only on a short-term basis.

Macrobiotic: a diet based closely on East Asian principles. Macrobiotic diets are restricted in animal food. Macrobiotic diets consist of relatively high amounts of brown rice, accompanied by smaller amounts of fruits, vegetables and pulses. Proponents of the macrobiotic diet claim that raw foods are difficult to digest, thus a macrobiotic diet consists almost exclusively of cooked foods. Processed foods and food from the Solanaceae (of or pertaining to the nightshade family) species—tomatoes, aubergines and potatoes—are also avoided. Fish is permitted, though most macrobiotics prefer to avoid them.

Lacto-Vegetarian: a diet incorporating dairy products into the Vegan dietary patterns.

Ovo-Lacto-Vegetarian: a diet which incorporates dairy products as well as eggs. This is the most common of the vegetarian diets.

Pollo-Vegetarian: a diet similar to Ovo-Lacto, but incorporating poultry.

Pesca-Vegetarian: a diet that incorporates fish and seafood into an Ovo-Lacto-vegetarian diet.

There are multiple health benefits that come with a vegetarian diet. Vegetarians eat lower levels of saturated fatty acids. In many cases, the majority of saturated fat consumed comes from animal products. Since vegetarians only consume the dairy and eggs from animals, their diets are almost always lower in overall saturated fat than those who eat red meat. Vegetarians also have a higher intake of dietary fiber. Vegetarians usually eat a greater number of high-fiber foods, especially legumes, since these are an excellent source of protein. A diet high in dietary fiber has been shown to decrease the probability of developing certain cancers, in particular colon cancer.

Vegetarians have a higher intake of antioxidant nutrients. Nutrients like vitamin C are found in certain fruits and vegetables, while vitamin E is found in plant oils. A vegetarian diet focuses on incorporating a wide variety of these fruits, vegetables and plant oils. Therefore, a vegetarian diet will almost always be higher in these nutrients than a diet that does not focus specifically on their intake.

Though there are many benefits associated with a vegetarian diet, there are also some potential dangers. Vegetarians are at risk for iron deficiency anemia, vitamin B12 and vitamin D deficiency, and complications resulting from a bulky diet.

Dietary iron is essential to avoid iron deficiency anemia. Females should make certain to obtain an adequate amount of absorbable iron. Food contains heme iron and non-heme iron; the body more easily absorbs heme iron. About 40 percent of the iron in meat, poultry and fish is heme iron, of which about 15 to 35 percent is absorbed. The iron in dairy, eggs and plant foods is largely non-heme, of which about 2 to 20 percent is absorbed. Non-heme iron comprises more than 80 percent of total dietary iron.

Vegetarians are also at risk for vitamin B12 deficiency. Vitamin B12 is generally obtained strictly from animal products. An individual following a Vegan diet should use supplements to obtain this vitamin. A primary symptom of a deficiency is a change in the nervous system (weak limbs, difficulty in walking and speaking, and jerking of limbs). If vitamin B12 deficiency is not treated, permanent mental deterioration and paralysis may result.

The human body can synthesize vitamin D from sunlight, but this is only possible when the sun reaches a certain intensity level. For many people who live in North America, this means that for a few months of the year they will have to seek other sources of vitamin D because the sun is not intense enough to cause the body to make enough of it. In Boston, Massachusetts, for example, vitamin D can only be synthesized from sunlight from April to November. Milk is generally fortified with vitamin D, but for Vegans who do not consume dairy products, supplements are necessary.

Lastly, vegetarians are at risk for complications associated with bulky diets. A bulky diet is high in dietary fiber. In some circumstances, this regimen can restrict energy intake in the first few years of life. This is also true for adults who consume large amounts of fiber to the extent that many other nutrients are not absorbed in the small intestine.

Weight-Loss Diets

Many of the weight-loss diets today are so new we do not yet know what complications may arise. In contrast, there are literally thousands of studies published on the healthy effects of a balanced diet full of fruits, grains and vegetables with dairy and meat products in moderation. These investigations have consistently and repeatedly shown that a balanced diet following the Food Pyramid guidelines provides long-term health. We are still learning why this is the case. Current research is now helping us to understand why a balanced diet is capable of meeting all the body's needs and why it prevents disease and cancer. We hope you will begin to look at your diet with much more in mind than just weight loss.

It also happens that a diet that encourages appropriate weight loss will keep the weight off and promote general health. We strongly encourage an overall, life-long lifestyle change that includes physical exercise and eating an appropriate, well-balanced diet stocked with a variety of fruits and vegetables. The key here is to make a lifestyle change that is balanced and appropriate for your body's nutritional needs.

Diets that meet RDAs are almost certain to ensure intake of enough essential nutrients. The Dietary Guidelines describe food choices that will help you meet these recommendations. Like the RDAs, the Dietary Guidelines apply to diets consumed over several days and not to single meals or foods.

Dieting and Diet Fads

What is dieting? The word "dieting" is often used to express a space of time in which we limit food consumption, change the composition of our diets or try a variety of other manipulative measures to induce weight loss. The dictionary defines the word *diet* as "what you eat." A diet is everything that is consumed by an organism to sustain life.

The need to lose weight and look great has generated many expensive diet fads that promise to make our dreams of being thin and healthy come true. But dieting is not a permanent answer. Dieting is not even a permanent problem, most often by the definition of diet fads, it is temporary. From temporary efforts you can expect temporary results. The weight will come right back with possible additions after the diet is terminated unless other changes are made. We all want permanent results, and that calls for permanent changes. The problem with many of these diets or diet fads is that they cannot be sustained without sacrificing your health.

Diets That Limit Variety

Any diet that limits the variety of foods you eat is going to have negative effects; for example, increased risk of disease and illness and decreased efficiency of body systems. Diets such as the grapefruit diet, the kiwi diet, the cottage cheese diet, the protein diet or any other diet that rests heavily on a single source of food is obviously unhealthy. Malnutrition and/or subtoxic levels of individual phytochemicals generally cause the weight loss experienced from these diets. Because the body is not getting what it needs from the foods that are being consumed, there is a natural inclination to break the diet because the body can feel that something is missing. Often people on these diets do not feel well and get no joy out of eating. Once the diet is discontinued and the urge to replace missing nutrients is relatively satisfied, all the weight comes back usually with a little more. Now we will discuss how the harms of these limited diets come about.

How does a limited diet increase your risk for disease and illness and decrease the efficiency of body systems? We can address this problem by studying the diets mentioned above. Any diet that excludes entire food groups or the variety of foods you eat is not good for you. The most dangerous diets are those that limit the variety of foods to a single food group, eliminate entire food groups or focus on a single food.

For instance, grapefruit is a wonderful fruit filled with vitamins and helpful phytochemicals; but by limiting a diet to nothing but grapefruit, you deprive your body of the benefits and nutrients offered by other fruits, vegetables, protein and fats and expose it to large doses of grapefruit composition. You can get too much of a good thing. Other types of fruit and foods have lots to offer that grapefruit lacks. If one stayed on this diet long enough their health and energy would fail; their immune system would be weakened, and their own body would begin to lose weight by destroying itself in search of the molecules that a single food source cannot provide.

This is also true for the protein diets in which people are instructed to eat large quantities of meat with the accompanying fat, small quantities of vegetables, even smaller quantities of fruits, either minuscule or no grains or carbohydrate sources at all. By eating nothing but meat, fat, a few vegetables and inadequate carbohydrates you miss out on the disease-preventative antioxidant molecules present in fruits and vegetables, as well as the fiber and energy of grains. By eating large quantities of proteins and fats, you force your body to use emergency pathways to generate the energy molecule glucose. This process does expend a great deal of energy, which causes weight loss, but also results in a lot of undesirable biological byproducts. These byproducts include ammonia, urea and elevated levels of ketone bodies and homocysteine (see section on homocysteine).

It is necessary for people on these diets to drink a large amount of water to dilute the toxic molecules and to facilitate their removal from the body via the liver and kidneys. If concentrations grow too high, these molecules can have toxic effects on internal organs and/or otherwise negatively affect the functions of the body. The situation in the body created by the combination of these chemicals and molecules results in an ideal disease-causing combination that should not be ignored. When increased cholesterol levels from fat intake accompany factors such as deficient antioxidants and increased oxidant production, they very likely result in a greatly increased risk for heart disease, arteriosclerosis, stroke and cancer.

These diets are quick fixes and should never be used for long periods of time due to the potential for negative consequences. Even in the short term, damage can result from these diets. People with liver and kidney problems should never attempt these diets. Quick-fix diets are, in a sense, purposeful malnutrition and will serve to further weight and health problems. Avoid these diets wherever possible. If you do try a quick fix, do it under the direction of a qualified physician or nutrition expert, make it a short-term trial, and follow it up with a permanent and sustainable program of good diet and exercise.

The worst thing you could possibly do is stay on one of these diets for a long period of time without expert care; this has the potential to cause you irreparable harm. The second worst thing you could do is repeatedly bounce on and off these diets causing your body to go through periods of weight gain and loss, like a yo-yo, which is definitely ineffective and eventually dangerous.

Diets That Use Pills

Just think about this one a little while. Most of the diet pills that have come out on the market have not only had questionable results, many of them have also turned out to be dangerous. Do you remember fen-phen? A lot of them are marketed as supplements; hence the government does not closely regulate them, and they are often not really proven safe and effective. These pills often contain substances that affect the speed and manner at which your body is functioning. They are often loaded with stimulants such as caffeine and ephedrine. These chemicals can cause your heart to race and your blood pressure to rise. They tend to make you very nervous and edgy. They can make it harder for you to sleep. They can become addicting and create a host of problems for you. In addition, they are only to be used in the short term, offer no permanent solution and may do damage if used for long periods of time.

These drugs should be avoided wherever possible. Buying weight-loss supplements from TV infomercials or grocery store shelves without learning a whole lot more information about the products from a more impartial source is a bad idea. Sometimes it may be necessary to use medications to get control of a serious weight problem. If you do decide to take a medicinal route to address a weight problem, it is best to consult a qualified physician or nutritionist for guidance. Often these drugs are only necessary to help you get started and should be taken with a good diet and with exercise, which will eventually become the permanent solution.

Diets That Limit Caloric Intake

Diets that limit caloric intake are not new. They were a great invention for those of us who do not know when to stop. Their use can be very healthy, if done appropriately. It is well known that if you eat too much and exercise too little, the most common result is fat. It is also known that by limiting dietary calories to the same number that a person uses, one can avoid getting fat, or at least fatter.

These diets can also be used to lose weight by calculating and sticking to a diet just below the calories that are used. Care must be taken in adjusting the diet appropriately. For some people, the temptation to be super thin could lead to eating disorders, which have their own list of negative health effects. This tendency should be watched for. The idea is to be healthy.

People who are on the restricted calorie diets have to calculate and figure out what intake is best for them at their energy expenditure to maintain body weight, energy and maximum health. You need to balance calories and nutrition; try to not go over or underweight, and glean all the nutrients you need to be healthy. This method of dieting requires self-control, patience and durability. Properly used, this diet can and should become a lifestyle as long as you monitor the quality and types of food you eat.

It is very important to know that even people who are of the same weight, height and energy expenditure may have very different metabolisms and very different energy requirements. Calculations of appropriate caloric intakes are very individual and should be flexible for changing situations. For this reason people who try calorie-control diets should not depend too much upon charts or graphs of information to tell them what their needs are. These are helpful to give a range to start in. Most importantly you should be perceptive to your body's needs and eat amounts that help you feel healthy. People who use this type of dieting should seek the help of a qualified physician or nutritionist to help them get started correctly. Calorie restriction should not take the place of exercise. It also should not be attempted during pregnancy without the close care of a physician, as a higher plane of nutrition is required in this circumstance.

Conclusion to Dieting

In order to get the results you want, not only in weight loss but also in increased health and quality and quantity of life, you need to change your whole lifestyle to include healthy nutrition and exercise. A good diet has been defined as one that contains all of the elements required to live a healthy, long, productive life. This includes eating a diet rich in many different kinds of fruits, vegetables and grains and eating a proper amount of appropriately balanced proteins and fats.

We have known the benefits of good diet and exercise for a long time. The scientific data just continues to add up. The only problem is practicing what we preach. We can only benefit if we use the information that we have gathered actively in our own lives. We now know that the answer for a good diet is variety.

There is such a variety of good things in the large variety of foods we have available to us, it only makes sense to take advantage of them. Eat as many different kinds of fruits and vegetables as is practical and possible. Vary the kinds of grains you consume. Eat whole grains and grain mixtures. If you choose to eat meat, which is an easy way to get many nutrients, eat different kinds of meats, and eat them in appropriate amounts. Consume a limited quantity and appropriate variety and quality of fats. Strictly limit the amount of refined sugars you consume. If you need to, restrict the calories in your diet to prevent obesity. This should all sound familiar. You've heard it all before. Dieting is not the end-all answer. What we really need to do is change our entire lifestyles to include good nutrition and healthy exercise.

References

American Cancer Society Dietary Guidelines May 8 1997. Cancer—Eating To Beat The Odds.

Carolyn Katzin. Cancer and Nutrition: What is the Connection? 1997–99. Copyright © 1998, 1999 [foodandlife.com].

Eleanor Noss Whitney, Sharon Rady Rolfes. Understanding Nutrition. West Publishing Company, New York 1996.

Fances Sizer , MS, RD, FADA and Eleanor Whitney, PhD. Nutrition Concepts and Controversies. West/ Wadsworth: An International Thomson Publishing Company, Washington 1997.

Getty T. Ambau. The Importance of Good Nutrition, Herbs, and Phytochemicals for your Health, Good Looks, and Longevity. Falcon Press International. CA, 1997.

Hegarty, Vincent Ph.D. Nutrition, Food, and the Environment. Minnesota: Eagan Press, 1993.

J. A. Milner. Functional Foods and Health Promotion. Nutrition Department and Graduate Program in Nutrition, The Pennsylvania State University, University Park, PA 16802.

Katherine Mitchell, BA. And Margaret Cowden Bernard BS. Food in Health and Disease. FA Davis Company, Philadelphia 1995.

LE Lloyd, BE McDonald, EW Crampton. Fundamentals in Nutrition. WH Freeman and Company, San Francisco 1978.

Martha Davis Dunn MS Public Health Nutrition, MPA. Fundamentals in Nutrition. CBI Publishing Company, INC. Mass 1983.

Martin Eastwood. Principles of Human Nutrition. University of Edinburgh, Western General Hospital, Edinburgh, UK. Chapman and Hall, UK 1997.

Maurice E Shils, James A. Olson, Moshe Shike, A. Catherine Ross. Modern Nutrition in Health and Diseases. Maryland: Williams and Wilkins, 1999.

Richard A. Knox. New Research Backs A Balanced Diet. Source: NY Times Syndicate Wednesday, April 26, 2000.

Ronald M Deutsch and Judi S Morrill, Ph.D. Realities of Nutrition. Bull publishing Company, California 1993.

Rosemary C. Fisher. Some Recent Research About Foods and Cancer.

Sam Graci and Harvey Diamond. The Power of Superfood. Prentice Hall Canada Inc. Ontario 1999.

Stephanie Beling, MD. Power Foods. Harper Perennial. New York 1998.

The American Dietetic Association. Excerpts from The American Dietetic Association's Complete Food & Nutrition Guide.OSU

The Functions of the Human Body

All forms of life on Earth share some basic characteristics. For instance, all living organisms are composed of the same basic atoms: carbon, oxygen, hydrogen, nitrogen, sulfur and other trace elements. In addition, all forms of life must obtain energy in some form from the environment in which they live. Finally, all life forms are made of the same basic "molecules of life": proteins, carbohydrates (sugars), fats and nucleic acids. These four basic molecules of life are then arranged, modified and assembled to make up basic structural units of living organisms called cells.

A major task of our body is to regulate the number of cells in the body through a process known as homeostasis. Each day our body produces ten billion new blood cells while at the same time it programs the death of ten billion old blood cells through a process called apoptosis.

Metabolism

The biochemical processes that generate and maintain life are generally referred to as *metabolism*. Metabolic processes can be divided into two general types: anabolic and catabolic.

ANABOLIC

Anabolic metabolism includes those biochemical reactions in which small precursor molecules are assembled into larger macromolecules. Thus anabolic metabolism may be thought of as a constructive process, just like large buildings are built from smaller materials like bricks and mortar.

CATABOLIC

Catabolic metabolism includes those biochemical reactions in which large molecules are degraded or "broken" down into smaller molecules. This is a destructive process. For example, the proteins in meat or legumes are degraded to their respective building blocks, which the body can then use to synthesize proteins needed for the maintenance and generation of new cells.

Chemistry of Molecules

ATOMS

At the most basic level, we are made of atoms. In this sense, a human is no different than any other mass of matter in the world—everything consists in one way or another of atoms. There are over 100 different kinds of atoms known as elements. Atoms, in turn are made of three basic particles: protons, neutrons and electrons.

It is important to understand how these three particles interact in atoms in order to better understand how the chemicals and nutrients in fruits and vegetables help prevent disease. Every atom

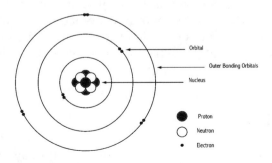

Figure 3.1 The Atom

shares the same basic structure. The difference between an atom of one element and an atom of another is often extremely small.

However, on an atomic level, small changes in structure account for major changes in function. In fact, every basic function of your body is dependent upon the structures of reacting atoms. Within the context of life, structure is function, and changing a structure will change or destroy the function associated with it.

In every atom there is a nucleus, or center, consisting of protons and neutrons. Protons carry a positive electrical charge, while neutrons do not carry any charge at all. Protons and neutrons remain in the nucleus while electrons orbit around them.

Electrons carry a negative charge. They are the most volatile part of an atom and determine in large measure how an atom interacts with other atoms. Electrons circle the nucleus much like planets circle the sun. Electrons prefer to run around the nucleus in pairs because it gives the atom greater stability. The path of the orbit of electrons is called an "orbital." Different atoms have different numbers of orbitals—thus carry varying numbers of electrons.

The orbitals furthest away from the nucleus are called "bonding orbitals." Bonding orbitals are so named because they make connections with orbitals from other atoms. When an atom has only one electron in a bonding orbital the atom looks for another electron and will react with another atom in order to take or share one of its electrons. When an atom exchanges or shares an electron with another atom, we say there has been a reaction.

When two atoms share the electrons in their bonding orbitals, the atoms are connected, or form a bond. When electrons are given and received, ions are formed. An ion is an atom that carries a charge because it either has an extra electron or is missing an electron. The essence of biological life on earth at the most fundamental level consists of atoms losing, gaining or sharing electrons. Life is thus a matter of making and breaking atomic bonds. This process is what takes place in the biochemical reactions involved in both anabolic and catabolic reactions.

Atoms vary in their reactivity, or readiness to interact with other atoms. Reactivity depends upon how strongly each atom pulls on its electrons and the electrons of other atoms. This property of atoms is known as electron affinity. Some atoms, such as oxygen, nitrogen and fluorine react with many other atoms because they have high electron affinities. Other atoms are very stable and much less reactive because their electron affinities are more moderate. This concept of electron affinity is very important to our later discussion of free radicals.

As we have discussed, individual atoms frequently react with each other to form bonds. Several atoms bonded together in a specific shape make up a molecule. Molecules can be very simple and small, such as oxygen molecules, which are composed merely of two atoms of the element oxygen. On the other hand, molecules can incorporate literally hundreds of thousands of individual atoms from many different elements. For example, there are twenty different amino acids that are used in all types of combinations and numbers in the biosynthesis of thousands and thousands of different proteins that become parts of our bodies. This type of molecular complexity is found regularly within the realm of biology where living organisms assemble atoms into huge conglomerates as a matter of day-to-day survival.

The distribution of electrons throughout a molecule is sometimes unequal and results in varying electric charges within the molecule. In some molecules there may be regions with a high concentration of electrons, causing a negative charge. On the other hand, within the same molecule there may be areas with few electrons, causing a positive charge.

Molecules that have both positive and negative charges on different parts of their structure are called polar molecules. Water, for example, is a polar molecule. Water is made up of two hydrogen atoms and a single oxygen atom (H_2O) arranged like a "V." Because the oxygen atom has a greater electron affinity than the hydrogen atoms it pulls harder on the electrons, concentrating them on the oxygen side of the molecule. This leaves the hydrogen side with a positive charge. All polar molecules are usually very soluble in water because they share this same type of charge.

While polar molecules have both positive and negative charges, nonpolar molecules may have either a positive, negative or neutral charge, but they do not have both positive and neutral charges simultaneously. Many molecules are nonpolar, especially molecules composed mainly of carbon and hydrogen atoms. These compounds are often referred to as hydrocarbons and include such things as oils, gasoline, and fats or lipids.

Polar and nonpolar molecules do not mix. Molecules that are attracted to water and dissolve well in it are said to be hydrophilic (water loving) while those that are not readily soluble in water are referred to as hydrophobic (water fearing). Though hydrophobic and hydrophilic molecules will not dissolve in each other, they will dissolve in substances that have similar properties. This concept of polarity becomes a significant factor in our later discussion of vitamins, herbs, and other phytochemicals because both hydrophobic and hydrophilic environments exist in our bodies.

Molecules of Life

The most frequent elements or atoms making up molecules found in the body are compounds of carbon, hydrogen, oxygen, nitrogen, and sulfur. There are four principle types of molecules produced and used in the body. They are fats, proteins, nucleic acids, and carbohydrates.

Cells: The Basic Unit of Life

All of these molecules and many others are organized to form cells. Cells are the basic units of life and are amazingly complex and intricate despite their microscopic size. Cells with particular qualities and abilities are given special arrangements within the body to perform specific functions. These arrangements of cells are called tissues. The muscle in your arm is an example of a tissue. A simple task like lifting your arm is possible only because there are billions of cells working in concert.

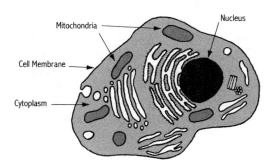

Figure 3.2 The Cell

Tissues themselves are arranged in specialized groups to form organs with greater functions. The heart, for instance, is a collection of several tissues working together to keep blood circulating through the body. Keep in mind that the tissues of the heart are also made up of billions of cells and the smooth functioning of your heart relies on the cooperation of all of them. Organs are arranged together into systems to perform even more complex functions. When an organ fails to work properly the problem comes down to the malfunction of many cells. On the other hand, when cells are functioning properly, the body works efficiently.

Metabolism

The average adult has about 100 trillion cells. The sheer number of cells that make up your body is mind boggling. At every given moment there are billions upon billions of reactions taking place. All of this activity requires macronutrients and micronutrients for the successful maintenance of life. The more readily the necessary nutrients are found, the more efficiently all of these reactions take place. This is why it is important to eat a balanced diet.

All of these reactions taken together as a whole are covered by the term *metabolism*. Sometimes it is helpful to think of metabolism as the simultaneous work of circulation, respiration, digestion, and other vital body processes. As we mentioned in the previous chapter, metabolism is the process of bringing essential nutrients to cells in order to give them the necessary chemicals to maintain and promote life.

However, when essential nutrients are missing or unavailable your body is forced to function with hampered cells. Often this leads to extensive cellular damage, causing cancer, disease, aging and death. The single greatest thing you can do to prevent chronic and lifestyle-related diseases and to forestall aging and death is to eat a diet rich in the nutrients that maintain the healthy life process of your cells. In this process, your cells perform three basic metabolic functions: respiration, circulation and digestion.

Respiration

Strictly speaking, the respiratory system consists of tissues and organs that bring oxygen into the body and into the blood. This is important because all of the cells of the body need oxygen and must discard carbon dioxide in order to live. The chief components of the respiratory system are: the nasal cavity, the trachea (windpipe), the bronchioles and other air ducts in the lungs, and the alveoli.

When we breathe, air passes through the nasal cavity and trachea where it is heated and moistened. Tiny particles like bacteria and other pollutants are trapped in the mucus lining of these tissues, keeping them from getting into the lungs. The air passes through the trachea, the bronchioles (the first main branches off the trachea), and then through progressively smaller and smaller channels in our lungs until it reaches tiny air sacs called alveoli. These little sacs are surrounded by tiny blood vessels called capillaries. Here oxygen enters the bloodstream while carbon dioxide is discarded through the very thin membranes between the alveoli and the capillaries. This is known as gas exchange. The heart then pumps high-oxygen blood to the rest of the body. The blood unloads its oxygen as it circulates through the body and picks up carbon dioxide on its way back to the lungs.

Circulation

The purpose of the circulatory system is to distribute oxygen and nutrients throughout the body while collecting cellular waste. It also shuttles the cells of our immune system from one part of the body to another as they protect us from infectious organisms. The circulatory system consists of the heart, the blood vessels, the lymphatic system, and, of course, the blood.

The function of the heart is to pump blood throughout the body. It is made up almost completely of muscle cells that contract rhythmically to move the blood through the blood vessels. Nerve cells coordinate the muscle cells in order to make sure that they all contract at the right time. Connective tissue holds everything together. The heart pumps the blood first to the lungs, where carbon dioxide is dropped off and oxygen is picked up. After exchanging gasses in the lungs, the blood returns to the heart so that it can be pumped into the rest of the body. Because the heart is always working, it needs a steady supply of oxygen and nutrients. When those supplies are impeded or cut off, serious problems such as heart attacks can occur. We will discuss later how eating a diet high in fruits and vegetables can avert such problems.

There are three main types of blood vessels: arteries, veins and capillaries. Arteries carry blood away from the heart and fan out into smaller and smaller vessels in order to deliver oxygen-rich blood to tissues. Veins carry blood back to the heart, collect blood from the tissues and merge into one another to make larger and larger vessels as they near the heart. Capillaries connect the arteries and veins, deliver oxygen and nutrients to cells, and pick up all of the carbon dioxide and cellular waste. Capillaries are so important that every cell in your body is within two cells of a capillary. If cells were any further away from a capillary they would die from lack of nutrients. Arteries and veins transport blood, while capillaries distribute oxygen and nutrients from the blood to tissues.

Blood is composed of two main parts or phases: the solid phase and the liquid phase. The solid phase of the blood consists primarily of red blood cells, white blood cells, and platelets. Red blood cells make up the vast majority of the cells in blood. They are disks, shaped to carry oxygen. Red blood cells are saturated with a protein called hemoglobin. Hemoglobin binds with oxygen in the lungs and releases it in the tissues. When hemoglobin binds to oxygen it turns bright red. Blood is so dense with red blood cells that it appears to be red because of the prevalence of hemoglobin. Red blood cells are so full of hemoglobin that there is little room for other cellular parts. In fact, red blood cells do without most of the organelles that other cells could not live without. They do not even have nuclei.

Although red blood cells outnumber white blood cells by a huge margin, the white blood cells are by no means unimportant. White blood cells are part of the body's immune system. Among other things, white blood cells protect the body from attack by invading bacteria and viruses. Without white blood cells, these malicious microscopic organisms would overrun us.

Most white blood cells use the blood as a system of transit to get from one area of the body to another. For example, when someone gets a cut on the arm, white blood cells leave the bone marrow where they are produced and travel through the blood until they get to capillaries near the area of the cut. The white blood cells will then slip out of the blood vessels and into the tissues of the skin to make sure that bacteria in the cut do not spread to other parts of the body.

Some white blood cells, however, stay in the blood and constantly protect the blood vessels. They serve as backup defense in case any bacteria get past the body's primary defenses in the tissues.

The last major component of the blood's solid phase is called platelets. Platelets are small noncellular disks that help the blood to clot. When blood vessels themselves have been damaged, the cells of the vessel wall release chemical distress signals called chemokines. These chemicals cause the platelets to clump together and stick to the damaged wall. They also initiate the formation of a thick fibrous mesh of proteins to plug the hole. This mesh of platelets and proteins is called a clot. Once the damage has been repaired, the body releases enzymes to dissolve the clot.

Without platelets and the clotting mechanism they initiate, small cuts and bruises could cause significant and even fatal damage. The blood has no other way of stopping itself from flowing out of damaged vessels. In fact, there are rare cases of people who lack the ability to clot blood. This is a disease known as hemophilia (literally "love of blood"). On the other hand, blood that clots too easily can cause heart attacks and strokes. We will discuss these conditions later, and the beneficial effects that fruits and vegetables can have on blood flow.

The liquid phase of blood is called plasma. Plasma is 85 percent water. It carries dissolved proteins, fats, sugars, nutrients, chemicals, chemical messengers, and important elements of the immune system, among other things. A very significant set of proteins and chemicals found in the plasma regulate the body's pH. The pH is a measure of acidity. The level of acidity affects the activity of every enzyme in the body as well as the function of most proteins. The body's normal pH is 7.4 on a scale of 0 to 14. A pH of "0" is most acidic, while a pH of "14" is most alkaline. Fluctuations in pH as small as 0.2 can cause serious illnesses. A change in pH of 0.4 is lethal. This concept of pH is important because what we eat affects our body's level of acidity. Some of the current fad diets, such as the popular low-carbohydrate/high-protein diets, cause changes in our pH that might be very detrimental over the long run.

Digestion

The digestive system consists of the mouth, stomach, and intestines. The pancreas, liver, and gall bladder also play very significant roles even though they are not directly involved with the transit of the food through the body. The digestive system breaks down the food we eat into its basic components. This is important because the cells of our various tissues cannot utilize nutrients unless they are in an appropriate form. By the time the digestive system finishes with food it will be broken down into miniscule bits of nutrients suitable for use within cells. Digestion begins in the mouth. The act of chewing begins the process of breaking food into smaller pieces. Saliva moistens the food so that it can be swallowed and begins to break down starches and proteins in the food into their respective amino acids and basic sugars.

The digestive process continues when food enters the acidic environment of the stomach. The stomach is essentially a large, muscular sac that has three primary functions: mix food, add acids and enzymes that continue to break food down, and then store food until the intestines are ready for it. As the stomach churns, acids and various enzymes decompose the food. Enzymes called proteases degrade the proteins while other enzymes called amylases chop up the various sugar chains. Still other enzymes degrade DNA and the rest of the molecules in the food. These enzymes function like molecular scissors, cutting the bonds linking molecules together. All of these processes occur at a much quicker rate in the stomach than in the mouth because of the strong acid and powerful enzymes there.

Food leaves the stomach and enters the intestines. Here the mixture is de-acidified so that different digestive enzymes can work at peak performance. This happens when bile is released into the intestines from the gall bladder. Bile is produced by the liver to aid in digestion and is stored in the gall bladder until needed. The pancreas also aids digestion by producing an assortment of enzymes. Some of these enzymes are called "lipases" because they catalyze the degradation of lipids and fats. The intestines are full of water, which poses some challenges for the digestion of fat.

Since fat and lipid molecules are hydrophobic they tend to attract one another in the intestines. This clumping together runs contradictory to the process of digestion—a process of breaking down rather than building up. When fat and lipid molecules clump together it makes it difficult for enzymes to cut the fat into digestible pieces. Besides de-acidifying the intestinal contents, bile has another very important function to compensate for this clumping activity. The bile emulsifies the fats, or in other words, it breaks the fat up into smaller pieces that are dissolvable in water. Much like a good squirt of dishwashing soap helps cut through tough grease, bile helps dissolve large clumps of fat in the intestines.

Once food is broken down nutrients are absorbed into the intestinal wall and then successively into the bloodstream. Sugars and amino acids dissolve readily in the blood and are transported easily. Because of their hydrophobic nature, fats and cholesterols first enter the blood as small clumps called chilomicrons, which are then converted into little balls of fat, cholesterol, and protein called lipoproteins. Fats and cholesterols circulate in the body as lipoproteins. There are several different kinds of lipoproteins, but the ones we hear the most about are low density lipoproteins (LDLs), and high density lipoproteins (HDLs). LDLs are often known as "bad" cholesterol because they can cause serious heart problems like atherosclerosis and heart attack if they are not managed appropriately with good diet and exercise. HDLs have been called "good" cholesterol because an increased level of HDLs in the blood has been correlated with decreased risk of these same diseases.

Although the exact mechanisms are not understood, it appears that LDLs promote the build-up of fatty plaques in the arteries that can block blood flow. HDLs appear to absorb fat in the blood vessels and carry it to the liver where it is broken down. We will discuss more about LDLs and HDLs and the diseases to which they contribute in Chapter 13.

The intestines have a muscular layer in their walls that contract rhythmically to push the food along the length of the digestive tract. This rhythmic contraction is known as peristalsis. As the food moves along the intestines, the intestinal walls absorb its nutrients. Once the food reaches the latter part of the intestines, an area called the large intestine, water is absorbed from the mixture and a semisolid paste is then ready for excretion.

Controlling Respiration, Circulation and Digestion

All of these systems work together in order to provide cells with the nutrients they need to remain healthy. These systems are controlled subconsciously by two principle methods.

First, the brain regulates many of these functions through signals it sends through nerves. For example, when the brain recognizes that the body is exercising it sends signals to the heart to speed up the pulse rate, tells the lungs to breath faster, and directs the blood to those muscles being used more heavily to provide them with the greater amounts of oxygen and energy they need.

Second, the brain, as well as other organs, produces hormones and other chemical messengers to communicate with each other and coordinate their various actions. Hormones are small molecules that are produced by one cell or organ to send a specific signal to another cell or organ. After they are produced, hormones and other chemical messengers are released in the bloodstream to be transported to target cells to perform a specific function. For example, when the small intestine senses that the food it is receiving from the stomach is laden with fat, it releases a hormone that tells the stomach to slow the rate at which it sends food into the intestines. After the fat in the small intestine is digested and absorbed, the hormone is no longer produced and the stomach sends food into the small intestine at a quicker rate.

The Immune System

The body is an intricate mesh of chemicals and chemical reactions. The human body is designed to sustain the life of literally trillions of cells. This is accomplished through the successful maintenance of a nutrient-rich environment. Of course this nutrient-rich environment is also very enticing to bacteria, viruses, and other organisms. In some cases these foreign organisms work to keep the body in good shape. Many bacteria in the intestines help digest food for us that we could not digest on our own, and other microbial inhabitants keep bad bacteria from getting inside of us. However in other cases these organisms are harmful and dangerous to our body. Bacteria that are harmful are known as pathogens.

In order to prevent pathogens from running rampant, your body is equipped with a powerful immune system. We will not dig too deeply into the complexity of the immune system. However, there are some important points that we wish to make in order to further persuade you to eat more fruits and vegetables. We will focus our discussion on the parts of the immune system that are bolstered by nutrients in plant food.

The immune system is divided into the cellular and humoral components. The cellular component is comprised mainly of white blood cells circulating throughout the body in blood and tissue. There are many different types of white blood cells, each with a specific function. For example, macrophages are large cells that engulf intruding pathogens ("macro" means "big" and "phage" means "eater"). Other white blood cells poison pathogens by releasing toxic chemicals, while still others police the cells of your body. If they find a cell housing a pathogen, they kill the cell before the pathogen becomes strong enough to cause serious trouble. This forces your body to excrete dead cells (and the pathogens with them) and replace them with healthy cells. Lastly, another type of white blood cell produces antibodies. Antibodies comprise a major portion of the humoral component of the immune system.

The humoral component of the immune system relies most heavily on antibodies and complement proteins. Antibodies search out foreign substances and attach themselves to them. This changes the structure of the pathogen, which also changes its function. Often this simple activity is sufficient to neutralize the potentially harmful effect of a pathogen. Yet there is another benefit derived from antibodies attaching (or binding) to pathogens. This makes it easier for macrophages to recognize and engulf the pathogen.

Antibodies are quite selective and will attach to only specific pathogens. Antibodies produced to attack a specific pathogen will generally only attack that pathogen. For example, when someone has chicken pox the body produces huge amounts of antibodies specifically attacking the chicken pox virus. Once the disease has been taken care of, the antibody remains in the blood. If the chicken pox virus enters again, the antibodies will attack and neutralize it so quickly that symptoms of a second infection almost never occur. The antibodies that were built to attack the chicken pox virus will not, however, recognize any other virus or pathogen.

For example, if a virus that causes a cold enters our bodies, the chicken pox antibody can do nothing against it and we get sick until the body's immune system adjusts and produces antibodies to it. The reason we can get colds many times is because there are literally hundreds of different kinds of cold viruses.

Antibodies defend the body from pathogens; however, there are unfortunate cases when antibodies recognize body tissues as pathogens. This is much more serious than a case of mistaken identity because antibodies will cause the body to attack itself. This is the chief problem in auto-immune diseases: the body thinks that its own cells are pathogens and tries to kill them. This can literally lead to self-destruction. Auto-immune disorders are believed to contribute to such illnesses as arthritis, Alzheimer's disease, multiple sclerosis, lupus erythematosis, AIDS, rheumatoid arthritis, and diabetes.

Complement proteins, which form the second part of the immune system, act in similar ways to antibodies but they are not as selective. Complement proteins will bind to all foreign objects, possibly neutralizing the ability of pathogens to do damage to the body as well as helping macrophages engulf them. One interesting property exclusive to the complement proteins is that they can bind together on the surface of bacteria and puncture the bacterial membrane. This ultimately kills the bacteria.

Fueling Cellular Metabolism: A Different Kind of Respiration

We obtain our energy from the nutrients in our diets. This energy originally comes from the sun. Plants capture the sun's energy in the process of photosynthesis in which water and carbon dioxide are converted to carbohydrates. We then eat these plants, or other animals that ate plants, in order to get energy.

Our cells create the energy they need to live and carry out their activities through a process called cellular respiration. On a large scale, respiration is the means by which oxygen is brought into the body; on a cellular level, respiration is the manner in which cells use oxygen to break down nutrients for energy.

As we have discussed, the cells of our bodies take in amino acids, fats, and other materials in order to produce proteins, lipids, and other molecules. The energy required for the cell to live and perform these functions comes ultimately from the nutrients we eat. The cells of our bodies prefer to use simple carbohydrates such as sucrose (table sugar) for fuel because they are easily broken down and provide the greatest amount of energy for the effort. Fat is used to produce energy only when sugars are not readily available. Sometimes the body is forced to use proteins as a source of energy, but such a course of action is both inefficient and undesirable. Proteins consumed in this manner come at a cost to the body itself and entail a wasting of the tissues. Proteins are used as an energy source only in cases of starvation where the body has no other option. (See Appendix A for more information on cell biology.)

A diet of fruits and vegetables provides an assortment of carbohydrates. Some are large complex carbohydrates, while others are simple sugars such as fructose and sucrose. In our cells, enzymes convert the different simple carbohydrates or sugars to glucose, which is the major source of energy used by the body. The breakdown or oxidation of glucose, which is a six-carbon sugar, into two three-carbon sugars called pyruvate occurs through a process called glycolysis. This process produces a relatively small amount of energy. By no means, however, can glycolysis provide for the huge power needs of an active cell. For that reason, pyruvate is transported from the cytoplasm into the mitochondria.

Within the mitochondria more enzymes ultimately convert pyruvate to carbon dioxide in a process of oxidation, or the removal of electrons from pyruvate. Thus, the six carbons from glucose end up as six molecules of carbon dioxide (CO_2) that are removed from the body when we exhale. Various electron carrier molecules gather up these high-energy electrons and ferry them to what is called the electron transport chain, or ETC. The ETC is found in the inner mitochondrial membrane. It is a series of protein complexes that accept electrons from electron carriers and transport them from one protein to another until they are "accepted" or bond with oxygen. This takes place like a series of linked waterfalls. As electrons "fall" from one pool to the next they release energy. The energy released by the "falling" electrons is harnessed by yet another enzyme that is found in the inner mitochondrial membrane. This enzyme uses the energy released to form ATP: the high-energy compound we need to survive. This is how the cell produces its primary source of energy.

Oxygen is essential to the process of electron transport in the ETC. It is located at the end of the chain and is the terminal acceptor for the electrons. At the end of the ETC one oxygen molecule

(O_2) is reduced to two water molecules (H_2O) through the addition of four electrons and four hydrogen ions. The water created in this fashion is called the water of metabolism.

If there were no oxygen to unload the electrons from the last protein of the ETC, the electrons would get backed up in the ETC. The stopping of electron flow through the ETC would halt the production of the high-energy compounds we need. If all of the ETCs in all of our cells were shut down in this manner at the same time, we would die in a matter of seconds. The reason we do not die so quickly when we hold our breath is because there is a great amount of oxygen already dissolved in our blood and tissues that can be used for several minutes before it is finally depleted. Oxygen is part of the ETC because it has a high electron affinity.

When water is made through the production of energy, millions of free radicals are also generated. We will discuss this in greater detail in chapter 4. Data from many scientific studies suggest that antioxidant activity in components of fruits and vegetables can significantly reduce the action of free radicals produced in this process and protect mitochondria and other cellular components from free-radical damage.

References

Raven and Johnson. 1995. Biology. 3rd edition. Wm. C. Brown Communications, Inc.

Tamarin. 1996. Principles of Genetics. 5th edition. WCB Publishers.

Voet and Voet. 1990. Biochemistry. John Wiley and Sons.

Stryer. 1988. Biochemistry. 3rd edition. W.H. Freeman and Company.

Voet, Voet and Pratt. 1999. Fundamentals of Biochemistry. John Wiley and Sons.

Goodwin. 1976. Chemistry and Biochemistry of Plant Pigments. Vol. 1 and 2. Academic Press.

Stryer. 1995. Biochemistry. 4th edition. W.H. Freeman and Company. New York.

CHAPTER 4

Free Radicals and Antioxidant Protection

As we discussed in the last chapter, oxygen is a molecule essential to life. Its high electron affinity keeps us alive and allows our cells to perform many functions. Oxygen maintains life by aiding the mitochondria in creating energy. However, oxygen's high electron affinity also contributes to the formation of free radicals. Free radicals cause oxidative damage, the damage that results when electrons are removed (oxidation) from a molecule or compound. Oxidative damage is a process that has been implicated in many lifestyle diseases such as coronary heart disease, heart attack, stroke, cancer and hypertension. (See Appendix B for more detailed information on free radicals.)

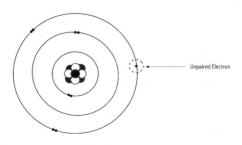

Figure 4.1 Free Radical

You may have heard of free radicals. A free radical is any atom with a single electron in its outermost bonding orbital. Electrons prefer to orbit the nucleus of atoms in pairs. When an electron is alone in its orbital it will try to take an electron away from another atom to become more stable. This is what makes oxygen atoms so dangerous. When they are free radicals, they will pull an electron from most other atoms in the body because oxygen has such a high electron affinity.

When an atom gains or loses an electron, several things happen. First, the atom that loses the electron becomes less stable and begins searching for another atom from which it can obtain an electron. This often causes a chain reaction, where several atoms begin stealing electrons from one another. This disrupts the normal functioning of many molecules, which disrupts cell functions and may cause irreparable damage to DNA, membrane lipids, mitochondria and cell proteins. Second, atoms that gain or lose electrons often lose the ability to perform vital functions. Vital functions are thus compromised by free radicals because they change the function of atoms, molecules and cells by removing electrons.

Where Do Free Radicals Come From?

The vast majority of destructive free radicals in your body come from oxygen atoms. In fact, free radicals of oxygen have a class of their own. They are often called reactive oxygen species, or "ROS" for short. The second most prevalent type of free radical comes from nitrogen atoms. These free radicals are also grouped under a blanket term. They are called reactive nitrogen species, or RNS. Both ROS and RNS can be found in various forms in the body.

Transition Metals

We will start our discussion of free radicals with transition metals because they frequently react with oxygen compounds to form free radicals. Transition metals received their name from the position they occupy on the periodic table of elements. They are located in the transition between alkali earth metals and nonmetals. The two most common transition metal ions in the human body

The Five Known Types of Free Radicals

superoxide ion	This free radical is essentially an oxygen molecule with an extra electron. Also known as reactive oxygen species, these free radicals can cause damage to the mitochondria and other important cellular components.
hydroxyl radical	This free radical is formed through the reduction of O_2 in the electron transport chain.
singlet oxygen	Singlet O_2 is generated by the immune system and is also produced by light. These free radicals can cause damage to double bonds between carbon atoms in saturated fatty acids.
hydrogen peroxide	Hydrogen peroxide itself is not a free radical, but it is an important ROS because it is involved in the generation of so many other ROS.
reactive nitrogen species	Nitric acid (the most important RNS) reacts with the superoxide ion to form peroxynitrite, which causes damage to body tissues.

are iron (Fe) and copper (Cu). Transition metals are classified as free radicals because they have varying numbers of unpaired electrons in their outer orbitals. These metals do not have sufficient electron affinity to pull electrons off of other atoms, but can act readily as electron donors and receivers. This attribute allows them to participate in reactions that involve the transfer of electrons.

Many enzymes use these important elements in their active sites to help catalyze reactions by shuttling electrons between reacting atoms. Proteins involved in the transport of electrons also use transition metals in a similar fashion. The proteins of the electron transport chain contain iron compounds that allow them to transfer electrons from one compound to another.

Some transition metal ions are able to catalyze the formation of free radicals from oxygen compounds when they are unbound in solution. In fact, these ions generate vast quantities of free radicals, which can present substantial oxidative hazards. Electrons are taken from these metals by oxygen molecules, for example, to produce superoxide ions, a type of oxygen free radical. In another reaction, hydroxyl radicals, the most damaging of all ROS, result from the reaction of iron or copper with hydrogen peroxide.

Oxidative Damage

Free radicals cause oxidative damage in four ways. In essence, free radicals will try to find another electron to pair with the single electron in its bonding orbital as quickly as possible. First, radicals can attach to other molecules, forming bonds. Second, radicals can give up their extra electron to another molecule. This is known as a reduction reaction. Third, radicals can take electrons from other molecules. Finally, radicals can take away an atom of hydrogen from a molecule it attacks. Rather than stealing just an electron, the free radical ends up with an entire atom of hydrogen.

As free radicals indiscriminately remove electrons from other atoms and molecules, the radical may become stable, while the molecule that was attacked becomes a radical itself and seeks to obtain an electron from other molecules. This creates a chain reaction where literally thousands of molecules can be damaged and altered by a process initiated by a single free radical. Bonds between atoms can be broken and molecular arrangements distorted. Chemical rings can be opened and helices disrupted. In short, compounds affected by oxidative damage can no longer perform their functions and must either be repaired or replaced.

The three most important types of molecules subject to oxidative damage are DNA, membrane lipid fatty acid chains, and proteins. Damage done to DNA molecules by free radicals can occur in a variety of ways. Free radicals can interfere with the normal electron interactions of the atoms that compose the bases. This can disrupt the replication and maintenance of the information safeguarded by the precise arrangement of the rings of the bases.

These rings can be broken open or broken off by free radicals. Entire bases can be completely lost from the molecule, causing a serious loss of genetic information. Radicals can attach themselves to DNA, altering its structure, thus altering its function. These changes and mutations to the structure of DNA, introduced by oxidative damage, can disrupt the normal function of the cell and cause many different diseases, most notable among them, cancer. If the damage is extensive enough, it can kill the cell outright.

The lipids found in our cell membranes are damaged by the same free radicals, but the processes and results are slightly different because the structures of the two molecules are not the same. Normally, if a molecule wants to get through the cellular membrane it needs the help of special proteins. However, small, uncharged particles like oxygen and some free radicals are able to pass through the cell membrane easily. For its part, oxygen prefers the lipid environment in the center of the cell membrane between the water on either side. The high concentration of oxygen inside the membrane creates a perfect setting for a particularly malicious form of oxidative damage known as lipid peroxidation.

These free radicals can, in turn, cause serious damage to the proteins embedded within the membrane acting to transport important molecules across the membrane to be used by the cell. When these proteins are damaged or destroyed cells risk malnutrition.

The process of lipid peroxidation and membrane protein damage causes the membrane to become brittle, leaky and increasingly immobile. Because many cellular processes necessitate that specific ions and compounds be kept out and others kept in, membrane leakage can disrupt cellular communication, metabolism and the structure of the cell's internal skeleton. If lipid peroxidation is extensive enough, all membrane integrity is lost and the cell dies.

Whether embedded in membranes or free in solution, proteins are often targets for free-radical attack. To completely disable a protein or an enzyme, a much greater degree of oxidative damage is usually required than for DNA or lipids.

Environmental Sources of Free Radicals

Free radicals contribute to and cause many diseases. In order to avoid as many free radicals as possible, it is important to know where they come from. As we have discussed, one of the principle sources of free radicals is the ETC found within every one of our cells. Even though we can't get away from the radicals originating there, the antioxidant defense mechanisms of our body usually take pretty good care of neutralizing those reactive species.

The ultraviolet light present in sunlight is also a source of free radicals. When UV light strikes our skin it generates free radicals by changing the oxygen molecules already there.

Burned food can also carry free radicals, especially meat that has been overcooked on a grill with a hot flame. Toxic chemicals, industrial pollutants and automotive exhaust fumes can also be sources of free radicals. Inordinate exposure to these substances in the workplace and at home should be avoided.

One of the largest sources of free radicals is cigarette smoke. There are few things more dangerous to the body than smoking because of the sheer quantity of reactive species sucked in from cigarette smoking. One researcher estimated the number of free radicals in just the gaseous portion (not counting the solids) of ONE puff of cigarette smoke to be on the order of $10^{17,}$ or 100,000,000,000,000,000. Perhaps this is one reason that stopping smoking would reduce the rate of cancer in a community by 30 percent!

Antioxidant Defenses

The body has many ways to protect itself from oxidative damage. These mechanisms can be divided into two general classes: enzymatic and molecular.

First, the body has enzymes in every cell that help neutralize some radicals. Often these enzymes work in pairs and teams. A particularly important team is superoxide dismutase (SOD) and catalase. SOD is an enzyme that converts superoxide ions to hydrogen peroxide. Catalase then consumes hydrogen peroxide and produces water and oxygen. One of the reasons a solution of hydrogen peroxide bubbles when poured on an open wound is because catalase is converting it to oxygen, gas and water. Even though superoxide itself is not extremely reactive, this system of superoxide disposal allows the body to avoid the more dangerous free radicals often produced by it.

Another family of enzymes known as glutathione peroxidase catalyzes the removal of hydrogen peroxide from the body.

Glutathione is a small molecule of three amino acids. Glutathione peroxidase enzymes bind two glutathione molecules together, converting hydrogen peroxide to water in the process. This prevents hydrogen peroxide from interacting with other molecules to form free radicals. Glutathione peroxidase uses the transition metal selenium in its active site to catalyze the reaction. This is the reason many people take selenium supplements.

Another important manner in which the body protects itself from oxidative damage is by producing proteins and compounds that bind metal ions preventing them from reacting with other molecules to form free radicals. When a molecule binds a metal ion in this way it is said to "chelate" (key-late) the metal ion. The molecule that does the chelating is called a chelator and the whole process is known as chelation. In the cells that line the intestines, iron is bound to the transferrin protein (the chelator) and then released into the bloodstream. In this manner the body can distribute iron obtained from the diet to all its tissues without creating oxidative stress.

Vitamins and other natural chemicals act in our system to tie up free radicals and stop the chain reactions they initiate. These are frequently called free-radical scavengers or antioxidants because when they react with radical species, they can neutralize them without becoming unstable radicals themselves. Notable among these are vitamins C and E. Vitamin C scavenges free radicals dissolved in water while vitamin E neutralizes lipid radicals within the plasma membranes of our cells.

A delicate balance exists between free radicals and the body's antioxidant defenses. When the defenses match the amount of attacking species, all is well and no significant harm is done. If, however, the quantity of free radicals increases above the body's capacity to neutralize them, the body undergoes oxidative stress and cellular components are rapidly damaged. Even when there is no oxidative stress, the body cannot dispose of every radical. Thus there will always be a minimum level of oxidative damage.

This is one of the biggest reasons the body has ways to repair and replace damaged molecules. When fats and proteins are damaged they are most often decomposed and replaced by new molecules. DNA, however, cannot be disposed of and replaced very easily because it contains the specific genetic information we need to live. Special repair enzymes exist that rejoin the breaks, fix the damaged bases, and accurately rewrite altered information. These repair mechanisms are very effective, but not fool-proof. Not every damaging event by a free radical will be repaired. Over time these unseen damages accumulate. Many think this is one of the principle reasons we age.

References

Bidlack, Omaye, Meskin and Topham. 2000. Phytochemicals as Bioactive Agents. Technomic Publishing Co., Inc. Lancaster, Basel.

Byung Pal Yu. 1993. Free Radicals and Aging. CRC Press.

Cadenas and Packer. 1996. Handbook of Antioxidants. Marcel Dekker, Inc.

Cerutti, Fridovich and McCord. 1988. Oxy-Radicals in Molecular Biology and Pathology. Alan R. Liss, Inc. New York.

Chow. 1988. Cellular Antoxidant Defense Mechansims Volume I–III. CRC Press.

Garewal. 1997. Antioxidants and Disease Prevention. CRC Press.

Halliwell and Gutteridge. 1999. Free Radicals in Biology and Medicine. 3rd edition. Oxford University Press.

Lin and Lonsdale. 1993. Free Radicals and Disease Prevention. Keats Publishing, Inc. New Canaan, Conn.

Matkovics and Kal. 1990. Radicals, Ions and Tissue Damage. AkadJmiai Kiad\, Budapest.

Miquel, Quintanilha, and Weber. 1989. Handbook of Free Radicals and Antioxidnats in Biomedicine Volume I–III. CRC Press.

Moslen and Smith. 1992. Free Radical Mechanisms of Tissue Injury. CRC Press.

Null. 1999. Gary Null's Ultimate Anti-Aging Program. Broadway Books. New York.

Packer and Colman. 1999. The Antioxidant Miracle. John Wiley and Sons, Inc.

Packer, Hiramatsu, and Yoshikawa.1999. Antioxidant Food Supplements in Human Health. Academic Press.

Papas. 1999. Antioxidant Status, Diet, Nutritionm and Health. CRC Press.

Shahidi. 1997. Natural Antioxidants. AOCS Press. Champaign, Illinois.

Smythies. 1998. Every Person's Guide to Antioxidants. Rutgers University Press.

CHAPTER 5

The Phytochemical Revolution

N ow it's time to tell you exactly how all of these compounds work. Following is some pretty technical information, but it's definitely useful information. From the reams of scientific data we've collected and studied, we've come up with all of the "hows" and "whys" of phytonutrition.

A Breakthrough Discovery

One of the most exciting and significant findings in the study of nutrition has been the discovery of phytochemicals. It has revolutionized our understanding of how the quality of life can be improved by taking care of our diets. It is becoming increasingly clear that phytochemicals are an important factor in nutrition. As we have already discussed, there are thousands of phytochemicals in fruits and vegetables and an untold number yet to be isolated and characterized.

In many cases, scientists have uncovered indisputable evidence of the benefits of fruits and vegetables without pinpointing the nutrients responsible. The recent discovery of phytochemicals has made it possible for scientists to determine how fruits and vegetables maintain health with greater accuracy. For example, in a recent study published in the scientific journal *Nature* on the antioxidant effect of fresh apples on tumor cell growth, the authors state the following: "Phytochemicals in apples other than ascorbic acid (vitamin C) seem significantly to enhance their antioxidant properties and their capacity to inhibit the proliferation of tumor cells. We suggest that this strong inhibition of tumor cell proliferation *in vitro* could be due to apples' combination of phytochemicals (phenolics acids and flavonoids)."

Despite the explosion in research on phytochemicals, we still have a long way to go in understanding how fruits and vegetables maintain health. For instance, a recent study published in the *American Journal of Clinical Nutrition* on the benefits of the antioxidant activity of a diet rich in fruits and vegetables, states, "based on this and other studies, it appears that compounds other than vitamin C and E and carotenoids contribute a major portion of the increase in antioxidant capacity." In other words, we are not exactly sure what chemicals are responsible for the increase in antioxidant activity we have noted, but we know that it isn't just vitamin C, vitamin E or carotenoids. Studies like this point the way for future research.

In addition to being powerful antioxidants, phytochemicals also exhibit other health-promoting potential. Phytochemicals found in broccoli and garlic produce enzymes that modify and detoxify many toxic chemicals, including some that appear to cause cancer. These enzymes are found in liver cells as part of a system known as the cytochrome P450 enzyme system. These cancer-preventing enzymes are also known as Phase II enzymes.

Another phytochemical found in garlic has been shown to inhibit cholesterol production. This chemical may account for lower cholesterol levels in individuals who consume dietary garlic in comparison to people who do not.

In this chapter, we will introduce and describe important features of major groups of phytochemicals. We will focus on those that have demonstrated powerful potential in improving the quality of life by improving health and preventing disease.

Carotenoids

Carotenoids are so named because they were first isolated in carrots, though they are found throughout the plant and animal kingdoms. Primarily, they are responsible for the red, yellow and orange colors of many flowers, birds, animals, insects and vegetables. Carotenoids give carrots their orange color. They are also found in leafy greens like spinach. Sometimes, carotenoids are called by different names like "phenolics" or "terpenoids."

Despite the fact that the first carotenoid was isolated from carrots in 1831, we still have a great deal of research to do to understand them. In 1955, a scientist named Sistrom and his team developed mutant plants that were unable to use carotenoids. When exposed to intense light, these plants died. They concluded that one of the functions of carotenoids was to protect plants from the damaging effects of the sun's visible light.

A few years later, in 1968, scientists began to think aging was the result of the combined affect of free radicals. These scientists also noted that carotenoids seemed capable of curtailing the damaging effects of free radicals.

In the 1970s, researchers found that many cancer patients had low plasma levels of many carotenoids. This research has sparked a great interest in carotenoids. Scientists now believe carotenoids may be instrumental in preventing many chronic diseases such as cancer, cardiovascular disease, and other neurodegenerative diseases. We are now seeking to confirm these ideas, as well as to develop an understanding of how carotenoids quench free radicals.

Both plants and animals use a five-carbon molecule called isoprene in the biosynthesis of a variety of compounds.

When two or three isoprene molecules are connected they form ten- or fifteen-carbon units called terpenes. Limonene, for example, is a terpene made up of ten carbon units.

When six isoprene molecules are connected they form a thirty-carbon chain called vitamin K2. When eight isoprene molecules are connected they form a forty-carbon chain called a carotenoid. For example, beta-carotene and lycopene are some of the most common of the large carotenoid family.

The long chain of carbon atoms is called an isoprene chain. There are actually several hundred different types of carotenoids. They are distinguished by differences in small molecules attached to the end of the forty-carbon chain.

Lycopene, found primarily in tomatoes, has a forty-carbon length chain, without an end on either side. B-carotene, on the other hand, is also forty-carbon units long, but both ends are capped with carbon rings. This subtle difference completely changes the function of these molecules. The shape of the atoms comprising a carotenoid further distinguishes them from one another. Some carotenoids are comprised of identical atoms, but in different shapes.

Even though molecules have exactly the same number of atoms, and are exactly in the same order, even this change can play an important role in the unique function they can have in our bodies.

Carotenoids and terpenes are often classed together because they share a similar structure. Some of the terpenes receiving scientific attention are limonene, myrcene, zingiberene, and natural rubber. (Refer to Appendix E to see these terpenes.) In general, these molecules share many of the characteristics of carotenoids, so we will not discuss them in further detail.

The structure of carotenoids makes them powerful antioxidants. The chemical structure found in Appendix E shows that the length of the carotenoids is spanned by a long isoprene chain. The characteristic feature of these isoprene chains is that they contain alternating double bonds, or conjugated bonds.

Isoprene Chain

Conjugated bonds are extremely stable. This stability makes carotenoids capable of quenching free radicals. The conjugated bonding pattern of carbon atoms in the isoprene chain makes carotenoids resilient and versatile. They can repeatedly give electrons to free radicals without becoming dangerous themselves. This converts free radicals into harmless molecules and averts potential damage to the cells of your body. Carotenoids do not become dangerous because the bonds between carbon atoms in the isoprene chain rearrange in ways to maintain stability despite the loss of an electron here and there. It is estimated that a single carotenoid may be capable of quenching one hundred to one thousand free radicals. Scientists continue to run tests with carotenoids to determine which free-radical species they quench.

The majority of the carotenoids in your body are beta-carotene. However, a total of thirty-four carotenoids have been found in human plasma, making the number of carotenoids actually used by humans only a fraction of the 700 carotenoids known. They are found throughout the body, but are concentrated in fats. As much as 80 percent of your body's supply of carotenoids is in your fat cells. Eight to twelve percent of your body's supply of carotenoids is in your liver. The remaining carotenoids are often concentrated in the ovaries of women or the testes of men, and in the adrenal gland.

The amounts and kinds of carotenoids absorbed by the body from the food you eat depend upon several factors. The tendency for a nutrient to be absorbed into the body is coined its bioavailability. The fact that a fruit or vegetable may be full of carotenoids may mean little if you do not have the right environment in your body to absorb them. Often people experience deficiency symptoms despite eating a nutrient-dense diet. This is possible because nutrients require specific environments to be absorbed by your body.

For instance, if a tomato is eaten with a little fat, lycopene will be absorbed more efficiently than if a tomato is eaten alone. This is because the absorption of lycopene requires fat to be absorbed by the body. Fat and fiber are the two biggest factors influencing carotenoid bioavailability. In order to get the most carotenoids out of the fruits and vegetables you eat, you ought to make sure you have adequate amounts of fiber and fat in your diet.

The manner in which carotenoid-rich foods are prepared also influences their bioavailability. For example, blood plasma measurements show that lycopene is more easily absorbed from blended tomato juice or paste than from eating a raw tomato. This may be because carotenoids in raw tomatoes are tied up in a matrix of proteins and carbohydrates that are broken up by processing. Often carotenoids are absorbed most efficiently when eaten in conjunction with other vitamins, minerals or phytochemicals. For example, beta-carotene seems to be absorbed more efficiently when with vitamin E. Many experts recommend eating whole fruits and vegetables because nature often provides effective combinations of vitamins, minerals, and phytochemicals to ensure maximum bioavailability.

Beta-carotene: Lung, Prostate, and Breast Cancer

Beta-carotene is found in carrots, pumpkin, squash, cantaloupe, apricots, sweet potatoes, pink grapefruit, spinach, and most dark green leafy vegetables. The more intense the yellow, orange or green color of the food, the more beta-carotene the vegetable or fruit contains. These foods are also good sources of alpha-carotene.

Low Carotenoid Levels Linked to Cancer Risk

A study published in the June 2002 issue of the *American Journal of Epidemiology* suggested, "These observations offer evidence that a low intake of carotenoids, through poor diet and/or lack of vitamin supplementation, may be associated with increased risk of breast cancer and may have public health relevance for people with markedly low intakes."

The slight change of the double bond at the end beta- and alpha-carotene can change the entire function of the molecule. Once in the body, carotenoids perform functions as varied as free-radical quenching to vitamin production. Many of the carotenoids are precursors of vitamin A, sometimes called provitamin A compounds.

Carotenoids may stimulate the body's immune system. For example, studies have shown that carotenoids play a key role in activating natural killer cells (NK), which naturally attack and kill cancer cells and certain virus-infected cells. Other studies correlate the increase in carotenoids in the diet with a lowered risk of certain types of cancer, theorizing that the stimulation of NK cells is responsible for these findings.

Many have thought carotenoids helped combat lung cancer, but tests have demonstrated surprising results. In 1994, a large study in Finland baffled scientists. Researchers supplemented the diets of 29,133 males who were heavy smokers with vitamin E or beta-carotene, or a combination of both vitamin E and beta-carotene. Scientists hoped to determine whether beta-carotene, vitamin E, or a combination of both molecules would help prevent lung cancer. The results were surprising.

They found no beneficial correlation between the supplementation of either or both of these compounds with incidences of lung cancer. In fact, contrary to previous claims and reports, the incidence of lung cancer and heart disease rose 18 percent. A few years later, the findings of the Finnish study were confirmed when the Carotene and Retinol Efficacy Trial (CARET) administered another experiment using 18,314 smokers and asbestos workers. The test was aborted after four years because the supplements appeared to be causing an increase in mortality. Lung cancer incidence rose 27 percent!

The reason for the increase in lung cancer among these individuals is not clear, but since these trials, many explanations have arisen. One theory is that beta-carotene acts as an antioxidant alone, but when converted into some of its other forms it becomes damaging. It is possible that the environment of the lungs in smokers and asbestos workers is saturated with free radicals such that beta-carotene is converted into a pro-oxidant, rather than an antioxidant. Whatever the answer is to these questions, the CARET study and the Finnish study have sparked the interest in supplemental beta-carotene, especially among the smoking population.

On the other hand, it appears that nonsmokers may benefit from beta-carotene supplements. In a 1994 study conducted by The Yale University School of Medicine, the diets of 413 nonsmoking lung cancer patients were compared with the diets of 413 noncancer patients. The results showed a statistical decrease in the risk of lung cancer among both women and men who had high dietary intake of fruits and vegetables rich in beta-carotene.

These findings were confirmed in a study done in Uruguay. Here, the diets of 541 lung cancer patients were also compared with the diets of 540 healthy individuals. Again, those with diets rich in carotenoids had significantly lower incidence of lung cancer.

In 1999, a study was published by the American Cancer Society. As part of *The Physicians' Health Study*, the research was to determine if beta-carotene supplementation would lower the risk for prostate cancer. Scientists analyzed blood samples of a total of 14,916 men. After twelve years of follow up, 631 of these men developed prostate cancer. Results showed a significant increase in risk among those men who had the least amount of beta-carotene in the blood.

In 1998, Italian researchers investigated the relationship between beta-carotene and the risk of breast cancer. They compared 2,569 women with breast cancer to a control group of 2,588 women who had never had cancer. They found that the healthy group of women had diets rich in foods with beta-carotene.

A study reported in 1997 by an Italian group of researchers indicates there is a beneficial relationship between carotenoids and the heart. Researchers compared 433 nonfatal heart attack patients to 869 people without heart disease. The study showed that those with high beta-carotene intakes were about half as likely to have a heart attack as people with low intakes of beta-carotene.

Dutch researchers studied the affect of beta-carotene on mental function among the elderly. Five thousand one hundred eighty-two people from the ages of fifty-five to ninety-five were tested for memory impairment and mental function. Subjects with diets providing less than 0.9 mg of beta-carotene were twice as likely to experience impaired memory, disorientation, and a decline in problem-solving abilities as those who had intakes of 2.1 mg or more.

Through such evidence, we can see that a diet rich in beta-carotene can prevent many diseases. It is best to receive your beta-carotene through your diet and not through supplementation.

Lycopene: Prostate Cancer and Heart Disease

Lycopene can be found in tomatoes, watermelon and pink grapefruit. It is more readily absorbed from tomato paste and other processed tomato products than from whole fruits and vegetables.

In 1999, studies attempted to determine whether lycopene could protect cells from DNA damage. Cells given lycopene had 33 percent less damage than cells with low lycopene concentrations. Another study divided ten women into two groups. The first group ate a tomato-free diet, while the second group drank a tomato puree every day for three weeks. At the end of the three weeks, researchers found that those in group one experienced considerably higher rates of DNA damage to lymphocyte cells than group two. Researchers concluded that the lycopene in the tomato puree significantly protected cells from DNA damage.

Tomatoes Linked with Lower Prostate Cancer Risk

Published in the March 2002 issue of the *Journal of the National Cancer Institute*, the Professionals Follow-Up Study (HPFS) performed from 1986 through 1998, suggests that frequent intake of tomato products or lycopene, a carotenoid from tomatoes, is associated with reduced risk of prostate cancer. "Results for the period from 1992 through 1998 confirmed our previous findings—that frequent tomato or lycopene intake was associated with a reduced risk of prostate cancer." Having studied over 47,000 people and their eating habits, the study concludes: "Frequent consumption of tomato products is associated with a lower risk of prostate cancer."

In a study reported in January 2000, 108 individuals diagnosed with atherosclerosis were compared with one another. Researchers measured the size of plaques in the abdominal aorta of each participant. They also measured the amounts of alpha-carotene, beta-carotene, lutein, lycopene, and zeaxanthin in the plasma of each participant. Those patients who had higher lycopene levels in their plasma were less susceptible to aortic atherosclerosis.

A study conducted by The Harvard Medical School, involving 48,000 men, found that men who ate large quantities of foods rich in lycopene were 34 percent less likely to develop prostate cancer than men who did not. More specifically, the 1995 study found that tomato-based foods seemed particularly effective in reducing the risk of prostate cancer.

Lutein and Zeaxanthin

Zeaxanthin is found in yellow corn, oranges, apricots, peaches, squash, mangos, papaya, spinach, kale, amaranth, and mustard greens. Lutein, similar to zeaxanthin, is also found in spinach, kale, peas, corn, potatoes, carrots, and tomatoes.

Lutein and zeaxanthin seem to be most beneficial because of their antioxidant properties. These carotenoids are particularly important to normal vision. There is a strong tendency for dangerous reactive oxygen species to form in the eye because the retina is exposed to light and oxygen so often. Many think that free radicals are one of the main reasons for blindness in the elderly. Lutein and zeaxanthin play a crucial role in quenching free radicals in the macula of the eye.

These carotenoids seem to be instrumental in reducing the risk of age-related macular degeneration (ARMD). ARMD is the biggest cause of blindness in the elderly, affecting approximately thirteen

Lycopene Reduces Risk of Breast Cancer

Results from a study published in the August 2001 issue of *Cancer Causes & Control* suggested "that lycopene and other plasma-carotenoids may reduce the risk of developing breast cancer and that menopausal status has an impact on the mechanisms involved."

to fourteen million people in the U.S., or about 30 percent of people over sixty-five. Although supplemental studies involving these compounds in isolation have yet to be significantly correlated to protection against ARMD, the consumption of dark green, leafy vegetables has been shown to reduce the risk of ARMD.

In the year 2001, the University of Utah Medical School published a study indicating that lutein prevents colon cancer. Examining data from 1,993 subjects who had had cancer of the colon and 2,410 case control subjects, they found that individuals with higher levels of lutein in their diet had a significantly lower risk of colon cancer. Levels of lutein were estimated based on reported diets from all of the individuals. Researchers concluded that those foods containing the most lutein, namely spinach, broccoli, lettuce, tomatoes, oranges, carrots, celery and other greens may help to reduce the risk of developing colon cancer.

Organosulfurs

Organosulfurs are primarily found in broccoli, cauliflower, onions and garlic. Organosulfurs contain large amounts of sulfur, a necessary element for maintaining good health. There are actually many different types of compounds called organosulfurs. Scientists are beginning to focus on organosulfurs because they seem to be anticarcinogenic. Many recent studies indicate that they may inhibit the growth of certain kinds of cancers. However, other studies indicate they actually may promote the growth of certain other cancers. Further research on organosulfurs is required to better understand how some can prevent cancers and others promote them. Organosulfurs may be effective in preventing cancers of the prostate, skin, gastrointestinal tract, liver and colon.

The organosulfur compound S-allylmercaptocysteine (SAMC) was indicated to inhibit the proliferation of actively dividing hormone responsive breast and prostate cancer cells. Cells that were not actively dividing were not susceptible to SAMC.

Diallyl disulfide (DADS), an organosulfur found in garlic, has been indicated to increase the activity of the Phase II enzymes quinone reductase (QR) and glutathionone transferase (GT) in the gastrointestinal tract. Increased activation of this enzyme system may lead to decreased risk for cancer in the GI tract. A second study indicated that DADS protects against chemically induced skin cancer in mice. DADS may be effective against skin cancer by suppressing an H-ras oncogene through the inhibition of p21H-ras membrane association. DADS has also been indicated to inhibit cytochrome P450 activation of toxic substances, thus giving a protective effect for the liver. The organosulfur anethole trithione seems to have even greater anticarcinogenic effects than DADS on the colon.

The organosulfurs S-methylcysteine (SMC) and cysteine tended to have the strongest inhibitory effects compared to other organosulfurs on the promotion and initiation stages of liver cancer formation. They appeared to have their effects through the enzymes glutathione S-transferase and ornithine decarbosylase.

The vegetable-derived organosulfur, S-methylmethanethiosulfonate, has been indicated to have a protective effect against chemically induced colon cancer.

S-allylcysteine (SAC) has been indicated to have significant antiproliferative effects on induced colon cancer formation during the initiation phase of carcinogenesis but not in the proliferation phase. It is said to have effects through activation of the detoxification enzyme glutathione S-transferase (GST). SAC also has been indicated to cause the reduction of reactive oxygen-induced DNA damage. SAC does not appear to inhibit the formation of breast cancer.

The organosulfur compound S-methylmethanethiosulfonate was indicated to not reduce the incidence of lung cancer when supplemented in the initiation phase of carcinogenesis.

The organosulfur compounds isothiocyanic acid isobutyl ester (IAIE), dipropyl trisulfide (DPT), and allyl mercapton (AM) were indicated to increase cell proliferation in the liver, possibly via polyamine synthesis, indicating the potential for liver cancer promoting effects.

Though the water-soluble organosulfur compounds diallyl disulfide, S-methylcysteine and cysteine were indicated to inhibit liver carcinogenesis, diallyl sulfide, diallyl trisulfide and allyl methyl trisulfide tended to enhance the formation of liver carcinogens.

An unusual organosulfur isolated from garlic, with an unbelievably long name (E-4, 5, 9-trithiadeca-1, 7-diene-9-oxide iso-E-10-devinylajoene, iso-E-10-DA) was indicated to have antimicrobial properties against gram-positive bacteria and yeast but not gram-negative bacteria.

Organosulfur compounds are used as nutrient sources of sulfur to feed and grow some of the same gram-positive bacterial strains whose growth was inhibited above. Obviously the activities of organosulfur compounds are highly variable and subject to the type and activities of each individual compound.

Flavonoids

Flavonoids are a group of health-promoting compounds found in all plants. We know of over 3,000 flavonoids. Like carotenoids, flavonoids give plants color. In fact, the name flavonoid is derived from the Latin word for yellow: *flavus*. Some flavonoids have antioxidant, antibacterial, antiviral, anti-inflammatory, and cardioprotective functions. Flavonoids may be the chemicals responsible for many of the results of herbal and folk medicinal therapies.

Flavonoid compounds are usually composed of three rings of carbon, oxygen, and hydrogen atoms. There are many different groups in the flavonoid family, each with a slightly different arrangement of the basic three-ringed structure. These different flavonoid groups are the flavones, flavonols, flavanols, flavonones, flavononols, anthrocyanidins, and the isoflavones. We won't treat each one of these groups individually.

Flavonoids have come under much recent scientific scrutiny because of their potential to promote health and combat disease. As with carotenoids and organosulfurs, flavonoids are powerful antioxidants. Like carotenoids, their molecular structure allows strength and versatility.

Flavonoids perform important functions in protecting against LDL oxidation, making them instrumental in preventing atherosclerosis, heart attacks and strokes. Some flavonoids are hydrophilic (water loving), likely remaining in the plasma, while others are more hydrophobic (water fearing), likely entering the fat and cholesterol of LDLs. Flavonoid molecules in both the plasma and LDLs can quench potentially dangerous free radicals and protect the body from the harmful effects of cholesterol accumulation in the arteries.

Flavonoids also seem instrumental in preventing oxidative damage by binding free metal ions in the body. As we discussed before, transition metal ions, especially iron and copper, create free radicals out of oxygen compounds normally circulating in the body. Your body generally controls metal ions with special proteins, preventing them from interacting with oxygen. Flavonoids can help prevent free metal ions from creating free radicals because they are structured like a pocket that holds metal ions between oxygen atoms. In the end, flavonoids may prevent the creation of thousands or millions of free radicals by helping control metal ions. They also seem to help regulate the activity of some antioxidant proteins and enzymes.

Recent studies have shown that genistein, an isoflavone, increases the amount of a metal-binding protein called metallothionein. Other studies have shown that flavonoids can inhibit the action of enzymes that generate free radicals. For instance, flavonoids may be able to prevent an enzyme known as xanthine oxidase from doing significant damage to tissues recovering from acute oxygen deficiency (stroke or heart attack). Low concentrations of common flavonoids such as kaempferol, quercetin, and myricetin appear to cut the activity of xanthine oxidase in half.

Flavonoids may also help increase the productivity of enzymes that combat free radicals, but thus far research has been inconclusive. We will need to wait until experimental methods are better

---

Citrus Fruits May Reduce Degenerative Disease

A new study published in the January 2002 issue of the *Asian Journal of Clinical Nutrition* states, "Accumulated evidence from experimental and epidemiological studies indicates that there is a low risk of degenerative diseases, cardiovascular disease, hypertension, cataract, stroke and, in particular, cancers in people with a high intake of fruit and vegetables. This protective effect is assumed to be associated mainly with the antioxidant activities of either individual or interacting bioactive components present in the fruits and vegetables, and with other biochemical and physical characteristics of the identified and unknown bioactive components. The implicated bioactive components present in citrus fruits include vitamin C, beta-carotene, flavonoids, limonoids, folic acid, and dietary fiber."

The study concludes: "A high intake of citrus fruits may reduce the risk of degenerative diseases."

capable of pinpointing how flavonoids affect many of the enzymes within our bodies.

Flavonoids may inhibit lipid peroxidation. A recent study conducted at Michigan State University suggests that various flavonoid molecules can affect the arrangement and packing of lipid fatty acid chains. It seems that some flavonoid compounds actually decrease molecular motion within the membrane of fatty acids, increasing lipid density. This increased density makes it much more difficult for free radicals to enter the membrane and start lipid-radical chain reactions.

For many years researchers have been perplexed about what is called the "French Paradox." The French people consume much greater quantities of foods high in fat and cholesterol than Americans do, but have an incidence of heart disease that is significantly lower than Americans. A higher intake of fat and cholesterol should increase the risk of heart disease, but this does not appear to be the case. Scientists suggest that one of the contributing factors of this paradox may be that the French people drink red wine more often than Americans. Red wine is a good source of flavonoids.

Red wine contains many flavonoids and other polyphenolic compounds that are not found in other alcoholic drinks because it is prepared from grapes with the skins and seeds. Purple grape juice has also been shown to have similar protective functions because it may contain the same or similar compounds. One of the ways scientists believe these molecules help to protect the body is by scavenging free radicals in the blood.

Flavonoids also perform another important function in the protection of cardiovascular health. They seem to inhibit platelet aggregation in the blood. Blood vessels ridden with atherosclerotic plaques can sometimes cause the spontaneous formation of blood clots. To avoid these complications many high-risk individuals take aspirin to inhibit platelet aggregation, or in other words, to thin the blood. Many initial studies have shown that flavonoids have the same effect as aspirin.

Quercetin, a flavonoid found abundantly in onions and apples, has particular potential for inhibiting platelet aggregation. Some researchers believe it prevents platelet aggregation by coating the platelets and preventing them from sticking together. Others think that quercetin inhibits the production of signal molecules that induce aggregation.

Flavonoids May Prevent Hormone-Related Cancers

A study published in the January 2002 issue of *Chemico-Biologic Interactions* came to the following conclusions: "Flavonoids in the human diet may reduce the risk of various cancers, especially hormone-dependent breast and prostate cancers." The study also found that flavonoids may also prevent menopausal symptoms.

Flavonoids may also help protect against heart disease by relaxing the arteries. When the body senses stress it often causes the muscular layer of the arteries to contract. This can compound conditions such as atherosclerosis where the blood vessels are already partially blocked. Apparently, flavonoids can cause the muscular layer of the arteries to relax, allowing more blood to pass through, and decreasing the risk of heart attack or stroke.

Several recent studies suggest that certain flavonoids may be able to prevent osteoporosis. Studies using rats have indicated that genistein, a flavonoid found in soy products, may enhance the process by which the body absorbs bone material. Normally the body builds bone material as quickly as it absorbs it. Osteoporosis occurs when bones are broken down, but not rebuilt. Women lose bone density after menopause because they stop producing estrogen, a hormone that helps regulate the density of bone matter in women. Genistein may do the same work as estrogen. Research will show whether foods high in genistein and other related flavonoids will prove to be an effective dietary treatment for osteoporosis.

Recent studies indicate that people with diets high in flavonoids have a lower risk of various forms of cancer. A study conducted in Spain with over 700 participants showed that individuals whose diet contained a high level of flavonoids were at a decreased risk for stomach cancer. A group of researchers in Hawaii conducting a study with over 1,000 participants reported that an increased intake of flavonoids is related to a decreased risk of lung cancer. Other studies indicate that flavonoids may also inhibit breast, prostate, and colon cancers.

Flavonoids stop cancers by inhibiting their growth and division. A great deal of research demonstrates that an increased concentration of flavonoids causes cancer cells to stop growing at crucial DNA checkpoints. There are two ways this is done:

First, it seems flavonoids can interrupt the growth signals that are transmitted from outside the cell to the nucleus telling it to grow. Normally, a protein called a receptor spans the cell membrane and receives a chemical signal from the cell's exterior. Receptors pass the signal on to other proteins within the cell, where the signal is passed from protein to protein until it reaches the nucleus. When the signal reaches the nucleus, the DNA responds by sending out commands allowing the cell to grow and divide. Some flavonoids such as apigenin and quercetin disrupt the passing of signals within the cell, preventing cancerous cells from growing and dividing.

Second, it seems flavonoids can shut down the machinery that makes the cell's proteins. When the nucleus receives the signal to grow, it sends out instructions to the ribosomes regarding what proteins need to be built and how to build them. Before the ribosomes can start putting together the amino acids encoded in the instructions, they need to bind another protein in the cell called an initiation factor (eIF-2). The flavonoids genistein and quercetin apparently interfere with the interaction of eIF-2 and the ribosomes, dramatically reducing the quantity of proteins produced in cancerous cells. The less protein produced within cancerous cells, the less they can grow and divide.

Some cancers require hormones to live and progress. For example, one-third of all breast cancers diagnosed are dependent upon estrogen and will regress when the estrogen is blocked or its level decreases in the body. Flavonoids have been shown to decrease the activity of the enzyme that produces estrogen. Another enzyme whose products contribute to the development of prostate cancer has also been shown to be effected in a similar way.

Flavonoids can also be a bit more aggressive in combating cancer. Studies have shown that a variety of flavonoids induce apoptosis, programmed cell death, in cancer cells.

Flavonoids appear to be helpful in combating diseases caused or compounded by the body's inflammatory responses. These diseases include arthritis and Alzheimer's. A molecule called nitric oxide and a class of compounds called prostaglandins are both involved in inflammatory responses. These compounds act as signal molecules to initiate inflammation. They cause the blood vessels of affected areas to widen, allowing an increase in blood flow to affected areas. Prostaglandins often cause blood vessel walls to become leaky, allowing more fluid to enter the inflamed area, causing swelling.

Prostaglandins also activate and recruit white blood cells, which release chemicals that can damage the cells of inflamed tissues. Though the inflammatory response is necessary to combat infections, when it is turned on the body it can cause serious damage.

The flavonoids apigenin, genistein and kaempferol have been shown to inhibit the production of prostaglandins. Apigenin and kaempferol also decrease the production of nitric oxide. Quercetin has also been shown to inhibit the production of a chemical that attracts white blood cells contributing to inflammation. The fact that these compounds may slow or ameliorate inflammatory diseases is still under investigation. Preliminary research on arthritic mice shows that flavonoids may help the body combat these diseases.

Unlike carotenoids, flavonoids do not need to be eaten in conjunction with other foods in order to be absorbed and used.

Phytochemicals in Soy

The soybean is relatively new in the West, but has a long history in Asia. The soybean was first used in the West for its oil and then as feed for animals. It wasn't until the 1950s that the soybean was used for food in the Western world. Today the soy industry is a booming business.

Soybeans are great sources of protein, surpassing other vegetables and rivaling animal products. Soy protein products are easily digested and are not accompanied by dangerous saturated fats and cholesterols, like the protein found in animals. Soy protein is also a wonderful source of dietary fibers. Fiber may play a role in controlling blood cholesterol, and may prevent colon cancer.

Soy protein has been known for its cholesterol-lowering effects for over eighty years. A recent study conducted by the University of Toronto confirmed that a diet rich in vegetable and soy protein lowers blood cholesterol levels. This is due to the fiber found in soybeans. Another study conducted by the University of Kentucky indicated that the consumption of soy protein significantly lowered levels of serum cholesterol, LDL (bad) cholesterol, and triglyceride concentration. There was also an insignificant increase in HDL (good) cholesterol.

Soy contains many phytochemicals that may help prevent hormone-sensitive cancers (breast and prostate). These phytochemicals may partly block receptors with plant estrogens known as genistein and daidzein. Many other studies have been conducted with soybeans and cancer. One such study conducted at the University of Alabama at Birmingham suggested that soybeans contain a chemical compound similar to tamoxifen, a drug generally used to treat breast cancer. Soy contains compounds that cause apoptosis.

In another study, diets rich in soy protein (Asian diet) were compared with diets that had no or little soy protein (American diet). Asians suffered from hormone-related cancers three to six times less than Americans. Interestingly enough, Asian-Americans suffered from hormone-related cancers just as much as Americans, ruling out the possibility that these rates were due to genetic factors.

Phytosterols

Phytosterols are sterols that come from plants. Sterols predominantly consist of unsaturated carbon rings and various attached side chains. Within the sterol family, there are many related molecules with highly variable functions. For instance, cholesterol is a sterol found throughout your body. Though cholesterol has gotten a lot of bad press, it's not all bad. Cholesterol and fats help form the cytoplasmic or cellular membranes of your cells and help maintain an appropriate balance between water inside cells and water outside cells. Unlike essential fatty acids, you don't have to worry too much about getting cholesterol from your diet. Your cells make 80 percent of the needed cholesterol out of other materials.

Steroid hormones are also sterols. In fact, they are manufactured from cholesterol in the body. Phytosterols, on the other hand, are slightly different than the sterols manufactured in your body, though it appears that they can augment their activities. Plants can make molecules that resemble the steroid hormones made by our bodies in form and/or function. Plant steroids can have hormone functions. Phytoestrogens are plant sterols that resemble the hormone estrogen, either in structure and/or function.

Phytoestrogens are found in a large number of plants. They are commonly found in high concentrations in soy products and various herbs. Phytoestrogens have been discovered in unexpected places like whole grains and beer.

Some research indicates that phytoestrogens will lower cholesterol and/or decrease the chances of developing heart disease. Other studies indicate they are ineffective. The results in experiments were highly variable. This lack of a definite pattern prevents scientists from drawing specific conclusions on the effectiveness of phytosterols or phytoestrogens on lipids and cholesterol. Thus, no conclusion can be made on the usefulness of phytosterols in heart disease.

A study involving fifty-one women indicated that soy phytoestrogen supplementation reduced total cholesterol by 6 percent and LDL cholesterol by 7 percent. During the six-week study researchers also observed a decline in diastolic blood pressure in the group eating soy-supplemented diets. These researchers concluded that soy could be good for lowering the risks associated with heart disease. Another study involving seven subjects concluded that soy sterol esters reduced cholesterol absorption in the small intestine.

The effects of soy phytoestrogens on LDL cholesterol oxidation in thirty-one hyperlipidemic subjects were studied during two one-month duration diets. They found that a diet higher in soy products decreased the levels of oxidized LDL cholesterol circulating in the subjects' blood, possibly reducing the risk of cardiovascular disease.

The supplementation of soymilk and its effect on cholesterol levels was researched using ten men as participants for a four-week study. There were no changes in cholesterol or triglyceride levels when compared to control groups.

Another study involving fourteen female subjects for four months, resulted in inconclusive data. Ingestion of isoflavonoid phytoestrogens did not change the total blood cholesterol, LDL cholesterol, or plasma triacylglycerol. There may have been a change in HDL metabolism but further studies were required for clarity.

In another study researchers used plant stanol ester spreads in addition to the diets of preschool children. The thirteen-week study was divided into a one-week lead-in period, followed by one of two four-week diet phases and a two-week washout and then a crossover to the second diet. The children showed a 12.4 percent reduction in total cholesterol and a 15.5 percent reduction in LDL cholesterol when on the plant stanol ester spread diet. There were no changes in HDL or triglyceride levels. No side effects were noted.

A study of plant sterol spreads, which lasted nine weeks and involved seventy-six healthy adults, also found that total and LDL cholesterol was lowered, but by a much more moderate degree of 3.8 and 6 percent respectively.

A study on phytosterol esters involving twenty-four subjects, twelve men and twelve women, found that supplementation (plus diet) caused 18 and 23 percent reductions in total and LDL cholesterol respectively. In this study it was found that the phytoestrogens biochanin, genistein, equol, diadzeiin, and formononetin (most to least effective) were found to inhibit proliferation of smooth muscle cells that had been stimulated by calf serum, collagen and protein synthesis, and migration and MAP kinase activity in a concentration dependant manner. These traits researchers believe will lead to a lower risk for heart disease.

In a recent report the phytoestrogens genistein, daidzein and 17 beta-estradiol were tested for their effects on the *in vitro* injured aortic walls of male and female rabbits. The object was to stop the proliferation of the injured cells. Genistein was shown to slow the proliferation, but decreased formation of the neointima only in the male rabbits' aortic rings, while it actually increased formation of the neointima in female rabbits' aortic rings. Daidzein was found to decrease formation of the neointima in both males and females.

This study showed that the soy phytoestrogens were incorporated into LDL cholesterol and resulted in a greatly reduced amount of cellular proliferation *in vitro* (36 to 43 percent for 4',7-dioleates of genistein and daidzein and 93 percent for daidzein 4',7-dilinoleate).

The effects of genistein on the cardiovascular pathology of myocardial ischaemia-reprofusion injuries were studied. Genistein was found to lower the incidence of cell death, to increase contractility of the heart and to decrease the occurrence of off-beat heartbeats. It also appeared to reduce the production of an inflammatory molecule called Tumor Necrosis Factor alpha (TNF-A) thus possibly reducing inflammation.

The research regarding phytoestrogens and cancer has been very promising. Some phytoestrogens may be helpful in reducing the risk of certain kinds of cancers. More research is necessary to solidify these trends, but data showing that phytoestrogen intake from fruits, vegetables and soy products may reduce the risk of developing cancers continues to increase.

A study that looked at the supplementation of soymilk used ten men as participants for the four-week study. The soy phytoestrogens genistein and daidzein were reflected in the plasma. Tests indicated that oxidative damage to DNA in lymphocytes was reduced during supplementation. A second study involving the phytoestrogens coumestrol, genistein and daidzein indicated that very high doses of the first two substances could actually cause DNA damage including chromatid breaks, gaps and interchanges in lymphocytes. Daidzein did not seem to induce any DNA damage, even at higher concentrations.

The effects of various phytoestrogens on DNA synthesis were investigated. Researchers found that the phytoestrogens coumestrol and genistein enhanced DNA synthesis at concentrations lower than 10 mM. Genistein also enhanced insulin and epidermal growth factor at this dose and smaller doses. Both of these phytoestrogens switched effects at higher doses. In fact in doses of 10 mM and higher, all of the phytoestrogen compounds studied inhibited DNA synthesis. This research indicated that the cancer effecting abilities of phytoestrogens are variable and dependent upon dosage.

In a nine-week study of nude mice with transplanted prostate cancer cells the effects of diet were ascertained. Nude mice are strains of mice that lack a thymus and that are mostly hairless. Without a thymus they are defective in many immune functions, which makes them very useful in tumor studies since they do not reject transplanted tumors. Animals supplemented with soy had reduced formation of tumors. Animals supplemented with rye bran had even greater tumor inhibition. The tumors that grew in the rye bran and soy test groups were smaller, fewer and underwent higher degrees of apoptosis (a genetic program used to kill cancer cells) than tumors seen in control mice, though cell proliferation was unchanged. When fat was added to the rye diet the beneficial effects were diminished.

In a study that compared the Western diet to the Asian diet it was found that consumption of the phytoestrogens coumestrol and daidzein decreased prostate cancer risk while campesterol and stigmasterol increased cancer risk.

Diets high in phytoestrogens are connected to a low risk for breast cancer. Decreased risk is also connected to the increase of not just phytoestrogens but other fruits and vegetables.

A recent *in vitro* study found that some phytoestrogens, namely genistein and quercetin, inhibited the growth of human breast cancer cells. The researchers determined that these two phytoestrogens have their effects through different means. Other phytoestrogens were found much less effective and even ineffective in reducing proliferation of breast cancer cells.

Another recent study indicated that the phytoestrogen beta-sitosterol inhibited the growth of breast cancer cells. It was also found to increase the rate of apoptosis of breast cancer cells via an unknown mechanism by six-fold when compared to a cholesterol control model. Another phytoestrogen, campesterol, was found ineffective.

The effects of a phytoestrogen named resveratrol were studied *in vitro* on several kinds of cancer cells. It was found to inhibit proliferation of pancreas, breast, and renal cancer cells. It inhibited the proliferation of colon and prostate cancer cells to a lesser degree. It stimulated the growth of normal fibroblasts in the lungs.

The phytoestrogen genistein, biochanin A, equol and coumestrol were tested *in vitro* for effects on pancreatic tumor cells from male or female donors. Equol and coumestrol served to inhibit cancer growth in the cells of females and stimulated cancer growth in the cells of males. These phytoestrogens were toxic in higher concentrations. The phytoestrogen genistein did not seem to effect cancer growth in female cells and also stimulated the growth of male cancer cells. Biochanin A inhibited both female and male cancer cells but it wasn't very effective. Each phytoestrogen appeared to work via different pathways.

Information regarding the use of phytoestrogens to remedy problems associated with menopause is also highly contradictive. Some studies seem to indicate it is effective, while others demonstrate there is no effect at all. The largest and best-designed studies indicate that phytoestrogens are ineffective in most of the estrogenic pathways, including hot flash reductions. The only benefit that appears likely is increased bone density. Pregnant women should avoid ingesting a lot of phytoestrogens during pregnancy as there is now evidence that phytoestrogens increase the risk for certain birth defects in male babies. Following are some of the studies on phytoestrogens and hormone therapy:

One well-designed study, including 177 women, concluded that soy supplementation was not effective in reducing menopausal hot flashes. Another study concluded that soy had no significant effect on the reproductive system in menstrual function or hormone levels. Another showed soy did not have an estrogenic effect on breasts, and that the soy phytoestrogen genistein did not have an effect on the uterus.

There are only a few reports indicating that soy phytoestrogens might have estrogenic activities. In one, groups of twenty female rats were either given soy supplements or used as controls. Researchers concluded that there were estrogenic effects related to soy when it was consumed in moderately concentrated doses. A third study concluded that the genistein had estrogenic action in bone, leading to greater bone volume.

A Few Notes of Caution

It is important to not overdo your phytoestrogen intakes. Heavy ingestion of phytoestrogens in a vegetarian diet during the first half of pregnancy has been connected to an increased risk for the birth defect hypospadias among male infants. Phytoestrogens may effect the normal development of male infants.

Phytoestrogens can have highly variable and complex effects on the brain. In some instances phytoestrogens act estrogenically, in other instances they act anti-estrogenically, and sometimes they have no effect at all. Obviously this area requires a great deal more research before any conclusions can be made about the overriding effects of phytoestrogens in the brain.

Pregnant women should be cautious when eating foods with high concentrations of phytoestrogens because they may cause alterations in the development of infant brains. For example, fifteen spayed rats were used to determine the effects of soy supplementation on mRNA levels of brain-derived neurotrophic factor (BDNF). Estradiol and soy had about the same effects compared to controls indicating that soy may have an estrogenic effect in the brain.

The phytoestrogen coumestrol may work as an anti-estrogen in the beta-estrogen receptors (Erbeta) in the brain. In a recent study coumestrol increased mRNA when it bound to Erbeta while estradiol, a true estrogen, did exactly the opposite.

Soy phytoestrogens may work as estrogen antagonists according to a study done on spayed rats. Phytoestrogens apparently have some estrogenic effects on nerve growth factor (NGF) and choline acetyltransferase (ChAT) in the brain. Soy effects on NGF were less than on estradiol-supplemented rats.

Another study looked at the effects of phytoestrogens on male rats. They found that there was no change in regulatory behaviors such as eating and drinking, brain aromatase activity, or reproductive factors such as prostate weight or testosterone levels when the rats ate phytoestrogens. There were changes in MBH-POA and amydala 5alpha-reductase activities when the rats consumed phytoestrogens.

The phytoestrogens genistein and daidzein decrease ACTH and cAMP stimulated cortisol release in the brain. They also inhibit the activity of 21-hydroxylase (P450c21), which causes an increase in DHEA/DHEA-S production by robbing the glucocorticoid pathway of metabolites. These effects indicate that phytoestrogens may decrease cortisol production and increase androgen (sex hormones) production in the brain.

Supplementation with phytoestrogens may also decrease the abundance of the calcium-binding protein calbindin in the brain. A recent study was carried out using male rats fed a phytoestrogen diet for five weeks. There were no effects found on the brain enzymes aromatase and 5alpha-reductase by phytoestrogens.

There are possible developmental problems that may result from consumption of phytoestrogens during pregnancy. In another study it was shown that normally Calbindin-D28K (CALB) levels are higher in female neonates and lower in males. If the mother consumes a phytoestrogen diet the levels of CALB in the sexes of infants are reversed and may result in sexually dimorphic brain structures in the neonates.

The phytoestrogens genistein and coumestrol have been indicated to inhibit the production of the thymic hormone thymosin-alpha 1 in the cells of the thymus.

There has also been research that shows that the phytoestrogen trans-resveratrol may interfere with clotting or platelet aggregation by inhibiting the activation of calcium channels in platelets.

The phytoestrogens genistein, daidzein and zearalenone have been indicated to inhibit hormone-induced lipid production in rat adipocytes (fat cells). Higher concentrations of genistein and daidzein also appeared to enhance lipolysis, or the breakdown of fat, in the adipocytes, though at the highest concentrations appeared inhibitory to lipolysis.

The phytoestrogens genistein and daidzein have also been implicated as glucose-uptake inhibitors in the intestine *in vitro*. They have also been indicated to reduce glucose-induced oxidation of LDL cholesterol *in vitro*. The first may have helpful use for diabetics. The second may have benefits related to heart disease.

Soy phytoestrogens have been indicated to reduce asthma-related inflammation but have a side effect of an increased leakage of protein into the airspace.

Alkaloids

Made primarily by plants, alkaloids are named such because they are a group of mildly alkaline compounds. Alkaloids can have strong effects on the body, even when ingested in small amounts. Over 3,000 alkaloids are known, including the following: quinone, nicotine, morphine and coniine.

Alkaloids are one of the most diverse groups of phytochemicals found in living organisms. Within the family of alkaloids there are multiple structures, biosynthetic pathways, and pharmacological activities. Alkaloids are traditionally isolated from plants, but they have been found in vertebrates, invertebrates, and marine animals. Alkaloids and alkaloid producing plants are well known for their toxic and at times psychomimetic, euphoric, and hallucinogenic properties.

Many alkaloids have been used for centuries in medicine, and some are still found in drugs today. The first crude drugs studied chemically were opium and morphine. These alkaloid products helped in the development of many pain medications used regularly under doctor supervision today.

Pelletier from the Faculty of Pharmacy of Paris classified an alkaloid as "a cyclic compound containing nitrogen in a negative oxidation state, which is of limited distribution in living organisms." In other words, alkaloids consist of rings containing nitrogen while lacking oxygen, and it is found in living organisms in small quantities. The Faculty of Pharmacy of Paris lab isolated many crude drugs from alkaloids.

Alkaloids have been found mainly in flowering plants, but in recent years a number of alkaloids are being found in animals, insects, marine organisms, microorganisms, and lower plants. Alkaloids are part of an elaborate chemical defense system in plants. However, most alkaloids can have a variety of toxic effects on some animals. Alkaloid plants have often been used as poisons for poisonous arrows. Alkaloids used in drugs generally affect the nervous system, especially the action of chemical transmitters (acetylcholine, epinephrine, norepinephrine, gamma-aminobutyric acid [GABA], dopamine, and serotonin). Thus they serve to prevent pain signals from transferring from nerve cells to the brain. In short, they dull or completely block sensations of pain.

Naturally occurring alkaloids often serve as models for the synthetic production of drugs. For example cocaine (*Erythroxylon coca*), morphine *(P. somniferum)*, and codeine *(Papaver somniferum)* are manufactured as a result of naturally occurring alkaloids. Alkaloids also have other pharmacological activities: antihypertensive effects, antiarrhythmic effects, antimalarial activity, and anticancer actions. Alkaloids also contain antibiotic properties and are used in antiseptics in medicine.

Here is a list of alkaloids and their therapeutic uses:

Atropine: Used as an antispasmodic in the treatment of gastrointestinal, urinary, and biliary colics. Atropine is also used in the general preparation of anesthesia, and to reduce bronchial and salivary secretion and bronchospams. It is also used in the local treatment of muscular rheumatism, sciatica, and neuralgia. Finally, it is used in ophthalmology as a mydriatic and cycloplegic drug.

Boldine: Used in the treatment of cholelithiasis, stomach disorders, vomiting, constipation, and dyspepsia.

Cocaine: Used as a local surface anesthetic, in ophthalmology for corneal anesthestheatic, and as a treatment of epistaxis.

Codeine: Used as a mild sedative and as an antitussive in the treatment of cough.

Ephedrine: Used as a nasal decongestant for the relief of cold symptoms and for the treatment of bronchial asthma.

Morphine: Used in the treatment of diarrhea and also to control pain in cancer patients.

Nicotine: Used as a natural insecticide and also used for stimulatory effects.

Tannins

Tannins are very large compounds that give color to many plant tissues. They are found in the purple skin of grapes, the color of the leaves in autumn, and in tree bark. Tannins received their name because they are used to tan leather.

Tannins do not have many helpful functions for humans. The body does not absorb them well. They often bind to proteins and prevent them from being absorbed. They can also inhibit the ability of digestive enzymes in the stomach hampering digestion. In fact, cattle eating feed with high tannin content put on considerably less weight than cattle eating a reduced tannin diet. Tannins may also cause headaches.

On the positive side, tannins can be used as an external treatment for varicose veins. They cause constriction of blood vessels, making them less visible.

Tannins come in two kinds: condensed tannins and hydrolysable tannins. Condensed tannins are a conglomeration of flavonoids strung together. They are sometimes called proanthocyanidins.

Saponins

Saponins are large molecules consisting of a multiple ring system composed mostly of carbons and hydrogens. Sugar chains are bound to the system of rings comprising saponins. There are three major classes of saponins, distinguishable by the arrangement of their carbon rings. They are called triterpene, steroid, and steroid alkaloid classes.

The steroid and steroid alkaloid classes are so named because of the structural similarity their ring systems have with cholesterol. Sugar chains are frequently bound to either or both ends of the molecules. Because the carbon rings are hydrophobic and the sugars hydrophilic, the molecule has great potential to work as an emulsifying agent. In fact, most of the saponins aid in the digestion of fats much like soap breaks up grease on dishes. Saponins get their name from the Latin word *sapo,* meaning soap. When dissolved in water and shaken, these chemicals form stable foams.

Saponins may be capable of lowering blood cholesterol levels because of this emulsifying potential. They can bind fat, cholesterol, and bile acids in the intestines preventing them from being digested. Theoretically, this would lead to increased excretion of cholesterol, and a subsequent lowering of cholesterol levels in the blood. It is also possible that this activity would also prevent fat-soluble vitamins from being absorbed. So far, however, little is known about the potential of saponins to decrease cholesterol levels.

Unfortunately, much like tannins, saponins do not appear to help much in human systems. Saponins are hemolytic. When they are highly concentrated they cause red blood cells to burst. Some think they destroy red blood cells by inserting themselves into the cellular membrane and dissolving it. Saponins are toxic to fish, snails, and other animals. They are also generally toxic to bacteria and fungus. They can inhibit some of the enzymes that viruses need to grow. Saponins seem to kill cancer cells but they also demonstrate toxicity to normal tissue, making it impractical to use them for chemotherapy. They generally irritate tissues they come in contact with, especially the mucous membranes that line the inside of our bodies. It is believed that plants have developed saponins in defense against organisms that cause them harm.

Fortunately, saponins are found in very low concentrations in fruits and vegetables. The intestines also absorb them poorly, reducing the risk of adverse affects resulting from saponin ingestion.

References

Albertazzi et al. 1999. Dietary Soy Supplementation and Phytoestrogen Levels. Obstet Gynecol. 94(2): 229–31.

Arora-A; Byrem-TM; Nair-MG; Strasburg-GM. Modulation of Liposomal Membrane Fluidity by Flavonoids and Isoflavonoids. Arch-Biochem-Biophys. 2000 Jan 1; 373(1): 102–9.

Awad, Downie and Fink. 2000. Inhibition of Growth and Stimulation of Apoptosis by Beta-Sitosterol Treatment of MDA-MB-231 Human Breast Cancer Cells in Culture. Int J Mol Med. 5(5): 541–5.

Ayesh, Weststrate, Drewitt and Hepburn. Safety Evaluation of Phytoesterol Eters. Part 5. Faecal Short-Chain Fatty Acid and Microflora Content, Faecal Baterial Enzyme Activity and Serum Female Sex Hormones in Healthy Normolipidaemic Volunteers Consuming a Controlled Diet Either with or without a Phytosterol Ester-Enriched Margarine. Food Chem Toxicol. 37(12):1127–38.

Balabhadrapathruni et al. 2000. Effects of Genistein and Structurally Related Phytoestrogens on Cell Cycle Kinetics and Apoptosis in MDA-MB-468 Human Breast Cancer Cells.

Bohm V, Bitsch R. Intestinal Absorption of Lycopene from Different Matrices and Interactions to Other Carotenoids, the Lipid Status, and the Antioxidant Capacity of Human Plasma. Eur J Nutr; 1999 Jun; 38(3): 118–25.

Bylund et al. 2000. Rye bran and Soy Protein Delay Growth and Increase Apoptosis of Human LNCaP Prostate Adenocarcinoma in Nude Mice. Prostate. 42(4): 304–14.

Carlos TF, Riondel J, Mathieu J, Guiraud P, Mestries JC, Favier A. b-carotene Enhances Natural Killer Cell Activity in Athymic Mice. In Vivo. 1997; 11: 87–91.

Casalini-C; Lodovici-M; Briani-C; Paganelli-G; Remy-S; Cheynier-V; Dolara-P. Effect of Complex Polyphenols and Tannins from Red Wine (WCPT) on Chemically Induced Oxidative DNA Damage in the Rat. Eur-J-Nutr. 1999 Aug; 38(4): 190–5.

Chan-EC; Pannangpetch-P; Woodman-OL. Relaxation to Flavones and Flavonols in Rat Isolated Thoracic Aorta: Mechanism of Action and Structure-Activity Relationships. J-Cardiovasc-Pharmacol. 2000 Feb; 35(2): 326–33.

Cherubini-A; Beal-MF; Frei-B. Black Tea Increases the Resistance of Human Plasma to Lipid Peroxidation in Vitro, But Not Ex vivo. Free-Radic-Biol-Med. 1999 Aug; 27(3–4): 381–7.

Choi-SU; Ryu-SY; Yoon-SK; Jung-NP; Park-SH; Kim-KH; Choi-EJ; Lee-CO. Effects of Favonoids on the Growth and Cell Cycle of Cancer Cells. Anticancer-Res.

1999 Nov–Dec; 19(6B): 5229–33.

Cohen, Zhao, Pittman and Lubet. 1999. S-allylcysteine, A Garlic Constituent, Fails to Inhibit N-methylnitrosourea-Induced Rat Mammary Tumorgenesis. Nutr Cancer. 35(1):58–63.

Cohen, Zhao, Pittman and Lubet. 1999. S-allylcysteine, A Garlic Constituent, Fails to Inhibit N-methylnitrosourea-induced rat mammary tumorgenesis. Nutr Cancer. 35(1):58–63.

Cook NR, Stampfer MJ, Ma J, Manson JE, Sacks FM, Buring JE, Charles HH. Beta-Carotene Supplementation for Patients with Low Baseline Levels and Decreased Risks of Total and Prostate Carcinoma. Cancer. November 1, 1999; 86(9): 1783–1792.

Dechaud. 1999. Xenoestrogen Interaction with Human Sex Hormone-Binding Globulin (hSHBG). Steroids. 64(5): 328–34.

Deodato et al. 1999. Cardioprotection by the Phytoestrogen Genistein I Experimental Myocardial Ischemia-reperfusion Injury. Br J Pharmacol. 128(8): 1683–90.

Dobrydneva, Williams and Blackmore. 1999. Trans-Resveratrol Inhibits Calcium Influx in Thrombin-Stimulated Human Platelets. Br J Pharmacol. 128(1): 149–57.

Dubey, Gillespie, Imthurn, Rosselli, Jackson and Keller. 1999. Phytoestrogens Inhibit growth and MAP Kinase Activity in Human Aortic Smooth Muscle Cells. Hypertension. 33(1 PT 2):177–82.

Fang-Rong Chang, Chang-Yi Chen, Po-Hsun Wu, Reen-Yen Kuo, Yuh-Chwen Chang, and Yang-Chang Wu. New Alkaloids from Annona purpurea. Graduate Institute of Natural Products, Kaohsiung Medical University, Taiwan, Republic of China. November 5, 1999

Fanti-P; Monier-Faugere-MC; Geng-Z; Schmidt-J; Morris-PE; Cohen-D; Malluche-HH. The Phytoestrogen Genistein Reduces Bone Loss in Short-Term Ovariectomized Rats. Osteoporos-Int. 1998; 8(3): 274–81.

Favero A, Parpinel M, Franceschi S. Diet and Risk of Breast Cancer: Major Findings From an Italian Case-Control Study. Biomed-Pharmacother. 1998; 52(3): 109–15.

Finking, Wholfrom, Lenz, Wolkenhauer, Eberle and Hanke. 1999. The Phytoestrogens Genisein and Daidzein, and 17 Beta-Estradiol Inhibit Development of Neointima in Aortas from Male and Female Rabbits In Vitro after Injury.

Foth, Cline and Romer. 2000. Effect of Isoflavoines on Mammory Gland and Endometrium of Postmenopausal Macaques (Macaca fascicularis). Zentralbl Gynakol. 122(2)96–102.

Fukushima, Takada, Hori and Wanibuchi. 1997. Cancer Prevention by Organosulfur Compounds from Garlic and Onions. J Cell Biochem Suppl. 27:100–5.

Fukushima, Takada, Hori and Wanibuchi. 1997. Cancer Prevention by Organosulfur Compounds From Garlic and Onions. J Cell Biochem Suppl. 27:100–5.

Gallo et al. 1999. Reproductive Effects of Dietary Soy in Female Wistar Rats. Food Chem Toxicol. 37(5):493–502.

Gao-YH; Yamaguchi-M. Inhibitory Effect of Genistein on Osteoclast-Like Cell Formation in Mouse Marrow Cultures. Biochem-Pharm. 1999; 58: 767–772.

Garcia-Closas R; Gonzalez-CA; Agudo-A; Riboli-E. Intake of Specific Carotenoids and Flavonoids and The Risk of Gastric Cancer in Spain. Cancer-Causes-Control. 1999 Feb; 10(1): 71–5.

Geleijnse-JM; Launer-LJ; Hofman-A; Pols-HA; Witteman-JC. Tea Flavonoids May Protect Against Atherosclerosis: The Rotterdam Study. Arch-Intern-Med. 1999 Oct 11; 159(18): 2170–4.

Giovannucci E, Ascherio A, Rimm EB, Stampfer MJ, Colditz GA, Willett WC. J Natl Cancer Inst. 1995 Dec; 87 (23):1767–76

Gupta-S; Ahmad-N; Mohan-RR; Husain-MM; Mukhtar-H. Prostate Cancer Chemoprevention by Green Tea: In Vitro and In Vivo Inhibition of Testosterone-mediated Induction of Ornithine decarboxylase. Cancer-Res. 1999 May 1; 59(9): 2115–20.

Hageman et al. 1997. Reducing Effects of Garlic Constituents on DNA Adduct Formation in Human Lymphocytes In Vitro. Nutr Cancer. 27(2):177–85.

Hageman et al. 1997. Reducing Effects of Garlic Constituents on DNA Adduct Formation in Human Lymphocytes In Vitro. Nutr Cancer. 27(2): 177–85.

Hallikainen, Sarkkinen and Uusitupa. 2000. Plant Stanol Esters Affect Serum Cholesterol Concentrations of Hypercholesterolemic Men and Women in a Dose Dependent Manner. J Nutr. 130(4): 767–76.

Haqqi-TM; Anthony-DD; Gupta-S; Ahmad-N; Lee MS; Kumar-GK; Mukhtar-H. Prevention of Collagen-Induced Arthritis in Mice by a Polyphenolic Fraction from Green Tea. Proc-Natl-Acad-Sci. 1999 Apr; 96: 4524–29.

Hargreaves et al. 1999. Two-week Dietary Soy Supplementation has an Etrogenic Effect on Premenopausal Breast. J Clin Endocrinol Metab. 84(11): 4017–24.

Hatono, Jimenez and Wargovich. 1996. Chemopreventive Effect of S-allylcysteine and It Relationship to the Detoxification Enzyme Glutathione S-transferase. Carcinogenesis. 17(5):1041–4.

Hatono, Jimenez and Wargovich. 1996. Chemopreventive Effect of S-allylcysteine and Its Relationship to the Detoxification Enzyme Glutathione S-transferase. Carcinogenesis. 17(5):1041–4.

Heinonen OP, Albenes D. The Effect of Vitamin E and Beta-Carotene on the Incidence of Lung Cancer and Other Cancers in Male Smokers. N Eng J Med. 1994 April; 330(15):1029–1035.

HF Linskens and JF Jackson. Modern Methods of Plant Analysis: Alkaloids. Springer-Verlag, Berlin 1994.

Hughes DA. Effects of Carotenoids on Human Immune Function. Proc Nutr Soc. 1999 Aug; 58(3): 713–8.

Ishikawa-Y; Sugiyama-H; Stylianou-E; Kitamura-M. Bioflavonoid Quercetin Inhibits Interleukin-1-Induced Transcriptional Expression of Monocyte Chemoattractant Protein-1 in Glomerular Cells Via Suppression of Nuclear Factor-kappaB. J-Am-Soc-Nephrol. 1999 Nov; 10(11): 2290–6.

Ishimi et al. 1999. Selective Effects of Genistein, a Soybean Isoflavones, on B-lymphopoiesis and Bone Loss Caused by Estrogen Deficiency. Endocrinology. 140(4): 1893–900.

Ishimi et al. 1999. Selective Effects of Genistein, a Soybean Isoflavones, on B-lymphopoiesis and Bone Loss Caused by Estrogen Deficiency. Endocrinology. 140(4): 1893–900.

Ishimi-Y; Miyaura-C; Ohmura-M; Onoe-Y; Sato-T; Uchiyama-Y; Ito-M; Wang-X; Suda-T; Ikegami-S. Selective Effects of Genistein, a Soybean Isoflavone, on B-lymphopoiesis and Bone Loss Caused by Estrogen Deficiency. Endocrinology. 1999 Apr; 140(4): 1893–900.

Ito-T; Warnken-SP; May-WS. Protein Synthesis Inhibition by Flavonoids: Roles of Eukaryotic Initiation Factor 2alpha Kinases. Biochem-Biophys-Res-Commun. 1999 Nov 19; 265(2): 589–94.

Jama JW, Launer LJ, Witteman JC, den-Breeijen JH, Breteler MM, Grobbee DE, Hofman A. Dietary Antioxidants and Cognitive Function in a Population-Based Sample of Older Persons. The Rotterdam Study. Am J Epidemiol. Aug 1996; 144(3): 275–80.

Janssen-K; Mensink-RP; Cox-FJ; Harryvan-JL; Hovenier-R; Hollman-PC; Katan-MB. Effects of the Flavonoids Quercetin and Apigenin on Hemostasis in Healthy Volunteers: Results From an In Vitro and a Dietary Supplemsent study.

Am-J-Clin-Nutr. 1998 Feb; 67(2): 255–62.

Jenkins et al. 2000. Effect of Soy Protein Foods on Low-Density Lipoprotein Oxidation and Ex vivo Sex Hormone Receptor Activity—A Controlled Crossover Trial. Metabolism. 49(4): 537–43.

Jeong-HJ; Shin-YG; Kim-IH; Pezzuto-JM. Inhibition of Aromatase Activity by Flavonoids. Arch-Pharm-Res. 1999 Jun; 22(3): 309–12.

Johnson, Thompson and Guthrie. 2000. Ongoing Research to Identify Environmental Risk Factors in Breast Carcinoma. Cancer. 88(5 suppl):1224–9.

Kameoka-S; Leavitt-P; Chang-C; Kuo-SM. Expression of Antioxidant Proteins in Human Intestinal Caco-2 Cells Treated With Dietary Flavonoids. Cancer-Lett. 1999 Nov 15; 146(2): 161–7.

Kandulska, Nogowski and Szkudelski. Effect of Some Phytoestrogens on Metabolism of Rat Adipocytes. Reprod Nutr Dev. 39(4): 497–501.

Keevil-JG; Osman-HE; Reed-JD; Folts-JD. Grape juice, But Not Orange Juice or Grapefruit Juice, Inhibits Human Platelet Aggregation. J-Nutr. 2000 Jan; 130(1)

Kertesz, Leisinger, and Cook. 1993. Protiens Induced by Sulfate Limitation in Esherichia coli, Pseudomonas Putida, or Staphylococcus Aureus. J Bacteriol. 175(4):1187–90.

Kertesz, Leisinger, and Cook. 1993. Protiens Induced By Sulfate Limitation in Esherichia coli, Pseudomonas putida, or Staphylococcus aureus. J Bacteriol. 175(4): 1187–90.

Khachik F, Spangler C, Smith JC Jr. Identification, Quantification and Relative Concentrations of Carotenoids and Their Metabolites in Human Milk and Serum. Anal Chem. 1997; 69(10): 1873–81.

Kim-HK; Cheon-BS; Kim-YH; Kim-SY; Kim-HP. Effects of Naturally Occurring Flavonoids on Nitric Oxide Production in the Macrophage Cell Line RAW 264.7 and Their Structure-Activity Relationships. Biochem-Pharmacol. 1999 Sep 1; 58(5): 759–65.

Klipstein Grobusch K, Launer LJ, Geleijns JM, Boeing H, Hofman A, Witterman JC. Serum Carotenoids and Atherosclerosis. The Rotterdam Study. Atherosclerosis. 2000 Jan; 148(1): 49–56.

Kulling, Rosenburg, Jacobs and Metzler. 1999. The Phytoestrogens Coumestrol and Genistein Induce Structural Chromosomal Aberrations in Cultured Human Peripheral Blood Lymphocytes. Arch Toxicol. 73(1): 50–4.

Kuntz-S; Wenzel-U; Daniel-H. Comparative Analysis of the Effects of Flavonoids on Proliferation, Cytotoxicity, and Apoptosis in Human Colon Cancer Cell lines. Eur-J-Nutr. 1999 Jun; 38(3): 133–42.

Kuo-SM; Leavitt-PS. Genistein Increases Metallothionein Expression in Human Intestinal Cells, Caco-2. Biochem-Cell-Biol. 1999; 77(2): 79–88.

Le-Marchand-L; Murphy-SP; Hankin-JH; Wilkens-LR; Kolonel-LN. Intake of Flavonoids and Lung Cancer. J-Natl-Cancer-Inst. 2000 Jan 19; 92(2): 154–60.

Lephart, Thompson, Setchell, Aldercreutz and Weber. 2000. Phytoestrogens Decrease Brain Calcium Binding Proteins but do not Alter Hypothalamic Androgen Metabolizing Enzymes in the Adult Male Rat. Brain Res. 859(1): 123–31.

Liang-YC; Huang-YT; Tsai-SH; Lin-Shiau-SY; Chen-CF; Lin-JK. Suppression of Inducible Cyclooxygenase and Inducible Nitric Oxide Synthase by Apigenin and Related Flavonoids in Mouse Macrophages. Carcinogenesis. 1999 Oct; 20(10): 1945–52.

Lowe GM Booth LA, Young AJ, Bilton RF. Lycopene and Beta-Carotene Protect Against Oxidative Damage in HT29 Cells at Low Concentrations but Rapidly Lose this Capacity at Higher Doses. Free Radic Res. 1999 Feb; 30(2): 141–51.

Lyn-Cook, Stottman, Yan, Blann, Kadlubar and Hammons. 1999. The Effects of Phytoestrogens on Human Pancreatic Tumor Cells In Vitro. Cancer Lett. 142(1): 111–9.

Margaret F. Roberts and Michael Wink. Alkaloids: Biochemistry, Ecology, and

Medicinal Applications. Plenum Press, New York 1998.

Martini et al. 1999. Effects of Soy Intake on Sex Hormone Metabolism in Premenopausal Women. Nutr Cancer. 34(2): 133–9.

Mayne ST, Janerich DT, Greenwald P, Chorost S, Tucci C, Zaman MB, Melamed MR, Kiely M, McKneally MF. Dietary Beta-Carotene and Lung Cancer Risk in U.S. Nonsmokers. J Natl Cancer Ints. 1994; 86(1):33–8.

Meng, Wahala, Adlercreutz and Tikkanen. 1999. Antiproliferative Efficacy of Lipophilic Soy Isoflavones Phytoestrogens Delivered by Low-Density Lipoprotein Particles in to Cultured U937 Cells. Life-Sci. 65(16): 1695–705.

Mitchell and Collins. 1999. Effects of a Soy Milk Supplementation on Plasma Cholesterol Levels and Oxidative DNA Damage in Men—A Pilot Study. Eur J Nutr. 38(3): 143–8.

Mitchell and Collins. 1999. Effects of a Soy Milk Supplementation on Plasma Cholesterol Levels and Oxidative DNA Damage in Men—A Pilot Study. Eur J Nutr. 38(3): 143–8.

Mitrocotsa-D; Bosch-S; Mitaku-S; Dimas-C; Skaltsounis-AL; Harvala-C; Briand-G; Roussakis-C. Cytotoxicity Against Human Leukemic Cell Lines, and the Activity on the Expression of Resistance Genes of Flavonoids from Platanus orientalis. Anticancer-Res. 1999 May-Jun; 19(3A): 2085–8.

Miyagi-Y; Miwa-K; Inoue-H. Inhibition of Human Low-Density Lipoprotein Oxidation by Flavonoids in Red Wine and Grape Juice. Am-J-Cardiol. 1997 Dec 15; 80(12): 1627–31.

Mori et al. 1997. Chemoprevention by Naturally Occurring and Synthetic Agents in Oral, Liver and Large Bowel Carcinogenesis. J Cell Biochem Suppl. 27:35–41.

Mori et al. 1997. Chemoprevention by Naturally Occurring and Synthetic Agents in Oral, Liver and Large Bowel Carcinogenesis. J Cell Biochem Suppl. 27:35–41.

Mori et al. 1999. Effects of Protocatechuic Acid, S-methylmethanethiosulfonate or 5-hydroxy-4-(2-phenyl-(E)ethenyl)-2(5H)-furanone(KYN-54) on 4-(methylni-trosamino)-1-butanone-Induced Pulmonary Carcinogenesis in Mice. Cancer Lett. 135(2):1123–7.

Mori et al. 1999. Effects of Protocatechuic Acid, S-methylmethanethiosulfonate or 5-hydroxy-4-(2-phenyl-(E)ethenyl)-2(5H)-furanone(KYN-54) on 4-(methylni-trosamino)-1-butanone-Induced Pulmonary Carcinogenesis in Mice. Cancer Lett. 135(2): 1123–7.

Munday and Munday. 1999. Low Doses of Diallyl Disulfide, A Compound Derived form Garlic,Increase Tissue Activities of Quinone Reductase and Glutathione Transferase in the Gastrointestinal Tract of the Rat. Nutr Cancer. 34(1):42–8.

Munday and Munday. Low Doses of Diallyl Disulfide, A Compound Derived form Garlic, Increase Tissue Activities of Quinone Reductase and Glutathione Transferase in the Gastrointestinal Tract of the Rat. Nutr Cancer. 1999; 34(1): 42–8.

Nagao-A; Seki-M; Kobayashi-H. Inhibition of Xanthine Oxidase by Flavonoids. Biosci-Biotechnol-Biochem. 1999 Oct; 63(10): 1787–90.

Nagata-H; Takekoshi-S; Takagi-T; Honma-T; Watanabe-K. Antioxidative Action of Flavonoids, Quercetin and Catechin, Mediated by the Activation of Glutathione Peroxidase. Tokai-J-Exp-Clin-Med. 1999 Apr; 24(1): 1–11.

Normen, Dutta, Lia and Andersson. 2000. Soy Sterol Esters and Beta-Sitostanol Ester as Inhibitors of Cholesterol Absorption in Human Small Bowel. Am J Clin Nutr. 71(4):908–13.

North and Golding. 2000. A maternal Vegetarian Diet in Pregnancy is Associated with Hypospadias. The ALSPAC Study Team. Avon Longitudinal Study of Pregnancy and Childhood. BJU Int. 85(1): 107–13.

Omenn GS, Goodman GE, Thornquist MD, et al. Effects of a Combination of Beta-

Carotene and Vitamin A on Lung Cancer and Cardiovascular Disease. N Engl J Med. 1996; 334:1150–5.

Pan, Anthony and Clarkson. 1999. Evidence for Up-Regulation of Brain-Derived Neurotrophic Factor mRNA by Soy Phytoestrogens in the Frontal Cortex of Retired Breeder Female Rats. Neurosci Lett. 261(1-2): 17–20.

Patisaul, Whitten and Young. 1999. Regulation of Estrogen Receptor Beta mRNA in the Brain: Opposite Effects of 17beta-Estradiol and the Phytoestrogen, Coumestrol. Brain Res Mol Brain Res. 67(1): 165–71.

Pryor WA, Stahl W, Rock CL. Beta-Carotene: From Biochemistry to Clinical Trials. Nutr-Rev. 2000 Feb; 58 (2 pt. 1): 39–53.

Quella. 2000. Evaluation of Soy Phytoestrogens for the Treatment of Hot Flashes in Breast Cancer Survivors: A North Central Treatment Group Trial. J Clin Oncol. 18(5):1068–74.

Reddy, Rao, Rivenson and Kellof. 1993. Chemoprevention of Colon Carcinogenesis by Organosulfur Compounds. Cancer Res. 53(15):3493–8.

Reddy, Rao, Rivenson and Kellof. 1993. Chemoprevention of Colon Carcinogenesis by Organosulfur Compounds. Cancer Res. 53(15): 3493–8.

Regal, Fraser, Weeks and Greenburg. 2000. Dietary Phytoestrogens have Anti-Inflammatory Activity in a Guinea Pig Model of Asthma. Proc Soc Exp Bio Med.

Reiners-JJ Jr; Clift-R; Mathieu-P. Suppression of Cell Cycle Progression by Flavonoids: Dependence on the Aryl Hydrocarbon Receptor. Carcinogenesis. 1999 Aug; 20(8): 1561–6.

Robert F Raffauf. Plant Alkaloids: A Guide to Their Discovery and Distribution. Food Products Press, New York 1996.

Ronco et al. 1999. Vegetables, Fruits, and Related Nutrients and Risk of Breast Cancer: A Case-Control Study in Uruguay. Nutr Cancer. 35(2): 111–9.

Rowe PM. Beta-carotene Takes a Collective Beating. The Lancet. 1996 Jan; 347:249

Sakabe et al. 1999. Inhibitory Effects of Natural and Environmental Estrogens on Thymic Hormone Production in Thymus Epithelial Cell Culture. Int J Immunopharmacol. 21(12): 861–8.

Sammon, Lyons-Wall, Chan, Smith and Petocz. 1999. The Effect of Supplementation with Isoflavonones on Plasma Women. Atherosclerosis. 147(2): 277–83.

Santos M, Meydani SN, Leka L, Wu D, Fotouhi N, Meydani M, Hennekens CH, Gaziano JM. Natural Killer Cell Activity in Elderly men is Enhanced by b-carotene Supplementation. Am J Clin Nut. 1996; 63:772–7.

Santos MS, Gaziano JM, Leka LS, Beharka AA, Hennekens CH, Meydani SN. Beta-Carotene-Induced Enhancement of Natural Killer Cell Activity in Elderly men: An Investigation of the Role of Cytokines. Am J Clin Nut. 1998; 68(1): 164–70.

Scambia et al. Clinical Effects of a Standardized Soy Extract In Postmenopausal Women: A Pilot Study. Menopause. 7(2): 105–11.

Segaert-S; Courtois-S; Garmyn-M; Degreef-H; Bouillon-R. The Flavonoid Apigenin Suppresses Vitamin D Receptor Expression and Viamin D Responsiveness in Normal Human Keratinocytes. Biochem-Biophys-Res-Commun. 2000 Feb 5; 268(1): 237–41.

Shih-H; Pickwell-GV; Quattrochi-LC. Differential Effects of Flavonoid Compounds on Tumor Promoter-Induced Activation of the Human CYP1A2 Enhancer. Arch-Biochem-Biophys. 2000 Jan 1; 373(1): 287–94.

Sierksma, Weststrate and Meijer. 1999. Spreads Enriched with Plant Sterols, Either Esterified 4,4-dimethylsterols or Free 4-desmethylsterols, and Plasma Total–and LDL-Cholesterol Concentrations. Br J Nutr. 82(4): 273–82.

Sigounas, Hooker, Anagnostou and Steiner. 1997. S-allylmercaptocysteine Inhibits Cell Proliferation and Reduces the Viability of Erythroleukemia, Breast, and Prostate Cancer Cell Lines. Nutr Cancer. 27(2):186–91.

Sigounas, Hooker, Anagnostou and Steiner. S-allylmercaptocysteine Inhibits Cell Proliferation and Reduces the Viability of Erythroleukemia, Breast, and Prostate Cancer Cell Lines. Nutr Cancer. 1997; 27(2): 186–91.

Singh et al. 1996. Novel Anti-Carcinogenic Activity of an Organosulfide from Garlic: Inhibition of H-RAS Oncogene Transformed Tumor Growth In Vivo by Diallyl Disulfide is Associated with Inhibitioin of p21H-ras Processing. Biochem Biophys Res Commun. 225(2):660–5.

Singh et al. 1996. Novel Anti-Carcinogenic Activity of an Organosulfide from Garlic: Inhibition of H-RAS Oncogene Transformed Tumor Growth In Vivo by Diallyl Disulfide is Associated with Inhibitioin of p21H-ras Processing. Biochem Biophys Res Commun. 225(2): 660–5.

Slattery ML, Benson J, Curtin K, Ma K-N, Schaeffer D, Potter JD. Carotenoids and Colon Cancer. Am J Clin Nutr. 2000; 71:575–82.

Slavin et al. 1999. Plausible Mechanisms for the Protectiveness of Whole Grains.

Stahl W, Nicolai S, Briviba K, Hanusch M, Broszeit D, Peters M, Martin HD, Sies H. Biological Activities of Natural and Synthetic Carotenoids: Induction of Gap Junctional Communication and Singlet Oxygen Quenching. Carcinogenesis. 1997; 18(1): 89–92.

Stefani ED, Boffetta P, Deneo Pellegrini H, Mendilaharsu M, Carzoglio JC, Ronco A, Olivera L. Dietary Antioxidants and Lung Cancer Risk: A Case-Control Study in Uruguay. Nutr Cancer; 1999; 34(1): 100–110.

Stein-JH; Keevil-JG; Wiebe-DA; Aeschlimann-S; Folts-JD. Purple Grape Juice Improves Endothelial Function and Reduces the Susceptibility of LDL Cholesterol to Oxidation in Patients with Coronary Artery Disease. Circulation. 1999 Sep 7; 100(10): 1050–5.

Strom et at. 1999. Phytoestrogen Intake and Prostate Cancer: A Case-Control Study Using a New Database. Nutr Cancer. 33(1):20–5.

Surh, Kim, Liem, Lee and Miller. 1999. Inhibitory Effects of Isopropyl-2-(1,3-dithietane-2-ylidene)-2-[N-(4-methylthiazol-2-yl)carbamoyl]Acetate (YH439) on Benzo[a]pyrene-induced Skin Carcinogenesis and Mironucleated Reticulocyte Formation in Mice. Mutat Res. 423(1–2):149–53.

Surh, Kim, Liem, Lee and Miller. Inhibitory Effects of Isopropyl-2-(1,3-dithietane-2-ylidene)-2-[N-(4-methylthiazol-2-yl)carbamoyl]Acetate (YH439) on Benzo[a]pyrene-Induced Skin Carcinogenesis and Mironucleated Reticulocyte Formation in Mice. Mutat Res. 1999; 423(1–2): 149–53.

Takada et al. 1994. 85(11): 1067–72. Enhancing Effects of Organosulfur Compounds From Garlic and Onions on Hepatocarcinogenesis in Rats: Association with Increased Cell Proliferation and Elevated Ornithine Decarboxylase Activity. Jpn J Cancer Res. 85(11): 1067–72.

Takada et al. 1994. 85(11):1067–72. Enhancing Effects of Organosulfur Compounds from Garlic and Onions on Hepatocarcinogenesis in Rats: Association with Increased Cell Proliferation and Elevated Ornithine Decarboxylase Activity. Jpn J Cancer Res. 85(11):1067–72.

Takada, Yano, Wanibuchi, Otani and Fukushima. 1997. S-methylcysteine and Cysteine are Inhibitors of Induction of Glutathione S-transferase Placental Form-Positive Foci During Initiation and Promotion Phases of Rat Hepatocarcinogenesis. Jpn J Cancer Res. 88(5):435–42.

Takada, Yano, Wanibuchi, Otani and Fukushima. 1997. S-methylcysteine and Cysteine are Inhibitors of Induction of Glutathione S-transferase Placental Form-Positive Foci During Initiation and Promotion Phases of Rat Hepatocarcinogenesis. Jpn J Cancer Res. 88(5):435–42.

Tavani A, Negri E, D'Avanzo B, La-Vecchia C. Beta-Carotene Intake and Risk of Nonfatal Acute Myocardial Infarction in Women. Eur J Epidemiol. Sept 1997; 13(6):631–7.

Taylor, Quintero, Iacopino and Lephart. 1999. Phytoestrogens Alter Hypothalamic

Calbindin-D28k Levels During Prenatal Development. Brain Res Dev Brain Res. 114(2) :277–81.

Tekel' et al. 1999. Determination of the Hop-Derived Phytoestrogen, 8-Prenylnaringenin, in Beer by Gas Chromatography/mass Spectrometry. J Agric Food Chem. 47(12): 5059–63.

Turnbell, Frankos, Leeman and Jonker. 1999. Short-Term Tests of Estrogenic Potential of Plant Stanols and Plant Stanol Esters. Regul Toxiocol Pharmacol. 29(2 pt 1): 211–5.

Ulsperger et al. 1999. Resveratrol Pretreatment Desensitizes AHTO-7 Human Osteoblasts to Growth Stimulation in Response to Carcinoma Cell Aupernatants. Int J Oncol. 15(5): 955–9.

Van Het Hof KH, West CE, Weststrate JA, Hautvast JG. Dietary Factors That Affect The Bioavailability of Carotenoids. J Nutr. 2000 Mar; 130(3): 503–6.

Vedavanam, Srijayanta, O'Reilly, Raman and Wiseman. 1999. Antioxidant Action and Potential Antidiabetic Properties of an Isoflavonoid-Containing Soyabean Phytochemical Extract (SPE). Phytother Res. 13(7): 601–8.

Wang and Kurzer. 1998. Effects of Phytoestrogens on DNA Synthesis in MCF-7Cells in the Presence of Etradiol or Growth Factors. Nutr Cancer. 31(2): 90–100.

Wang et al. 1996. Protective Effects of Garlic and Related Organosulfur Compounds on Acetaminophen-Induced Hepatotoxicity in Mice. Toxicol Appl Pharmacol. 136(1):146–54.

Wang et al. 1996. Protective Effects of Garlic and Related Organosulfur Compounds on Acetaminophen-Induced HepAtotoxicity in Mice. Toxicol Appl Pharmacol. 136(1): 146–54.

Wang W-D. Russell RM. Procarcinogenic and Anticarcinogenic Effects of Beta Carotene. Nutrition Reviews, 57(9): 263–273.

Washburn, Burke, Morgan and Anthony. 1999. Effect of Soy Protein Supplementation on Serum Lipoproteins, Blood Pressure, and Menopausal Symptoms in Perimenopausal Women. Menopause. 6(1):7–13.

Weber et al. 1999. Brain Aromatasse and 5alpha-reductase, Regulatory Behaviors and Testosterone Levels in Adult Rats on Phytoestrogen Diets. Proc Soc Exp Biol Med. 221(2): 135–5.

Williams, Boooella, Strobino, Boccia and Campanaro. 1999. Plant Stanol Ester and Bran Fiber in Childhood: Effects on Lipids, Stool Weight and Stool Frequency in Preschool Children. J Am Coll Nutr. 18(6):572–81.

Yoshida et al. 1999. An Organosulfur Compound Isolated Form Oil-Macerated Garlic Extract, and Its Antimicrobial Effect. Biosci Biotechnol Biochem. 63(3): 588–90.

Yoshida et al. 1999. An Organosulfur Compud Isolated Form Oil-Macerated Garlic Extract, and Its Antimicrobial Effect. Biosci Biotechnol Biochem. 63(3):588–90.

Yoshida-H; Ishikawa-T; Hosoai-H; Suzukawa-M; Ayaori-M; Hisada-T; Sawada-S; Yonemura-A; Higashi-K; Ito-T; Nakajima-K; Yamashita-T; Tomiyasu-K; Nishiwaki-M; Ohsuzu-F; Nakamura-H. Inhibitory Effect of Tea Flavonoids on the Ability of Cells to Oxidize Low Density Lipoprotein. Biochem-Pharmacol. 1999 Dec 1; 58(11): 1695–703.

223(4): 372–8.

CHAPTER 6

Vitamins and the Chemistry of Life

T here are thirteen vitamins: A, B, C, D, E, and K, with eight types of B vitamins. Initially, vitamins were named as they were discovered. The first discovered was named *vitamin A*; the second was named *B*, and so forth. However, scientists later recognized that the compound initially called vitamin B was actually a variety of different molecules with different structures and functions. These six B vitamins were then named individually based on their composition and function.

When we limit the number of vitamins to thirteen, it is important to understand that we are not just speaking about thirteen different compounds or molecules. The names now represent thirteen different families of molecules. Some scientists like to call the different compounds in vitamin families "vitamers." Vitamers function in different ways to promote and regulate various functions of the body.

The Chemistry of Life

Our bodies function through chemical reactions. Life can be thought of as a symphony of perfectly ordered and designed chemical reactions. The simple act of lifting an arm is actually a complex team-effort on the part of literally millions of cells and billions of reactions. In order to keep all of these cells and reactions working together, the body uses enzymes.

Enzymes are the directors of the chemical reaction symphony. Each of these enzymes (or proteins), with its unique composition and structure, catalyze, or cause, reactions that otherwise would have almost no chance of occurring. Some vitamins, such as vitamin A, K and C, thiamin, niacin, riboflavin, vitamin B6, biotin, pantothenic acid, folate and B12, function as coenzymes. A coenzyme is an organic compound that binds to an enzyme and increases or enables its activity. Vitamins thus help to activate or inactivate the enzymatic reactions that occur throughout our bodies.

Vitamins are studied for more reasons than to understand their roles as cofactors. They are of great interest because many act as antioxidants. This chapter and the one that follows will teach you the practical basics of all of the vitamins. First we will cover the vitamins that dissolve in water; and in the next chapter we will discuss those that dissolve in fat. The importance of this difference will become apparent. We will discuss how some of the vitamins, much like phytochemicals, are able to protect the body against oxidative damage.

Some vitamins are involved in electron transfers. For instance, niacin and riboflavin aid the body by helping move electrons from atom to atom safely. Some vitamins are also recognized as important signaling molecules that can travel throughout the body, evoking a specific response from certain cells. The best example of this is a derivative of vitamin A. This derivative, known as retinoid acid, helps to protect against cancer. Some vitamins help to stabilize cellular membranes so they remain resilient. Each of these vitamin functions and more will be discussed in greater detail as we investigate the specific properties of each vitamin.

The Vitamin Families

As mentioned, there are thirteen families of vitamins. Four are fat soluble and nine are water soluble. Fat-soluble vitamins look and act like fat molecules, and do not dissolve in water. These include vitamin A, vitamin D, vitamin E, and vitamin K. On the other hand vitamin C, and the B vitamins (thiamin, riboflavin, niacin, vitamin B6, folic acid, biotin, pantothenic acid, and vitamin B12) are water soluble because they are polar.

Because of the charges of polar molecules and nonpolar molecules, they will never dissolve into each other. This is important because our bodies are both polar and nonpolar in different places. Even an individual cell has components that are fat soluble and some that are water soluble. Fat-soluble compounds are also called hydrophobic (fearing water), and water-soluble compounds are called hydrophilic (water loving). Fat-soluble vitamins circulate through the watery environment of the blood by attaching to fats and enter the lipid environment of the cellular membrane comfortably. On the other hand, water-soluble vitamins circulate easily through the blood but need help to pass through the lipid layer of cellular membranes.

The Role of Vitamins in Health

Vitamins play an important role in helping us stay healthy, aiding our cells in the production of energy, and protecting the tissues in our body from damage. Science has invested considerable time, talent, energy and money in understanding the role of vitamins in health. We can now better understand how vitamins are absorbed from the digestive tract into the bloodstream, how they are transported in the blood, where they are stored, where they function, and how they are excreted from the body.

Although vitamins are commonly available in most of the foods we eat, we end up using only about 40 to 90 percent of the vitamins we actually eat. In fact, it is possible to suffer from a deficiency of a particular vitamin even if you eat plenty of foods containing it. This is because vitamins require an appropriate environment to be usable. For example, eating a slice of tomato on buttered toast is more beneficial than eating a slice of tomato on toast alone. The butter's fat helps the body utilize the tomato's fat-soluble phytochemicals and vitamins. The amount of a vitamin that we are able to use depends on other components of our diet.

As we discuss the vitamins we will try to indicate good sources of various vitamins. We will also spend a significant amount of time discussing how and why vitamins do the work they do to maintain health. We feel that understanding how vitamins work will better enable you to make good choices about your diet.

Vitamins in the Right Amount

As we have already discussed, too little of a particular vitamin will cause specific deficiency syndromes, and possibly lead to chronic diseases. Also, contrary to the popular idea that you can't get too much of a good thing, vitamins can be toxic if they are present in extreme amounts in the body. It is therefore important that we store and excrete vitamins. This provides us the ability to regulate the amounts of vitamins present in our bodies. After absorption, the fat-soluble vitamins are taken to the various tissues in which they function, or they can be taken to the liver or fatty tissue to be stored. Because these vitamins are stored in our fatty tissue, it takes longer to develop deficiency symptoms than for water-soluble vitamins.

In cases where you eat too much of a fat-soluble vitamin, the body has to work much harder to excrete the excess in comparison to water-soluble vitamins. Fat-soluble vitamins aren't freely soluble in the blood, so they are not normally excreted in the urine. Instead, they are carried to the intestine and are excreted in the feces.

The water-soluble vitamins, unlike their nonpolar counterparts, are not stored in the body to any great extent. They are rapidly depleted from the body, and therefore must be regularly consumed so that adequate levels of these vitamins are maintained throughout the body. These vitamins are filtered from the blood by the kidneys and are excreted in the urine either as intact vitamins, as in the case of riboflavin and pantothenic acid, or as metabolized forms of the initial vitamin, as in the case of vitamin C, thiamin, niacin, riboflavin, biotin, folate, and vitamin B12.

Disease Prevention through Vitamins

Presently, there is a lot of discussion and research being done to determine the role that certain vitamins play in disease prevention. As we discuss each vitamin, we will talk about the amounts of each vitamin that we have been advised to take each day. Because many terms such as RDA and DRI are unfamiliar to most of us and can be confusing, we would like to take a moment to explain where these nutritional recommendations came from and what they mean.

Nutrition a Vital Part of Determining Cancer Risk

A study published in the March 2002 issue of *Current Opinion in Gastroenterology* states, "Evidence emerging from many different types of experimental designs continues to support the concept that dietary habits and nutritional status play important roles in determining the risk of colorectal cancer.

"Although the inconsistencies in this field make it tempting to minimize its import, there is little question that diet has a major impact on colorectal cancer risk; diligent attention to the rigorous conduct of studies and their interpretation will likely clarify these relationships over the next decade, much to the benefit of public health."

In 1863, the United States government established an institution called the National Academy of Sciences. This academy consisted of a group of individuals who were experts in various fields of science, who could advise national leaders on governmental affairs that involved scientific issues. As time progressed and scientific advancements were made, the National Academy of Science expanded in order to include newer areas of national scientific interest.

Recommended Dietary Allowances

The Food and Nutrition Board was one of these many programs created. Established in 1940, the Food and Nutrition Board (FNB) was commissioned to study issues pertaining to the national food supply, to create nutritional guidelines, and to determine the relationship between food intake, nutrition, and health. As part of their job, the Food and Nutrition Board established the amount of vitamins that we need to include in our diets. These suggestions were previously given as Recommended Dietary Allowances (RDAs). Today, the FNB has revised these guidelines in line with more current research. They are now called Dietary Reference Intakes (DRIs).

In 1943, Recommended Dietary Allowances were established. These were viewed as reliable sources, indicating the daily amounts of essential vitamins and minerals that healthy individuals should eat. RDAs were published, describing the nutritional needs of groups of a given gender at a given age. The RDAs were designed to indicate the amount of a nutrient that would meet the needs of most of the individuals in a specific group. This standard was updated as knowledge increased. The last update was made in 1989.

Since the formation of the RDA system, understanding about the role of the various nutrients has increased. The original RDAs were formed to prevent deficiency-related diseases. However, at present, nutrient deficiencies do not pose much of a threat to the majority of the U.S. population. Researchers are realizing that many nutrients not only prevent deficiency-related diseases, but also play an important role in reducing the risk of chronic diseases such as cancer and heart disease. These nutritional insights have prompted the Food and Nutrition Board to create a new way of evaluating nutrient reference values. This new approach to nutrition inspired the formation of the Dietary Reference Intakes, or DRIs.

Using the DRIs, we are given four different dosages arranged by age and sex to plan our daily intakes of various nutrients. DRIs are indexes that give four different reference values. The DRI includes: EAR, RDA, UL, and AI. The first reference value is the Estimated Average Requirement, or the EAR. Basically, the EAR is the minimum amount of a nutrient we should eat per day. Typically, we will want to eat much more. The second reference value contains the RDAs, or Recommended Dietary Allowances. The RDAs are the amounts that are sufficient to meet the needs of most (97 to 98 percent) of the individuals in a given group. (See Table D1 in Appendix D on page 362 for nutrient RDAs organized by age.)

Tolerable Upper Intake Levels, or ULs, are listed third. ULs represent the maximum amount of a given nutrient that we can eat without experiencing any of the toxic side effects from having too much of that nutrient. It would probably be unwise to exceed these values in your diet.

The last reference value is Adequate Intakes, or AIs. This category is estimated when there is not enough scientific information to establish an EAR and calculate an RDA. The AIs are determined by observing the average intake of a given nutrient by a healthy population. The mere fact that AIs exist tells us that more studies need to be done on a given nutrient. However, AIs can be considered to be the amount recommended to meet the needs of a healthy individual.

Although DRIs offer more nutritional information, the general suggestion remains that healthy individuals should maintain their intake levels at about the RDAs and AIs. If we take much more than these values, we may be approaching the UI, and that can be toxic. Because the new system of DRI is still being developed, most tables and charts still only list the AI or the RDA instead of all four of the categories. Most people just pay attention to the RDA, and in the future, we will see increased awareness of the term *DRI*. We have included a table of RDAs for each of the vitamins in Appendix D.

CHAPTER 7

Water-Soluble Vitamins

Water-soluble vitamins include vitamin C and the B vitamins, which consist of folic acid, vitamin B12, vitamin B6, pantothenic acid, thiamin, niacin, riboflavin and biotin.

All of the water-soluble vitamins except vitamin C function as precursors for coenzymes. For example when pantothenic acid is bonded to two other organic groups, it is called coenzyme A. Without this B vitamin, however, the coenzyme would not function, and not all of the reactions would occur that require this coenzyme A. In short, the B vitamins help enzymes do their jobs. Coenzymes can be used over and over again. Over time, they wear out and need to be replenished. We will touch on all eight of the B vitamins, providing a brief history of their discovery and explaining what symptoms arise from deficiency and from overdose. We will focus on discussing how these vitamins work in the body, and the evidence of recent studies.

Vitamin Transport in the Body

Each vitamin must cross the intestinal wall and then move on into the bloodstream either through diffusion or active transport. Molecules often move from place to place through diffusion. The tendency of molecules to move from areas of high concentration to areas of low concentration is diffusion. Diffusion allows the water-soluble vitamins to move in and out of cells and spread throughout the blood. Diffusion is an effective way to move molecules from one place to another because it doesn't use any energy. However, it is also very slow. When the body must move water-soluble vitamin molecules quickly, it turns to more active means.

Active transport uses protein channels to move molecules. To move a vitamin from the intestinal wall and into the bloodstream, it must pass through the cells of the intestine. These cells have tiny protein channels in their cellular membranes. These channels are designed to allow only certain molecules in and out. They employ active transporters that allow certain vitamins to cross. Active transport is different from diffusion because the active transporters burn energy in order to move vitamins through the protein channels across the intestinal wall. However, the speed with which the vitamins are carried into the bloodstream is well worth the energy investment.

Vitamin Storage

Unlike fat-soluble vitamins, water-soluble vitamins are not stored in the body. Excess vitamins are filtered in the kidneys and discarded in the urine. This means that water-soluble vitamins must be replenished on a regular basis. It also means that it is much more difficult to have any toxic side effects from these vitamins. The body simply doesn't hold on to them long enough to create toxic build-up. However, in cases of extreme megadosing it is possible to suffer from water-soluble vitamin toxicity. Therefore, we will include recommendations for the daily intake of these vitamins. We'll begin with a closer look at the structure and function of the B vitamins, and then discuss vitamin C.

Thiamin

The importance of many of the water-soluble vitamins has been better understood as science has begun to recognize the structure and functions of enzymes. Thiamin is a cofactor for a coenzyme called thiamin pyrophosphate (TPP).

To be more precise, thiamin pyrophosphate is a derivative of thiamin. TPP is simply a thiamin vitamin with some other functional groups added on to it. TPP is an essential cofactor with five different enzymes involved in critical cellular metabolic pathways. These pathways are involved in the biosynthesis of components required for cells and organs to maintain life.

Historically, the lack of thiamin is associated with a deficiency disease called beriberi. The symptoms of beriberi include: wasting of the muscular tissues, edema (swelling of the tissues), pain, paralysis, energy deprivation, mental confusion, and ultimately death. The disease became more and more prominent in the early 1900s in Southeast Asia and was accompanied by the newly popular process of polishing rice (this meant that the husks of the rice were being shucked off, leaving only the white kernel). A scientist named Christian Eijkman discovered that the husk contained something that prevented beriberi. In time the vitamin thiamin was discovered as the molecule capable of preventing beriberi.

Because some of the important metabolic pathways require TPP, they cannot operate if the diet does not include thiamin. However, supplementation of polished rice with thiamin has made thiamin deficiency uncommon in the United States. Thiamin deficiency is more likely to be seen in a strict vegetarian diet because the more commonly eaten thiamin foods are meat. However, sunflower seeds, wheat germ, and beans are among the few nonmeat foods that do contain thiamin.

Many have claimed that megadoses of thiamin could improve the performance of athletes. Studies do not seem to substantiate these claims. A few years ago, six highly trained cyclists were given either a placebo or a 1.8 gram supplement of thiamin every day prior to a workout for seven days. Then they were given equal workloads on a steady-state cycle ergometer (stationary bike) to measure their performance. During the ride, measures of heart rate, breathing rates, and perceived exertion were recorded. Blood samples were also taken after every 10 km to measure different chemical changes in the blood. This same experiment was done on two different occasions using the same cyclists. The results showed no significant differences in the abilities of those supplemented with thiamin from those who were not.

The RDA for thiamin is about 1.5 mg for men and 1.1 mg for women. Toxicity has been seen only in individuals who have consumed well over one hundred times the RDA for this nutrient.

Riboflavin

Riboflavin is important because it is an essential component of a larger coenzyme known as flavin adenine dinucleotide (FAD). FAD is a coenzyme for hundreds of biochemical reactions, especially those involved in electron transport and oxidation-reduction reactions. Oxidation may be thought of as the process of removal of electrons (and hydrogen) from an atom or molecule while reduction is the process of adding electrons (or hydrogen) to an atom or molecule. Oxidation and reduction reactions are coupled. If one atom is oxidized, it is because another atom is reduced. FAD is one of a group of essential electron carriers involved in oxidation-reduction reactions and functions as a necessary coenzyme for these reactions.

Deficiency in riboflavin is characterized by burning and itching of the eyes and mouth. In addition, it also may cause the loss of visual acuity. These symptoms are easily remedied by eating foods rich in riboflavin: meat and dairy products. Although riboflavin's importance has been recognized for over one hundred years, the understanding of its biological role had not been elucidated until 1932. As we study the role of one vitamin in causing or preventing certain diseases it is important to remember that many of the vitamins work together. In addition, riboflavin can actually help produce niacin if necessary. Although most of the niacin required by the body comes from the diet, the body can produce some, provided there are adequate levels of riboflavin.

Again, here FAD is a coenzyme that aids the enzymatic pathways needed to make niacin. The relationship between riboflavin and niacin demonstrates how a balanced diet is necessary to ensure overall health. It is important to think of the vitamins in terms of relationships with one another rather than as individual molecules. Some studies help to illustrate.

In January of 1999, researchers at the St. Joan University Hospital in Reus, Spain studied the nutritional content of the blood of recent mothers and newborns to determine how well nutrients were transferred from mother to child prior to birth. One hundred thirty-one mothers were monitored along with their newly born babies. Blood was taken from both the mother and from the umbilical chord at the time of delivery. Following a micro nutritional analysis, researchers reported an interesting finding. The majority of the women and infants were deficient in thiamin, vitamin B6, and riboflavin. But most interesting was the link researchers found between these vitamins. Lower levels in one proved to be an indicator of lower levels in the others. Researchers suggest that these three vitamins are necessary in a group to ensure proper absorption of all of them. The RDA for riboflavin is between 1 and 2 mg for adults. It can be found in seafood, nuts, dairy products and many leafy greens such as spinach.

Niacin

Niacin (nicotinic acid) is converted to nicotinamide, which then becomes part of the vital coenzyme nicotinamide adenine dinucleotide (NAD).

Like FAD, NAD transports electrons and hydrogen atoms in oxidation-reduction reactions. Again, NAD participates as a coenzyme in hundreds of biochemical reactions affecting many essential cellular functions. In addition to NAD, a related coenzyme NADP also functions as an electron carrier, though it generally participates in different enzyme reactions.

The first signs of niacin deficiency are muscular weakness and anorexia, followed by diarrhea and tremors. These symptoms are often signs of Pellagra, a disease that had scientists and physicians dumbfounded until 1918. A scientist named Goldbereger noticed that in populations having low-protein diets, the disease was more prevalent. This was the case in the southern states particularly where the staple diet was cornmeal. He traced the disease down to a deficiency of niacin.

You should closely follow recommended daily allowances for niacin because megadoses are toxic. When 1 or 2 grams are taken three times a day, the liver is adversely affected, and the skin becomes flushed as if by an allergic reaction. Niacin is used in high dosages as a medicine for treating certain diseases, but should not be used as a supplementation. Niacin is most famous for its therapeutic use in preventing heart disease.

The largest of the studies, done by the Coronary Drug Project, monitored the effect of niacin alone on the frequency of myocardial infarction and cerebrovascular events. After a long-term follow up (fifteen years), patients treated with niacin were significantly less likely to suffer from cardiovascular problems. Even the total mortality was decreased.

Niacin has also been shown to have some anticancer properties. A group of researchers tested the effect of niacin supplementation on rats to understand its role in preventing tumors. We all know that exposure to UV light from the sun or from tanning beds increases our risk for skin cancer. This is because it damages the DNA, causing mutations to occur faster than the cell can repair them. This group hypothesizes that an increased amount of niacin raises the level of NAD in the skin. They say that NAD is critical in modulating the function of certain proteins in the cell responsible for DNA damage surveillance. For twenty-two weeks, the rats were placed for thirty minutes under UV irradiated sunlamps, while being fed 0.1, 0.5, or 1.0 percent niacin in their food. The results showed a reduced incidence of skin cancer ranging from 28 to 68 percent.

Pantothenic Acid

Pantothenic acid is a component of coenzyme A (CoA), a vital coenzyme involved in enzyme reaction in which a two-carbon acetyl molecule (acyl group) is transferred.

Acyl transfer reactions occur when glucose is oxidized to produce energy and when fatty acids are being "burned" as an energy source. Although deficiencies of pantothenic acid are rare, those who experience them show signs of fatigue, depression, and insomnia. It is recommended that adults receive about 4 to 5 mg per day.

Vitamin B6 (Pyridoxine)

The coenzyme form of vitamin B6 is pyridoxal phosphate (PLP) or pyridoxamine phosphate (PMP).

PLP acts as a coenzyme and has very diverse biochemical pathways involving amino acid biosynthesis and metabolism, glycogen metabolism, and nitrogen metabolism.

For instance, in some reactions, PLP and an enzyme called transaminase produce essential amino acids (or amino acids we do not get from food). One of the very important roles of PLP (vitamin B6) is in the biochemical conversion of the amino acid homocysteine to another amino acid, cysteine. High levels of homocysteine have been associated with the etiology of cardiovascular diseases and the impairment of mental awareness in aging. The role of homocysteine in lifestyle diseases is covered in later chapters, but in a recent study published by the American Heart Association, it was shown that those who are deficient in vitamin B6 have two times the risk of heart disease and stroke. Apparently, this is because of vitamin B6's role in the conversion of homocysteine to cysteine.

Biotin

Biotin functions as a coenzyme in cellular biochemical reactions called "one carbon metabolism." An example is a reaction in which CO_2 is transported from one molecule to another molecule. This occurs, for example, during the breakdown of glucose to carbon dioxide. Another example is the degradation of some fatty acids. Biotin is involved with burning up fats with an odd number of carbon atoms. The majority of fat in the body has an even number of carbon atoms. However, there is a need for fat with odd numbers of carbon atoms. These fats require a different pathway to be used for energy. Because of the vitamin role that biotin plays in the metabolism of glucose, biotin supplementation may help to improve the blood glucose control in diabetics.

Biotin deficiency is extremely rare because the microflora of the gut produce it and it can be directly absorbed into the bloodstream. A variety of red and white meats supply biotin, but so do peanuts, hazel nuts, and chocolates.

Vitamin B12

Vitamin B12 is also known as coenzyme B12 or cobalamin. It is one of the rare organic molecules using cobalt in its actual structure. Cobalt is at the center of eight rings and is also connected above and below to other atoms of the molecule.

Neither plants nor animals have the enzyme systems needed to synthesize vitamin B12 and only certain microorganisms have the capacity to produce it. We obtain our vitamin B12 from our diet, most of it from meat or dairy products. Herbivores acquire vitamin B12 from bacteria that are part of their gut microflora. There are only a few known functions of vitamin B12 in humans. One involves the transfer of a methyl group (in conjunction with folic acid) to homocysteine in the biosynthesis of the amino acid methionine. As mentioned above in the discussion of vitamin B6, it is essential for good health to control the amount of homocysteine in the body. Recent data from scientific studies associates high levels of homocysteine with cardiovascular diseases and decreased mental capacity as we age.

We metabolize fatty acids with both odd and even numbers of carbon atoms. Both of these processes require and produce energy, but they do not utilize the same enzymes to do the job. Additional enzymes are needed to break down fatty acids with an odd number of carbons. Vitamin B12 is also a coenzyme in the oxidation of odd-numbered carbon chains in fatty acids that contain an odd number of carbon atoms.

Vitamin B12 was first recognized in 1926 when it was associated with pernicious anemia, which is often a fatal disease in the elderly. Pernicious anemia results in a decrease in the number of red blood cells, low hemoglobin levels, and the slow onset of neurological dysfunction. The bone marrow, the intestinal mucosa, and even the brain can show signs of this cell division impairment. Symptoms include tingling in the feet and generalized weakness in the bones. Even further damage may include an enlarged red beefy tongue, jaundice and brain damage. Studies on pernicious anemia as a dietary deficiency disease have shown that the disease does not result from lack of dietary vitamin B12, rather it results from a defect in absorption of vitamin B12 from the intestine. Normally, in the intestine a protein called intrinsic factor, which is produced in the stomach, binds to vitamin B12 and this complex is then absorbed across the intestinal mucosa.

Vitamin B12 was isolated in 1948, but it wasn't until 1979 that it was synthesized, and research is only beginning to be done on the relatively "new" nutrient. It is found mostly in meats and dairy products.

Folic Acid

Folate, as well as a compound made from folate called tetrahydrafolate, is actively involved in "one carbon" metabolism.

Tetrahydrafolate is used in the synthesis of DNA. Also, proteins depend on tetrahydrafolate in order to synthesize some of the amino acids. Serine for example has one more carbon atom than does glycine (these are both common amino acids). Tetrahydrafolate is involved in removing one of the carbon atoms from serine to make glycine, or to add a carbon to glycine to produce serine. And as with vitamin B12, folic tetrahydrafolate is involved in the biosynthesis of methionine, another amino acid derived from homocytsiene.

There are about one hundred vitamers in the folate family. Folate is named after its food source: foliage. Deficiencies of folate result in an inability to synthesize DNA. This inability is particularly critical in cells that divide rapidly because they require DNA to divide. The cells most affected by folate deficiency are red blood cells, leukocytes, and cells in the digestive tract. Folate deficiency can inhibit growth in children. Folate deficiency causes anemia: a low blood cell count.

FOLIC ACID AND PREGNANCY

Women trying to get pregnant, or who are already pregnant, should make sure they are eating foods high in folate or taking a folate supplement. A recent study took 123 healthy pregnant women who had experienced at least two consecutive pregnancy losses and compared folate concentrations in their blood with 104 healthy control women. The women who had had pregnancy losses had a significantly lower concentration of folate in the blood than did the control group. The ability of folate in aiding the pregnancy may be explained at least in part by its breakdown of a molecule called homocysteine.

Homocysteine is a very important precursor to a few of the amino acids, and it is most infamous for its association with cardiovascular disease. If the body does not convert this molecule into these amino acids, it can cause deadly build-up of arterial plaques. We will talk much more about this molecule in chapter 12. Beyond contributing to cardiovascular disease, high levels of homocysteine in the blood might have deleterious effects as well on the developing fetus in pregnancy.

Studies have shown that increased levels of homocysteine are related to an elevated incidence of several common pregnancy complications. A publication recently released in the *American Journal of Clinical Nutrition* reported on a study of nearly 6,000 women and almost 14,500 pregnancies in those same women. The study showed that women who had high levels of homocysteine experience much greater risk for preeclampsia, prematurity, very low birth weight, clubfoot, and neural tube defects, or NTDs. Researchers are currently seeking to understand the relationship between NTDs and homocysteine.

NTDs result when the tissues of the brain, spinal cord, and the tissues that surround them fail to develop properly. There are three principle types of NTDs. The first is called anencephaly, which is underdevelopment of the brain and parts of the skull. Most babies born with anencephaly do not live more than a couple hours after birth. The second kind of NTD, known as encephalocele, results in a hole in the baby's skull through which brain tissue protrudes. Children with this disorder are highly unlikely to live. If they do they will be severely retarded.

The last NTD is by far and away the most prevalent of the three and overall is the most frequently occurring, permanently disabling birth defect. It is known as spina bifida and results in the failure of the spine to close properly around the spinal cord. In the most severe cases the spinal cord actually protrudes out of the back. These complications bring with them an assortment of attendant physical and neurological difficulties such as varying levels of paralysis, incontinence, and some mild learning disabilities. As a result of these and other health problems due to folate deficiency, the FDA now mandates that dietary foods (breads) be fortified with folate.

Vitamin C

Scurvy was a problem for voyagers for hundreds of years. Scurvy is characterized by edema, hemorrhage, weakness and softness in the bones, the teeth, the cartilage and all the connective tissues, lesions on the skin, and discolored spots. Captain Cook had success in preventing scurvy because he required all the men to take every opportunity to eat the grasses and fruits of islands they passed. Soon, sailors realized they could prevent scurvy by eating limes. They began keeping provisions of limes on board. Soon British sailors became known as "limeys." Of course, scurvy was not just a risk for sailors with poor diets. It was a common disease during the Civil War in America among soldiers. Any time a diet is lacking in fruits, more especially citrus fruits, there is a great risk of scurvy.

Only a few animals need to get vitamin C from their diets: humans, primates, and guinea pigs, to name a few. Since the 1940s, the vitamin has had many advocates and critics, some claiming that it would completely cure the common cold, and others warning against excess dosages. Linus Pauling, a famous British chemist wrote a book claiming that you couldn't get enough vitamin C. Pauling recommended people take from 12,000 to 40,000 mg per day. He claimed vitamin C was the cure for the common cold. We will try to help separate the fact from fiction about vitamin C. After describing the need for vitamin C, we will explore the most modern research done on this exciting nutrient.

Vitamin C becomes both ascorbic acid (AA), and dehydroascorbic acid (DHAA) in the body.

Both forms of vitamin C have a five-membered ring of four carbons and one oxygen. The most important parts of the molecule are its hydroxyl arms (these are OHs). These arms allow ascorbic acid to easily become dehydroascorbic acid. This makes vitamin C capable of becoming an effective antioxidant. Free radicals readily steal electrons from the hydroxyl arms, satisfying their need for an electron, while vitamin C itself remains stable. Vitamin C works much like vitamin E as an antioxidant with one major difference: vitamin C functions in water while vitamin E functions in fat. We will discuss how vitamin C works as an antioxidant in a moment.

VITAMIN C AND COLLAGEN BIOSYNTHESIS

Vitamin C is an essential cofactor for enzymes that synthesize collagen proteins. Collagen molecules are long, slightly twisted chains forming strong materials for bones and other connective tissues. Collagen helps to form strong bones, teeth, and cartilage. When the body lacks vitamin C it becomes increasingly difficult to create collagen, causing the symptoms known as scurvy. At a bare minimum, small amounts of vitamin C in the diet can prevent scurvy. However, in large amounts it appears that vitamin C can help prevent other conditions associated with bones and connective tissues.

Reflex sympathetic dystrophy (RSD) is a condition that occurs after injuries are sustained in the connective tissues. This condition is characterized by spells of hot and cold in the recently injured joints and tissues. In December 1999, researchers at the Department of Orthopaedics in Lyenburg Hospital, the Netherlands, studied whether vitamin C would prevent the occurrence of RSD in people with wrist fractures. One hundred twenty-three adults with 127 wrist fractures were chosen randomly and divided into two groups. Group 1, the test group, received 500 mg

of vitamin C daily. Group 2, the control group, were given a placebo. Researchers followed the two groups for a year to see if vitamin
C influenced the occurrence of RSD. In the placebo group, RSD
occurred in 22 percent of wrist fractures. In group 1, RSD occurred
in only 7 percent of wrist fractures. The hypothesis was that vitamin C was an effective treatment for injuries relating to trauma.

VITAMIN C AND CANCER

Many believe vitamin C acts as an anticancer agent in three
ways. First, it augments the activity of the immune response
against cancer. The activity of certain cells of the immune response
depends upon proper signaling. When activated, these cells, such
as the natural killer cells, go around and destroy anything they recognize as a threat. Vitamin C aids in the proliferation of some of
these cells. Second, vitamin C is able to inactivate certain mutagens. *In vitro*, ascorbic acid has been shown to detoxify the following carcinogens: benzpyrene, organochlorine pesticides,
anthracene, and heavy metals. Third, it is an effective antioxidant.
As a free-radical scavenger, the vitamin goes around "taking the
bullet" for DNA. One study indicated that diets rich in vitamin C
could help prevent oxidative damage to sperm cells in men.

VITAMIN C AND THE IMMUNE SYSTEM

Vitamin C appears to play an integral role in strengthening the
immune system. Although not completely understood, many think
vitamin C is a cofactor in the enzymes involved in making an
important chemical called interferon. When a cell is under attack
it sends a message to the immune system for help. Interferon is
this chemical signal. Vitamin C may be necessary to help cells produce this alert. Interferon molecules are involved in initiating an
inflammatory reaction. They are also involved in the stimulation of
leukocytes to proliferate. All of these jobs of interferon, as aided by
vitamin C, help strengthen the immune response.

For many years, researchers have attempted to demonstrate a
connection between vitamin C and the common cold. Studies and
experiments have yielded inconsistent results. To date, it appears
that there is consensus among researchers and scientists that vitamin C cannot actually prevent a cold, but it appears to have the
ability to reduce the severity and duration of a cold by 23 percent
on average. Still much research is being done, and the results are
becoming more positive.

In October 1999, a group of researchers studied "the effect of megadose vitamin C in preventing and relieving cold and flu symptoms." The group tested two groups, giving group one large doses of vitamin C daily. This group consisted of 242 students between the ages eighteen to thirty years. The control group consisted of a group of 463 students from the same college, ages eighteen to thirty-two years. For one year, group two was allowed to take decongestants and pain relievers to fight cold and flu symptoms. The following year, the test group was followed. They were administered a megadose of 1,000 mg of vitamin C three times a day for the year. If any cold or flu symptoms were reported, they were given the same dosage every hour for the first six hours and then continued with the normal daily dosage. They concluded, "overall, reported flu and cold symptoms in the test group decreased 85 percent compared with the control group after the administration of megadose vitamin C."

This study is one that seems to be opening current scientific thought on the power of vitamin C. The megadose of vitamin C not only relieved cold and flu symptoms once they had already hit, but it also seemed to have prevented the onset of these sicknesses to begin with.

Another study conducted in Italy, in April of 2000, confirmed that vitamin C seems to aid in the suppression of wheezing. The parents of 18,737 children, ages six to seven were asked to fill out questionnaires to determine how often their children ate citrus fruit. The groups were divided by the frequency with which they ate citrus fruit (one to two fruits a week, three to four per week, and five to seven per week). Researchers, having folowed 4,104 children for one yea, repored the following: "After controlling several confounders (sex, study area, paternal education, household density, maternal smoking, paternal smoking, dampness or mold in the child's bedroom, parental asthma), intake of citrus fruit or kiwi fruit was a highly significant protective factor for wheeze in the last twelve months."

VITAMIN C AND CARDIOVASCULAR DISEASES

In November 1999, a study was done to see if vitamin C helped to prevent heart disease. The study found that a dose of 2,000 mg of vitamin C significantly reduced the "augmentation index," which is a measure of arterial stiffness. Some believe that vitamin C may help prevent heart disease because it is an effective antioxidant.

Vitamin C may help control the number and damage of free radicals in the blood system. In particular, vitamin C may prevent free radicals from destroying nitric oxide gas. Nitric oxide seems to be necessary in maintaining the health of blood vessels. People with atherosclerosis have reduced levels of nitric oxide in their bloodstream compared to people with healthy blood vessels. When vitamin C is able to prevent the oxidation of nitric oxide, perhaps the blood vessels are able to remain clear of damaging plaques. In this study, the thickness of the arterial wall was measured using ultrasound. Those men who did not receive vitamin C supplementation had arteries that thickened significantly faster than those men who did receive 2 grams of vitamin C supplementation per day. This is much more than the RDA for merely preventing scurvy.

In another study, researchers tested the blood of 6,600 men and women to determine their vitamin C plasma level. After monitoring them for several years, it was determined that those with the highest levels of vitamin C in the blood were about 25 percent less likely to have a heart attack or a stroke than those who had the lowest levels.

OTHER THERAPEUTIC ASPECTS BEING INVESTIGATED

High doses of vitamin C have also been associated with protection against free radicals linked to senile dementia and Parkinson's disease. Other studies have positively linked vitamin C with prevention of age-related eye diseases such as macular degeneration, and cataracts. Vitamin C is also associated with degradation of histamine, and may therefore have anti-allergic properties. The improvement of wound healing, fertility and diabetes conditions are currently being studied.

RECOMMENDED DOSAGE

It is easy for any of us to look up the RDA for a particular nutrient and stick to that recommendation. Remember, however, that these amounts are based on known associations of the vitamin in merely preventing nutritional deficiencies. For example, in order to stop scurvy, only about 10 mg per day of vitamin C is sufficient. The RDA for adults is then geared towards preventing this disease. The RDA however does not list amounts to be taken if some of the preventative effects of higher dosages are to be obtained. If you remember the studies we just described, the dosages required to get positive correlations were much more than 10 mg. They were more like 1,000, 2,000, even 6,000 mg per day in some cases. As far as supplements go, a recent article published in *Nature,* one of the most prominent of scientific journals, reads:

"Vitamin C is used as a dietary supplement because of its antioxidant activity, although a high dose may act as a pro-oxidant in the body. Here we show that 100 g of fresh apples has an antioxidant activity equivalent to 1,500 mg of vitamin C, and that whole-apple extracts inhibit the growth of colon and liver cancer cells *in vitro* in a dose-dependent manner. Our results indicate that natural antioxidants from fresh fruit could be more effective than a dietary supplement."

In this study, Dr. Eberhardt and colleagues tested the effect of apple extracts on cancer cell lines, as compared to vitamin C, and found that the synergistic effects of the vitamin C in the apple with other phytochemicals was more effective than vitamin C by itself. Again, this goes to show that fruits and vegetables are very powerful in disease prevention because of their rich combinations of antioxidant compounds. To take in the same amounts of these compounds in the right combinations from supplements alone may not only prove to be expensive for you, but impossible. "An apple a day keeps the doctor away."

Vitamin C is found in citrus fruits and some vegetables. Broccoli and Brussels sprouts are excellent sources of vitamin C. Strawberries, lemons, oranges, grapefruit, pineapple, etc. also have plenty. (See Appendix D for nutrient tables.)

Toxicity has been suggested, but not proven. Because ascorbic acid can be degraded into oxalic acid, concerns have been raised as to the possibility of megadose vitamin C leading to kidney stones. Therefore we recommend that patients with kidney stones or renal disease avoid such megadoses above 1,000 mg.

References

Eberhardt MV, Lee CY, Liu RH. Antioxidant Activity of Fresh Apples. June 2000; Nature. 405:903–904.

Forastiere F, Pistelli R, Sestini P, Fortes C, Renzoni E, Rusconi F, Dell'Orco V, Ciccone G, Bisanti L. Consumption of Fresh Fruit Rich in Vitamin C and Wheezing Symptoms in Children. SIDRIA Collaborative Group, Italy (Italian Studies on Respiratory Disorders in Children and the environment.) Thorax. 2000 Apr; 55(4): 283–88.

Gensler HL, Williams T, Huang AC, Jacobson EL. Oral Niacin Prevents Photocarinogenesis and Photoimmunosuppression in Mice. Nutr Cancer. 1999;

34(1): 36– 41.

Gorton HC, Jarvis K. The Effectiveness of Vitamin C in Preventing and Relieving the Symptoms of Virus-Induced Respiratory Infections. J Manipulative Physiol Ther. 1999 Oct; 22(8): 530–3.

Guyton JR. Effect of Niacin on Atherosclerotic Cardiovascular Disease. Am J Cardiol. 1998 Dec. 17; 82(12A): 18U– 23U.

Wilkinson IB, Megson IL, MacCallum H, Sogo N, Cockcroft JR, Webb DJ. Oral Vitamin C Reduces Arterial Stiffness and Platelet Aggregation in Humans. J Cardiovasc Pharmacol. 1999 Nov; 34(5): 690–3.

Zollinger PE, Tuinebreijer WE, Kreis RW, Breederveld RS. Effect of Vitamin C on Frequency of Reflex Sympathetic Dystrophy in Wrist Fractures: A Randomized Trial. Lancet. 1999 Dec. 11; 354(9195): 2025–8.

CHAPTER 8

Fat-Soluble Vitamins

In the early 1900s, vitamins grew in importance to the scientific community. Some diseases were linked to dietary deficiencies, and many researchers began to take an interest in identifying these vital nutrients. As we have already mentioned, the term "vitamin" was coined in 1912, referring to a group of nutrients necessary to prevent specific deficiencies. The more we have grown to understand the nature of nutrition the more diseases we are recognizing as deficiencies. This is an important trend because it places greater emphasis on the possibility of prevention rather than on the search for cures. The more diseases we recognize as caused by something missing from our diets the more important proper nutrition will become in scientific circles.

In 1913, Drs. McCollum and Davis at the University of Wisconsin and Drs. Osborne and Mendel at Yale, independently, yet almost simultaneously, identified a compound known as "fat-soluble A." These researchers noticed that rats would not grow normally unless "fat-soluble A" was in their diet. They knew the compound was in butter and egg yolk. Quickly this essential nutrient was named "vitamin A." Vitamin A was the first vitamin to be discovered and so was given the letter A. Seventeen years later, in 1930, the structure of vitamin A was discovered (see Appendix E), and research began to discover the function of vitamin A in our bodies.

Provitamin vs. Preformed Vitamin A

Like many vitamins, vitamin A is not just the name given to one compound. Vitamin A is actually the name for a family of related compounds with similar structures, affecting the body in a similar fashion. There are two types of vitamin A: provitamin A and preformed vitamin A.

In the end there is no difference between preformed vitamin A and provitamin A. The difference, however, is in how you get it. You can get preformed vitamin A by eating animals that have already eaten enough other compounds to make it for you. Preformed vitamin A seems appropriately named because it is already formed by the time you get it. On the other hand we can also make vitamin A for ourselves. In order to make vitamin A we must eat precursors called provitamins. Vitamin A precursors are produced by plants and are widely available in a number of fruits and vegetables. Thus, provitamin A is the same as preformed vitamin A except that it is formed from various components of plants and vegetables by your body.

Retinoids: Retinol, Retinal, and Retinoic Acid

Vitamin A is actually a molecule known as retinol. Retinol can be modified to form an acid derivative of vitamin A. These acids are called retinoids. In some cases retinoids are turned into retinol, and in some cases retinoids are made from retinol. Retinoids are a group of three related molecules that act similarly in the body. These three molecules—retinol, retinal, and retinoic acid—are almost identical.

They look like tadpoles with round heads and skinny tails. The head is composed of six carbons in a ring, while the tail is made of a carbon chain with an oxygen molecule on the end. Retinol, retinal, and retinoic acid differ only in the way that the oxygen molecule is bound to the end of the carbon tail.

Retinol was originally isolated from the retina of the eye and was therefore named "retinol." Retinoids are found in animal products such as liver, fish, egg yolk, and dairy products. We'll discuss them in greater detail momentarily.

Vitamin A Increases Absorption of Other Fat-Soluble Vitamins

Vitamins A, D, E, and K can only be digested if eaten in combination with some form of fat. We will discuss the basics of fat-soluble vitamin digestion in order to better help you plan a healthy diet.

To begin, all of the vitamin A found in our diet, whether it is preformed or provitamin A, is initially bound to important proteins until released in the stomach. In the small intestine they are converted into retinol (or vitamin A).

Fatty matter tends to clump together in the stomach much like the grease from a pan in a sink of water. Bile acts as an emulsifier, or detergent, to break up the clumps of fat and help them dissolve. This increases the absorption of fats and fat-soluble vitamins. Your liver is an important organ in the efficient digestion of vitamin A. It must produce correct amounts of bile to break up fatty particles in your food. This is because vitamin A tends to hide in fatty matter because it is hydrophobic, or nonpolar, while the juices in the stomach are composed mainly of water.

Bile is an amphipathic molecule, which means that there are both polar and nonpolar regions on the molecule. Fat-soluble, or nonpolar, regions group with the fat in our diet, and surround it with the hydrophobic ends of their molecules. The water-soluble ends of the bile molecules thus stick outward into the water-based juices of the digestive system. This creates small balls or droplets of fat surrounded by bile. These droplets are called "micelles." Eventually the micelle is dissolved in the water-like juices of the digestive system. The nutrients in the fatty matter are then carried to the small intestine. In the small intestine, protein carriers known as chilomicrons pick up fat-soluble vitamins and other nonpolar molecules and carry them into the bloodstream. The bloodstream then carries them throughout the body.

Vitamin A molecules are used in bone marrow, blood cells, the spleen, muscles, the kidney, lungs, fat cells and the liver. The majority of vitamin A goes to the liver. Here, vitamin A is stored and carotenoids are transformed into retinol. The liver thus stores vitamin A in order to prevent a deficiency if our diet fails to take in enough vitamin A for a short time. From the liver, stored vitamin A can be mobilized and delivered to various tissues throughout the body.

Before discussing the various functions of vitamin A it is important to note that the fat-soluble vitamins pose some unique challenges to people seeking to ensure they are getting enough of them. You may be eating enough of the fat-soluble vitamins, A, D, E, and K, and yet have a vitamin deficiency if there is a breakdown in any of the components of this chain. In fact, fat-soluble vitamins are very poorly absorbed into the small intestine if the diet of an individual is low in fat. Taking fat substitutes such as Olestra can be one of the causes of fat-soluble vitamin deficiency. Olestra is a grease-like substance that can be used in foods in place of fat. However, unlike normal dietary fats, Olestra cannot be digested or absorbed by your body. Olestra passes right through you taking with it many other fat-soluble molecules. Because of this, vitamins A, D, E, K and carotenoids are not absorbed well if eaten with foods containing Olestra.

Functions in the Body

Vitamin A and other closely related retinoids have a variety of important functions. Vitamin A contributes to sight, the health and maintenance of skin and tissues lining internal cavities, as well as being vital in reproduction, growth, and immunity.

VISION

Vitamin A plays an elementary role in vision. Retinol is transported through the blood to rod and cone cells in the retina at the back of the eyes. In the eyes, the retinol form of vitamin A is converted into retinal. The carbon tail of retinal bends, and a protein already in the rod or cone cell called "opsin" sticks to it. This combination is called "rhodopsin." Rhodopsin sits in the back of the eye and waits for light. When light enters the eye, it passes through the pupil and into the retina. The bent tails of the rhodopsin then shift and straighten out as a result of the light. The conversion of vitamin A from a bent shape to a straight shape (or from cis to trans) sends a nerve impulse to the brain interpreted as vision. The opsin and retinal then separate and the straight-tailed retinal returns to its bent-tailed form and again combines with opsin to form rhodopsin.

When there is a shortage of vitamin A, one of the first symptoms experienced is night blindness. Night blindness occurs when

Antioxidants Linked to Reduced Breast Cancer Risk

Scientists perfoming a recent study published in the February 2002 issue of the *Journal of Nutrition* state, "We conclude that increased serum levels of beta-carotene, retinol, bilirubin and total antioxidant status are associated with reductions in breast cancer risk."

we are unable to adjust quickly from bright to dim lighting conditions. For instance, when driving down a two-lane road in the dark, an oncoming car may fail to dim its bright headlights, making it difficult to see even after it has passed. Though to some degree it is normal to experience momentary "blindness" due to such severe and sudden changes in lighting, night blindness is characterized by an inability to readjust without great difficulty. Night blindness is a symptom of vitamin A deficiency because without enough of it the cells in the retina will not cycle into rhodopsin and back into retinol fast enough to allow sight under changing lighting characteristic of night time. Specifically, the straight retinal can't be transformed into the bent-shaped retinal quick enough, creating a shortage of the necessary rhodopsin and resulting in the inability to see. Increased vitamin A levels speed up the reactions involved in seeing, and night vision is restored. Thousands of years ago, early physicians knew this and treated night blindness by feeding deficient patients liver: a great source of vitamin A.

VITAMIN A AND GENE REGULATION

Vitamin A plays an important role in cell replication: the process of cell reproduction. A form of vitamin A called retinoic acid, helps to control which genes are read and expressed as proteins. Retinoic acid enters the nucleus of specific target cells, joins with an assisting protein and acts as a transcription factor. This means that it binds to regions of DNA to either enhance or inhibit gene expression. In fact, retinoic acid is used as a chemotherapeutic agent because of its ability to act as a transcription factor for important genes such as the gene for HAT. In other words, retinoic acid may help prevent and treat some cancers because it helps regulate gene expression. In the end it may prevent genes from getting out of control, causing uncontrolled cell proliferation.

VITAMIN A IMPROVES THE IMMUNE SYSTEM

Vitamin A plays a key role in the development of our immune system. Our skin and digestive lining provides a physical barrier against invading microorganisms. The epithelium is a very important tissue in our body because it comprises the skin and lines our internal cavities and organs, such as our eyes, intestines, lungs and bladder. If our epithelial tissue is healthy, microbes are not allowed to infect the other tissues of our body. However, during vitamin A deficiency, the epithelium becomes dry and hard, and the physical barrier provided by our epithelium is weakened. Bacteria, viruses and parasites are more able to penetrate the protective epithelium and infect other tissues. Vitamin A helps keep your skin and other epithelial tissue healthy.

In addition to guarding against infection, the epithelial tissues are needed for a variety of reasons. Many areas of our epithelium have cells that produce mucus to lubricate and protect areas of our body. However, without vitamin A, immature epithelial cells are unable to grow into mucus-secreting cells. Instead, they produce a protein known as keratin. Keratin is the hard substance that makes hair and fingernails. Vitamin A deficient individuals often have skin that is hard, scaly, and dry due to the keratin that is being produced and deposited in the outer epithelium.

However, the skin is not the only place where a lack of vitamin A is noticeable. The eye is an organ whose epithelium is extremely sensitive to decreased amounts of vitamin A. During a deficiency of vitamin A, the front of the eye, which is moist and protected in normal individuals, becomes dry and susceptible to infection. This condition is known as "xerophthalmia." Keratin can also build up in the eye, causing the eye to become soft, resulting in possible blindness.

VITAMIN A AS AN ANTIOXIDANT

A lot of research has been done recently to identify the natural inhibitors of free-radical oxidation. Vitamin A is an antioxidant. Because vitamin A is a fat-soluble compound, it provides its oxidative protection in lipid membranes surrounding cells, and in other lipid environments. Although it is not as potent as vitamin E (covered in the next section), retinol, however, is more effective at stopping free radicals once oxidation has occurred in the membrane. It is thought that retinol is able to move more freely through the lipid membrane, and is more centered in the lipid membrane than alpha-tocopherol. Although it is not the major antioxidant protector, vitamin A has also been shown to reduce the oxidation of LDLs in our blood. The antioxidant protection that vitamin A provides our LDLs is important because it is currently thought that oxidative damage to LDLs is a major contributor in the initiation of atherosclerosis and heart disease.

We know for certain that there are ailments associated with vitamin A deficiency; but as far as showing its ability to prevent lifestyle diseases, vitamin A research has been somewhat discouraging. Some research has given evidence that the vitamin may cause decreased risk of head, neck and breast cancer, and also heart disease. All of this literature advocates the need for continued research to make more conclusive studies.

HOW MUCH DO WE NEED?

Because it can be difficult to quantify the amount of vitamin A in our diets, a unit of vitamin A "currency" was established that attempts to evaluate vitamin A on the quality of its effect, not its quantity. This vitamin currency attempts to determine how much of the food we eat actually acts like pure vitamin A once in the body. The first unit established was the international unit, or IU. The IU was established by experiments with rats, and scientists later realized that rats are more efficient at making vitamin A out of beta-carotene than we are. So, the IU is a little bit inaccurate. This was corrected in 1980 when the IU was replaced by RE, or retinol equivalents. Using the RE, the effects of provitamin and preformed vitamin A are compared to the effects of pure retinol in our bodies. One RE is equal to 1 mg of retinol. Because provitamins aren't as easily absorbed as preformed vitamin A, and because not all absorbed carotenes are actually converted into vitamin A, a large quantity of vitamin A precursors must be eaten to equal the activity of 1 mg of pure retinol. It takes 6 mg of beta-carotene and 12 mg of other provitamins to equal 1 RE.

1 retinol equivalent equals 1 mg of retinol
- which equals 6 mg of beta-carotene
- which equals 12 mg of other provitamins
- which equals 3.33 IF of retinol
- which equals 10 IF of beta-carotene

The most recent RDAs for vitamin A were established in 1989 and are given in units of retinol equivalents per day. DRIs have not yet been made for vitamin A or beta-carotene because of contradictory results of various tests. As you can tell, science still has a long way to go in figuring out how much vitamin A needs to be in a healthy diet. For this reason, the Food and Nutrition Board cautions against high doses. See Appendix D for the RDA values for vitamin A. Generally, men are recommended to include about 1,000 retinol equivalents, or 1,000 mg, of retinol per day.

Taking vitamins can be a tricky business. Not enough vitamin A can cause a variety of deficiency symptoms, while taking too much can be toxic. Vitamin A deficiency can cause poor growth in children and increases the chance of infection due to a weakened immune system. Hard, dry skin, poor sight, and blindness are also among results of vitamin A deficiency.

Vitamin A deficiency, or VAD, is a serious and common problem in the world, particularly among children in developing countries. For years, the World Health Organization (WHO) and the United Nation's Children's Fund, in conjunction with many other organizations have worked to alleviate VAD. In fact, in 1990, a goal was endorsed to completely eliminate VAD by the year 2000. Although many countries have achieved this goal, many more have not.

VAD is characterized by early childhood blindness, and is often followed by death. Measles also affects this same unfortunate large population, and even works synergistically in causing death of children. Alfred Sommer, one of the principle experts in this area of research, has found that supplementation of young children could reduce the death rate by as much as 30 percent! One of the keys to preventing infant VAD is for mothers to breastfeed. It is estimated that over a million children die as a result of VAD with measles, and that as much as one half of these measles deaths could be prevented if these children were supplemented with vitamin A.

In developed countries, such as the U.S., the risk of vitamin A deficiency is not very high because we benefit from the fruits and vegetables that are readily available. However, it is still possible to be at risk of vitamin A deficiency if you do not eat enough fruits and vegetables. A staple of burgers and fries won't provide much vitamin A.

Preformed vitamin A is toxic at doses significantly above the RDA. Stories are told of Arctic explorers who died from vitamin A overdose after eating polar bear meat. They would often eat as much of the bear as possible, including the liver. Unfortunately, polar bear liver contains extremely high amounts of vitamin A. As a result, some explorers have died. Many assert that it takes persistent doses of around 100 times the RDA to cause coma or death. At these high concentrations, the liver cannot store all the vitamin A coming into it, resulting in nausea, vomiting, headache, dizziness, blurred vision, and a lack of muscle coordination.

Lower doses, around ten times the RDA, taken for several months, can result in liver damage, muscle or joint pain, visual defects, skin irritation and dry lips. Birth defects have also been associated with the toxicity of vitamin A. One particular form of retinoic acid has been shown to work great in treating acne, but has proven to be harmful to unborn babies. Because supplements can easily contain the amounts of preformed vitamin A needed to be harmful to a fetus, it is normally suggested that pregnant women only use vitamin A supplements that contain carotenoids, which are not harmful to the fetus. Carotenoids are also nontoxic. These vitamin A precursors have been shown to have little or no toxic effects on the body. However, if large amounts of carotenoids are taken, such as beta-carotene, the skin can turn a yellow-orange color. As we have discussed, vitamin A and other carotenoid precursors are lipid soluble, and can accumulate in the fatty tissue close to the skin.

Vitamin E

In 1922, a group of researchers at the University of California at Berkley began a research project and unwittingly stumbled onto a compound destined for fame. Dr. Herbert Evans and Dr. Katharine Bishop were feeding rats a special diet. On this altered diet, the rats grew well and maintained seemingly normal health, though females were unable to carry pups to full term. In addition, some damage was done to various reproductive organs of the male and female rats. They determined that these abnormalities must be the result of some deficiency in the rat's diet. The scientists set out to identify this factor, which they termed Factor X. Eventually Factor X was identified in lettuce leaves. Because of the characteristics displayed by Factor X, Drs. Evans and Bishop realized that they might be on the trail of a vitamin. Eventually they decided that Factor X was indeed a vitamin.

Vitamins A, B, C, and D had already been identified and named, so in 1925 they named Factor X "vitamin E."

Simultaneously, research was done on this same vitamin by researchers at the Universities of Iowa and Arkansas, who observed similar problems in the reproductive systems of rats. They even suggested that the missing factor in the rat's diet be called vitamin E, using the same logic as Drs. Evans and Bishop.

Researchers wanted to know how vitamin E affected tissues other than the reproductive systems of rats. They were particularly interested in the role of vitamin E in humans. Unfortunately, research on vitamin E was quite tedious. This is because a vitamin E deficiency can go unnoticed for years, displaying no obvious symptoms. Slowly, however, the efforts of research began to pay off. Evidence began to appear correlating vitamin E deficiencies with damage to muscles and the nervous system in animals, and scientists began recognizing how vitamin E worked as an antioxidant. Later, the chemical structures were identified for the various molecules in the vitamin E family and methods of extracting vitamin E from vegetable byproducts were developed, along with ways to measure the amount of vitamin E in foods, body tissues, and body fluids.

While early research was done on vitamin E, a controversy arose concerning its role in treating various diseases. In the 1940s two Canadian brothers, Drs. Evan and Wilfred Shute, treated heart disease, skin disease, and burns with vitamin E, claiming that patients had made remarkable recoveries and that vitamin E had tremendous therapeutic properties. Most of the medical world thought that it was impossible that a mere vitamin could have such an impact on disease. The Shute brothers were soundly rebuffed by their medical colleagues. They were essentially blacklisted, unable to publish in the top medical journals of the day, or find employment with mainstream hospitals. Serious research concerning vitamin E slowed until the '90s.

Researchers seem to be making up for lost time. Since 1990 there has been an explosion of research and information on vitamin E. Its antioxidant functions are better understood, the method of absorption and transport of vitamin E within the body has been identified, and much research has been done, and is currently in progress, to identify how different molecules in the vitamin E family interact to protect our bodies from diseases. Vitamin E is linked to the prevention of heart disease, cancer, aging, Alzheimer's, cataracts and other diseases. Mainstream agencies such as the National Institute of Health are currently taking a great interest in vitamin E. As the information comes rolling in, it seems that the greatest benefits from vitamin E come from its ability to prevent, rather than treat, disease.

TEAM OF EIGHT

Vitamin E is a family of sixteen different compounds. They can be separated into two groups of eight: eight tocopherols and eight tocotrienols. The initial name given to vitamin E, "tocopherol," is Greek for "birth-bringing" tocos and ferin. Later on, several other relating compounds were discovered and given the name of tocotrienol, based on a key difference in their molecular structure. The eight common molecules of the vitamin E family are alpha-tocopherol, beta-tocopherol, gamma-tocopherol, delta-tocopherol, alpha-tocotrienol, beta-tocotrienol, gamma-tocotrienol and delta-tocotrienol. The chemical structure of each of these individual compounds is found in Appendix E.

All of these compounds have a similar structure. Each has a round head, known as a chroman ring, consisting of carbon atoms bound together to make a cyclic structure. Tocopherols all have what are known as phytyl tails or long strings of carbon atoms. The tocotrienols have a tail that is just as long as the tocopherol tail, and has just as many carbons, but the tocotrienol tail has three double bonds in it. The name "tri en" means "three double bonds."

The Greek prefixes alpha, beta, gamma, and delta are used to distinguish different arrangements of carbon atoms. All sixteen of these molecules work together as a vitamin E team, to benefit the body in a variety of ways.

SUPPLEMENTS CAN HELP

For years in the literature and common opinion, vitamin E has been synonymous with only one of these eight common compounds: alpha-tocopherol. The other seven compounds were considered to be extra compounds that had similar functions of alpha-tocopherol, but were less active and present in bodies in lower concentrations. Thus they were often ignored. For example, many vitamin E supplement pills contain only alpha-tocopherol, and many foods are fortified with only alpha-tocopherol. The inordinate emphasis placed on alpha-tocopherol results primarily because alpha-tocopherol is the most abundant of the eight compounds in our bodies. Alpha-tocopherol is also the

---

Vitamin E Linked to Reduced Cervical Cancer Risk

A recent study published in the June 2001 issue of *Revista Medica de Chile* states, "Cervical cancer is associated with reproductive and food consumption behaviors. A higher intake of vegetables and foods rich in vitamin E can reduce its risk."

---

most biologically active of the vitamin-E vitamers. However, recent studies have shown that the other seven compounds that make up the vitamin E family may play a very important role in aiding alpha-tocopherol in its antioxidant activities. It also appears that the other tocopherols and tocotrienols have their own important effects on the body.

For example, it seems that tocotrienols play a significant role in maintaining appropriate cholesterol levels. As the medical establishment works to find answers to cardiovascular disease, cholesterol has been an area of diligent interest. The general public gets plenty of pressure from the medical field to reduce cholesterol levels in our blood. In response to this, we choose diets that are lower in cholesterol. However only 20 percent of the cholesterol in our blood is from our diets. The liver produces the other 80 percent. Researchers are finding that tocotrienols are able to reduce the activity of the enzyme that produces cholesterol in the liver. Other studies indicate that the narrowing of the carotid artery, a condition common in cardiovascular diseases, is reduced or reversed when treated with a mixture of tocotrienols and tocopherols.

In addition, gamma-tocopherol seems to be the major antioxidant form of vitamin E against nitrogen radicals. Nitrogen radicals are the major damaging factors in arthritis, multiple sclerosis, and diseases of the brain such as Alzheimer's.

Also, a certain derivative of gamma-tocopherol seems to be involved in regulating the quantity of fluids filtered through the kidneys. This means that gamma-tocopherol could impact blood pressure, congestive heart failure, and cirrhosis of the liver. Also, gamma-tocopherol is used before alpha-tocopherol when there are a lot of free radicals or other reactive oxygen molecules present in our tissues. Thus, alpha-tocopherol is conserved, and the body is better protected from oxidative damage.

These examples illustrate that our bodies benefit most by the presence of all eight of the tocopherols and the eight tocotrienols rather than alpha-tocopherol alone.

We have discussed the history of vitamin E, the different molecules that make up the vitamin E family, and a few of the benefits this vitamin provides. It is not hard to see why companies are fortifying foods and products with vitamin E. In fact, fifteen thousand tons of vitamin E is produced each year to satisfy this demand. Vitamin E fortifies foods as well as cosmetics.

SYNTHETIC VERSUS NATURAL VITAMIN E

Vitamin E is manufactured in two ways: naturally and synthetically. For most of the vitamins, synthetic production does not alter the chemical structure of the vitamin, or the effect that the vitamin has on our bodies. Synthetically produced vitamins are usually identical to natural vitamins we find in fruits and vegetables. However, alpha-tocopherol is the only member of the vitamin E family produced synthetically, and it acts a little bit differently than natural vitamin E. The other seven tocopherols and tocotrienols are only produced naturally, and are not available synthetically. Supplements utilizing natural vitamin E pass vegetable products through extraction processes to remove all eight of the tocopherols and tocotrienols. Vegetable products such as corn oil, soybean oil, canola oil, rice bran oil, and palm oil are all great natural sources of the compounds in the vitamin E family. (Of course, remember that canola oil is the best of these because it does not contain large quantities of saturated fat.) These natural extracts are then normally used to make dietary supplements.

Natural vitamin E is better than synthetic vitamin E because natural alpha-tocopherol is created in plants by enzymes in a precise manner difficult to duplicate in a laboratory. When these enzymes add atom upon atom to make alpha-tocopherol, not only are the correct atoms added in the right sequence, they are added from the correct direction. This small detail results in molecules that contain all of the correct atoms in a proper sequence. However, the synthetic production of alpha-tocopherol is not as precise.

The chemical reactions induced to make alpha-tocopherol add the right atoms in the correct sequence to make a given compound, but the direction from which the atoms are added is not as tightly controlled as it is in plants.

Thus, synthetically produced alpha-tocopherol appears the

same, but some of the atoms have been added to the molecule from one side, while other atoms have been added from another side. Molecules that have the same overall structure, but may differ in the direction that their atoms have been added, are called sterioisomers. Synthetic production of alpha-tocopherol results in the production of eight different sterioisomers, only one of which is actually present in nature. The other seven differ only in the arrangement of their atoms. Natural alpha-tocopherol is commonly called RRR-alpha-tocopherol, or more commonly d-alpha-tocopherol. The synthetic alpha-tocopherol, which consists of its eight sterioisomers, is known as all-rac-alpha-tocopherol or more commonly dl-alpha-tocopherol.

We eat a lot of synthetic vitamin E (dl-alpha-tocopherol). It is used in many dietary supplements, and is used to fortify cereals and other foods. It's a good thing you get so much synthetic vitamin E, because the small difference between natural and synthetic vitamin E makes it twice as difficult for your body to use it. To say it another way, you must have twice the amount of synthetic alpha-tocopherol to do the work of natural alpha-tocopherol. Other studies have shown that the RRR-alpha-tocopherol passes from the mother through the placenta to the fetus three times more efficiently than dl-alpha-tocopherol. Your body is designed to use the natural, or d-alpha-tocopherol. When in doubt, look for the triple Rs.

A LONGER SHELF LIFE

Vitamin E is a particularly effective antioxidant because it consists of molecules with relatively low electron affinities. This means that molecules with strong electron affinities (like oxygen free radicals) will happily steal one of their electrons. When free radicals steal an electron from vitamin E, a chain reaction is averted because vitamin E remains stable despite losing one of its electrons. Thus vitamin E prevents serious damage from oxidation by being sacrificed in place of other molecules in your body.

This great benefit, however, also leads to problems in packaging supplemental vitamin E. Vitamin E will readily give up electrons to oxygen anywhere, not just in your body. As a result, vitamin E will not last long in a potent form if it is packaged without special precautions. In other words, unless vitamin E supplements are carefully packaged they will have a short shelf life.

Vitamin E can be packaged a number of ways to increase shelf life. First, it can be bound to other molecules like succinate, acetate, linolate, or nicotate before being packaged. This forces the vitamin E molecule to share electrons with other molecules, preventing oxygen from stealing them. Alpha-tocopherol packaged in this way is known as esterified alpha-tocopherol. When it is eaten, the added compound is easily broken away, leaving alpha-tocopherol ready and able to get to work. Alpha tocopherol is the only vitamin E vitamer made in an esterified form. The seven other vitamers must be packaged for supplementation in other ways. The idea is to keep the vitamin E family away from oxygen, other free radicals, bright light, and heat.

To do this, supplement manufacturers will often use gelatin capsules and dark bottles. This reduces exposure to light and oxygen, and the vitamin E supplement can maintain a shelf life of many years. Manufacturers have also found ways to make vitamin E accessible to people who cannot absorb fat very well, thus having difficulty absorbing fat-soluble vitamins like vitamin E. A special form of vitamin E, known as TPGS (or d-alpha-tocopherol polyethylene glycol 1000 succinate), is an esterified form of alpha-tocopherol, which will dissolve in water. People with liver diseases that prevent the production of bile or that have other diseases of the gut that interfere with absorption can use TPGS, and are thus able to avoid the problems that are caused by vitamin E deficiency.

Esterified vitamin E is very common. It is an effective way to prevent the degradation of vitamin E before it is ingested and used by the body. However, it is important to keep in mind that supplements often contain only alpha-tocopherol and do not provide all the compounds in the vitamin E family. It is important to get all eight vitamers of vitamin E. We will provide a few concrete suggestions in a moment. But first we'll discuss what vitamin E actually does in a little more detail. We hope this information will help motivate you to eat foods that will give you the appropriate amount and variety of vitamin E.

BIOLOGICAL EFFECTS

Vitamin E's primary role in the body is to act as an antioxidant. Antioxidants, such as vitamin E, have electrons that can easily be donated to a reactive free radical. In this process, vitamin E will itself become a free radical, yet it remains stable because of its structure. It can thus exist as a free radical without trying to take an electron from neighboring molecules, causing further tissue damage.

MORE ON VITAMIN E AS AN ANTIOXIDANT

Vitamin E is the most important fat-soluble antioxidant in our bodies, and works in a number of ways to protect our bodies from oxidative damage.

A lipid membrane surrounds our cells. It is important to keep the membranes surrounding our cells healthy in order to maintain normal tissue development and function. However, the long carbon chains that make up the inner portion of our cellular membranes are quite susceptible to free radicals and oxidative damage. Much like a bundle of dry branches and grass is susceptible to fires, these carbon chains can be easily enflamed in chemical reactions that will destroy the cellular membrane. A free radical in the wrong spot could cause the destruction of the entire cell. Vitamin E has been coined "nature's master antioxidant" because it is such an effective protector against lipid peroxidation.

The structure of vitamin E gives it this great ability to prevent oxidation. Recall how the tocopherols and tocotrienols have long carbon tails, attached to a cyclic head. There is a hydroxyl group (OH) attached to the head that readily donates an electron to other free radicals. The long carbon tail anchors the vitamin in the center, while the hydroxyl group on the head of the vitamin hovers near the surface of the cellular membrane. The positioning of the head of vitamin E allows it to react with and stop free radicals both outside and inside the cell membrane. Alpha-tocopherol is the vitamin E vitamer that is most abundant and biologically active in human cellular membranes.

Vitamin E is a particularly powerful antioxidant because of its efficiency in quenching free radicals. Studies have shown that during the process of lipid peroxidation, alpha-tocopherol will react ten times faster with the harmful radical than normal lipid molecules will, and that one alpha-tocopherol molecule will protect one thousand lipid molecules in our cell membranes. This powerful antioxidant activity makes vitamin E an important member of our bodies' complete antioxidant defense system.

Vitamin E is essential in protecting cellular membranes. In particular, vitamin E is essential to preventing oxidation in the tissues of the nervous system, such as the brain. Vitamin E also prevents the oxidation of LDLs and may therefore help prevent atherosclerosis and other cardiovascular diseases.

WHAT IS PKC?

Cells communicate with each other through proteins that readily shuttle between cells. There is a protein inside our cells called protein kinase C, or PKC, which is involved in a number of these important pathways. If PKC is stimulated too much, however, it can become overactive and actually cause damage to the cells it is supposed to help. PKC is an important regulator of the growth and division of cells. Therefore if PKC is overactive, the growth and division of the cells is overactive, potentially causing cancer. Vitamin E helps regulate PKC, preventing it from becoming overactive.

NEURODEGENERATIVE DISEASE

We discussed how vitamin E is a valuable fat-soluble antioxidant, protecting fatty tissue (like cells of the brain) from oxidative damage. In 1998, Mary Sano and her associates studied 341 moderate stage Alzheimer's patients. They were split into groups randomly and placed either on a placebo pill or vitamin E for two years. Vitamin E was given at 2,000 IU per day (1,300 mg). These researchers hoped to find out if vitamin E would help slow Alzheimer's in its progression. Results showed that vitamin E slowed the natural progress of dementia and death associated with Alzheimer's disease.

In July of 1999, however, a study of 3,385 Japanese-American men from Hawaii added some important details to our understanding of the connection between vitamin E and dementia. Researchers interviewed participants to determine how much vitamin E and C they were consuming. They were 88 percent less prone to vascular dementia.

Finally in March 2001, researchers from the Honolulu Heart Program studied 8,006 Japanese Americans and found that the risk of vascular dementia decreased by 68 percent in those men who took vitamin E supplements.

CORONARY HEART DISEASE

There has been considerable evidence in the past decade supporting the possibility that vitamin E lowers the risk of coronary heart disease, especially atherosclerosis. It is thought that the damaging effects of free radicals on circulating LDL levels can be somewhat curbed by vitamin E because it is an effective antioxidant.

In 1993, two studies were reported in the same edition of *The New England Journal of Medicine*. One was a study on coronary heart disease and men, and the other was on women. The study examined dietary questionnaires from 87,245 women and 39,910 men, neither of which had any previous history of heart disease. The results? The men who consumed the most vitamin E in the diet had a 36 percent lower chance for fatal or nonfatal heart attacks and disease than those who consumed the least. The women in the same group had 34 percent less risk! Since this time, both doctors and commercial supplement companies have urged us to save our hearts by taking vitamin E.

However, another study by Karen Woodson failed to demonstrate the same dramatic results. Woodson's study was a little bit different because the individuals participating, 2,545 women and 6,996 men, were at a high risk for heart disease. This meant that each of them had had a previous history of a cardiac event in addition to a high risk factor, such as being heavy smokers or having family history of heart disease.

Katalin Glosonczy et al examined 11,178 elderly people between the ages of 67 to 105 as to their vitamin E and C supplement use. The study was conducted from 1984 to 1993. They found that "use of vitamin E reduced the risk of all-cause mortality. . . and risk of coronary disease mortality."

The American Heart Association sent out a statement for healthcare professionals concerning the consumption of a variety of vitamins and their help in fighting against heart disease. They referred to a prevention trial done by The Cambridge Heart Antioxidant Study. They studied the effects of very high doses of alpha-tocopherol on patients that had angiographic evidence of atherosclerosis. Their results were a decrease in the risks of myocardial infarction by 77 percent. All other cardiovascular events were reduced by 47 percent.

The bottom line with heart disease, then, seems to be to guard against it in your future by eating plenty of vitamin E rich foods.

SOURCES OF VITAMIN E

Vitamin E is found in foods with fat in them. Our bodies do not make vitamin E, and neither do animals, so the majority of vitamin E must come from plants. There is a small amount of vitamin E in meat, provided the animal ate plants rich in vitamin E before you eat it. But remember vitamin E in meat was initially from a plant. Meat is, therefore, a rather poor source of vitamin E.

Fruits and vegetables are not a great source of vitamin E either. To really increase your intake of vitamin E you need to eat a lot of plant products high in fat, or eat natural supplements. Fat-rich plant products can be grouped into three basic groups: vegetable oils, nuts, and grains and legumes.

Vegetable oils are generally a great source of vitamin E. The amounts of tocopherols and tocotrienols present depend largely on what type of vegetable oil it is, and how the oil was processed. Sunflower oil contains mostly alpha-tocopherol, while soy and corn oils contain mostly gamma-tocopherol. Rice bran oil and palm oil are good sources of tocotrienols.

While vegetable oils easily fulfill the Recommended Daily Allowances (RDA) for vitamin E, 22 IU of natural source vitamin E, it is difficult to consume large amounts of vitamin E strictly from our diet without consuming a lot of extra fat. As we have mentioned, studies have shown that vitamin E can prevent many diseases, but the different studies that have reported these results used high doses of vitamin E, between 100 and 400 IU a day. On the heels of these results, many experts recommend taking 100 IU a day plus 100 mg of the other tocopherols and tocotrienols in order to profit from the preventative attributes of vitamin E. However, to get this much vitamin E from average vegetable oil, we would have to eat a few hundred grams of vegetable oil a day, which might lead to obesity and other dangerous health conditions that would outweigh the benefits of all that extra vitamin E. A great alternative to normal vegetable oils is wheat germ oil. It is loaded with tocopherols and tocotrienols. Most vegetable oils average around 30 IU of vitamin E per 100 g of oil, but wheat germ oil has 233 IU per 100 g. To get the recommended 100 IU and 100 mg of other tocopherols and tocotrienols a day, you need only 45 g of wheat germ oil. Generally, if one wants to boost vitamin E intake without taking supplemental pills, wheat germ oil is a great way to do it without consuming large amounts of fat.

Vitamin E is not destroyed when the vegetable oils are cooked as long as the oils are not repeatedly used. Margarine has more vitamin E than butter because it is made from vegetable oils. In addition, vitamin E is often added to margarine to protect it from going bad. However, the amount of margarine you would need to eat in order to meet recommended levels of vitamin E make margarine a rather poor choice of vitamin E for your diet.

Nuts are another good source of vitamin E. Though nuts are high in fat content, it is not saturated fat, and is thus less prone to clog your arteries. Nuts generally have a lot of other good things for us, like proteins, minerals and other phytochemicals. Like the vegetable oils, nuts also have various amounts of tocopherols and tocotrienols, depending on the type of nut. Almonds, for example are a great source of alpha-tocopherol. Pistachios, hazel nuts, and peanuts are also packed with tocopherols.

Seeds are another great natural source of vitamin E. Whole seeds tend to have more vitamin E in them than seeds or kernels that have been crushed, or had the oil removed. When the seeds are crushed, any oil that is lost also carries with it a large portion of vitamin E. Also, the crushed seeds leave vitamin E open to oxygen radicals, causing oxidation. The vitamin E that is destroyed fighting oxidation outside of your body will not be able to prevent oxidation inside your body.

Whole grains and legumes are some of the healthiest foods available. They have tremendous overall nutritional benefits: high vitamin content, good fiber, little fat, protein, and a lot of phytonutrients, to name a few. Grains and legumes are a good source of vitamin E. A wide range of tocopherols and tocotrienols can be consumed from various grains; rice, barley and oats, for example, are good sources of tocotrienols. Wheat germ is packed with vitamin E. It contains 27 mg of tocopherols and tocotrienols for every 100 g of wheat germ. If you are opposed to taking supplement pills, eating wheat germ can be a great way to bolster a diet with all the tocopherols and tocotrienols.

In planning a proper diet you will be faced with a few difficulties with regard to vitamin E. There are currently a number of ways of measuring vitamin E content in foods and supplements. The IU (international unit) is the oldest method and is hampered by its inability to account for the fact that vitamin E comes in eight different forms. The IU was established when alpha-tocopherol was considered the only vitamin E vitamer worthy of attention. It provides a good means of measurement between synthetic and natural alpha-tocopherol, however, and for this reason, consumers and producers alike have adopted the IU as the standard for measuring the amount of vitamin E in food products and dietary supplements.

Another unit has also been used in the past called the alpha-tocopherol equivalent or alpha-TE. It is an improvement on the IU because it takes into consideration the presence of beta and gamma-tocopherol and alpha-tocotrienol in natural foods, but still ignores everything but alpha-tocopherol in supplements. The alpha-TE is also a flawed system because it does not completely express the amounts of all of the tocopherols and tocotrienols present in products.

To best evaluate the vitamin E content in a product, we need to try and find the actual amount of the different tocopherols and tocotrienols in a product. These amounts will usually be represented in milligrams of a given tocopherol or tocotrienol per 100 grams of the product. Knowing the actual amount of vitamin E in our food or supplements allows us to see exactly what tocopherols and tocotrienols are present.

As was mentioned, the IU dominates the vitamin E industry right now. Thus, most of the literature available regarding the health benefits of vitamin E gives suggested doses in IUs. Other methods prescribe suggested doses of vitamin E in unique units of IU/mg. These IU/mg units actually represent the suggested amount of alpha-tocopherol, represented in IU, followed by the recommended amount of other tocopherols and tocotrienols in milligrams, or mg.

RECOMMENDED DOSAGE

It is hard to overdose on vitamin E. The Dietary Reference Intake, which can be thought of as the minimum amount that should be consumed, is a relatively low 22 IU. Most sources of information place the maximum level of vitamin E intake at about 3,200 IU per day, while warning of possible side effects at 1,200 IU.

We can try and evaluate the minimal amount of vitamin E that we can consume without showing signs of a deficiency, or we can try to estimate how much vitamin E we need to take to prevent various diseases. Many scientific studies have attempted to find a correlation between vitamin E intake and disease prevention. These studies generally establish that the amount of vitamin E needed in our diets to cause any significant preventative effects is much higher than the suggested DRI.

In 1989 the Recommended Daily Allowance (RDA) for vitamin E was established as 15 IU for men and 12 IU for women. In April 2000, the Food and Nutrition Board released a report increasing the DRI for vitamin E for men and women. The new recommendation is 15 mg for women and 22 mg for men. You may want to take a look at the different recommendations for different age groups in the table provided in Appendix D. However, although the DRI for vitamin E is only two years old, it still falls well below the amounts tested to prevent heart disease, cancer, and other diseases. It seems that the standard amount of vitamin E used in tests correlating vitamin E with disease prevention is around 100 IU daily. The average diet supplies between 7 to 20 IU per day. Therefore, in order to get higher levels of vitamin E we need to focus on eating foods rich in vitamin E or take natural vitamin E supplements.

Unfortunately, we are not getting enough of vitamin E. Government surveys report that only one in four women, and four in ten men consume the RDA of vitamin E.

Vitamin D

Rickets, a malformation of the bones, became more and more prevalent as the Industrial Revolution swept across Europe. Physicians were baffled by it because they could not determine its cause.

Rickets is characterized by bending of the spine and bowing of the legs. It causes pain in all of the bones but especially in the long bones of the legs. Patients with rickets develop a pigeon breast and deformation of the head. Cesarean sections became more common because rickets had deformed the pelvic bones of many women during the Industrial Revolution. In adults, this same bone disease is referred to as osteomalacia.

Sniadecki, a Warsaw physician, noted that children living in the city had a much higher incidence of rickets than those living in the farmlands. Soon it was found that cod liver oil was effective in many cases for curing rickets. Soon many foods were said to have antirachitic behavior. Was there a lack of vitamin A? McCollum was a scientist who believed it was some other factor. He heated cod oil and oxidized it until all the vitamin A was destroyed. Vitamin A is very sensitive to heat. After this process he found that there was still an antirachitic factor in the oil. In another experiment, Powers et al. put children under a mercury lamp and claimed they were cured.

Seeing that the middle class of modern industrial cities suffered more from rickets than did children in farmlands, scientists proposed that a lack of exposure to sunlight caused the disease. In the 1930s, a patent for vitamin D was established and the United States required it to be used to fortify all milk. Today, rickets is no longer a health problem in the United States or Canada.

It is argued that vitamin D is not a vitamin after all. Technically, a vitamin is a molecule the body needs and must get from the diet. But the skin can produce its own vitamin D with help from the sun. It is true that we can get vitamin D from animals and plants that have already gone through this photochemical process. Most of us do not get enough sun in our busy lives to make adequate amounts of vitamin D without turning to foods for help. Because vitamin D is not really a vitamin in the truest sense of the definition, it is often called prohormone D.

A form of cholesterol relatively abundant in your skin is transformed by ultraviolet light and heat into vitamin D. This cholesterol is called dehydrocholestrol, and it consists of four carbon and hydrogen rings. When exposed to ultraviolet light, one of the rings breaks leaving the dehydrocholesterol transformed into a three-ring structure called provitamin 3. Body heat converts provitamin 3 into vitamin D3.

In the section on vitamin A, we discussed the role of chilomicrons in delivering certain digestible bits to the different tissues of the body. Vitamin D3 is taken by chilomicrons through the lymphatic system on to the liver where it undergoes an important reaction. The liver contains a special enzyme called vitamin D-25-hydroxylase. It is responsible for changing the vitamin into hormone 25-hydroxyvitamin. From there, another enzyme in the kidney changes this to 1,25 dihydroxyvitamin D. It is 1,25-dihydroxyvitamin, or 1,25(OH)2D, that will do the rest of the work.

The cause for bone malformation and weakening in rickets is a lack of calcium and phosphorous. 1,25(OH)2D is a molecule that activates particular genes to produce a section of DNA called a Calcium Binding Protein. It also activates a section called the Acid Phoshetase Protein. When these proteins are activated, the small intestines take calcium from our food and carry it into the bloodstream. If there is a lack of vitamin D, 1,25(OH)2D is not produced, and the bones will never receive calcium and phosphorous.

Two studies show the importance of vitamin D in ensuring healthy bones. The first has to do with infants who take vitamin D supplementation beyond the recommended values. The second study shows that vitamin D supplementation from infancy notably increases bone strength.

A study was done in which thirty infants were chosen randomly to receive vitamin D up to a maximum of either 400 IU/day or 960 IU/day until they were three months old. The results showed that infants who received 960 IU daily did not have any better bone mineral content than did 400 IU given daily. Both groups had the same content and strength in their bones. This study therefore recommends caution when administering vitamin D. Vitamin D is a potent hormone in many of the organs of the body, and excess dosage can be toxic.

In 1999 Samuel A. Zamora et al. conducted a retrospective study on 106 young girls between the ages of seven and nine. The girls were classified into two groups: those who had not been supplemented with vitamin D during the first year of infancy, and those who had been supplemented during their first year of infancy. The groups were similar in many important variables (seasons of birth, growth during the first year of life, calcium intake at the time of the testing, and age). The testing used an x-ray absorptiometer to measure areal bone mineral content (aBMC). ABMC is similar to bone density. All of the girls were measured in the same six spots. The results showed that the girls who had taken vitamin D supplementation during the first year of life had higher aBMC at all six points of bone measured.

Cellular Differentiation and Cancer

The life of the body is a process of constant cell growth. Old cells die and new cells replace them at incredible rates. The constant nature of cellular growth also increases the risk of cells growing out of control. Cells that grow beyond the body's ability to regulate seem to take on a life of their own, and may kill neighboring cells. Cells that grow out of control are called "cancerous." Colon cancer is one of the deadliest forms of cancer in men, as is breast cancer for women. A historical study reported in 1999 compared colon cancer to rickets and suggested that geographic location was a significant factor in breast cancer.

The study found that: "The geographic distribution of colon cancer is similar to the historical geographic distribution of rickets. The highest death rates from colon cancer occur in areas that had high prevalence rates of rickets. . . . The geographic distribution of colon cancer mortality rates reveals significantly low death rates at low latitudes in the United States and significantly high rates in the industrialized Northeast. . . . Breast cancer death rates in white women also rise with distance from the equator and are highest in areas with long vitamin D winters."

Because vitamin D helps to regulate the growth and divisions of cells, it is an important nutrient in the prevention of cancer. What then does cancer mortality have to do with low latitudes? How does cancer mortality relate to rickets? All these have to do with having sufficient vitamin D in the blood, and this in turn has to do with the amount of sunlight our body is exposed to.

It may seem odd to connect incidences of cancer with geographic location, just as rickets baffled seventeenth century physicians. However, these seemingly unrelated statistics are connected by our knowledge of vitamin D. How does vitamin D act as an anticancer agent? We will discuss two of the hypotheses, and support them each with a study.

Like all tissues of the body, tumors need nutrients in order to survive. Tumors receive nutrients from the blood supply. The ability of a tumor to create blood vessels is called angiogenesis. Many anticancer drugs are being tested and developed in hopes of disabling angiogenesis in tumors. 1,25(OH)2D is a natural inhibitor of angiogenesis. Many would-be cancer cells never become tumors because of 1,25(OH)2D.

Dr. Ahonen et al. described the effect of a combination of vitamin D and androgen on human ovarian cancer cells. Androgen is a human growth hormone that regulates the growth of cells in the body. In a cell line, this growth can be measured. Cancer cells grown *in vitro* are called cell lines and are very useful in understanding cancer. This group of researchers demonstrated that 1,25(OH)2D and androgen regulate the growth of ovarian cancer cells. They reported that after nine days of treatment of their cell lines with 100 nM (a small unit of liquid concentration) of 1,25(OH)2D resulted in 73 percent growth inhibition of cancer. The same concentration of androgen alone however resulted in 43 percent growth in the cell line. When androgen and vitamin D were used together, the vitamin D blocked much of the growth hormone's ability to cause an increase in cells. This means that vitamin D is an effective growth regulator and makes it a great candidate for future cancer treatment.

Besides inhibiting cancer cell growth, vitamin D plays a role in the cellular growth regulation of the immune system. Another group's study helps further explain vitamin D's role in cell growth regulation. Robert J. Wilkinson et al. studied ninety-one Asian patients who had tuberculosis. They were also tested for a vitamin D derivative concentration in their serum. The results showed that active tuberculosis was associated with vitamin D deficiency. They found that more than half were vitamin D deficient. Tuberculosis is an infection from bacteria *(Mycobacterium tuberculosis)*. This study shows that in order to maintain a strong immune response, we must assure we are receiving enough vitamin D. Because vitamin D plays an active role in helping the phagocytes of the immune system become activated, they are able more active against the tuberculosis infection. This is significant because this disease is predicted to be the largest single infectious cause of death for at least the next two decades. Our body fights these germs by attacking them with the immune system.

SOURCE AND RECOMMENDATION

Because milk in the United States is usually fortified with vitamin D, brief and casual exposure to sunlight is usually sufficient to maintain the RDA value of 200 IU for adults (this equals about 5 mg per day). Those with the highest risk of vitamin D deficiency are the elderly and infants. For them it is often difficult to supply the needed amounts because they don't go into the sun as much. In fact newborns are often placed under a mercury lamp to prevent vitamin D deficiency. To see the RDAs for all of the other age groups, check Appendix D.

Vitamin K

In 1929, Frederich Dam, a scientist working in Copenhagen, observed that chicks that were fed fat-free diets were bleeding to death. Ten years later, in 1939, the same man isolated a compound from alfalfa that seemed to prevent hemorrhagic death in these animals. The compound was called vitamin K (the K is for coagulation).

Vitamin K deficiency is a particular danger for newborns and the elderly. Because it is crucial in blood clotting, a deficiency of vitamin K can cause people to bleed to death from the slightest of injuries. It seems that vitamin K will not cross the placenta efficiently, leaving newborns in need. In addition, breast milk does not contain much vitamin K. Newborns therefore are often given vitamin K supplement intramuscularly. This seems to prevent intracranial bleeding and death. Vitamin K's ability to prevent bleeding has been its major medicinal interest in the past. As we proceed with this section, we want to explain the molecular activity of the vitamin so as to understand how it is involved in bone formation and the prevention of heart disease.

THE VITAMIN K FAMILY AND STRUCTURES

There are three different types of molecules in the vitamin K family: the phylloquinones, the menaquinones, and the metadiones. All three types of the vitamin have a two-ring system involving ten carbon atoms. Protruding from one of these rings are two oxygen molecules. These molecules are responsible for the name "quinines." The difference in the three is in the length of the tail extending between the two oxygen molecules. Saturated tails are called phylloquinone (also vitamin K1), and the menaquinones (vitamin K2) are less saturated.

It is estimated that metadione (vitamin K3) is two times as potent than the other K quinones. The phyloquinones are found and synthesized primarily in plants, especially in leafy greens.

The second type is the menaquinones. These are produced in the gut by the bacteria that grow there. These bacteria grow naturally in the digestive tract. They are essential to our existence, and vitamin K production is one of their biggest benefits to us. The menaquinones are numbered seven through thirteen, each having a slightly different shape and functioning in a slightly different manner. The metadiones are not produced naturally, but are made synthetically by pharmaceuticals.

ABSORPTION INTO THE BLOOD

Dietary vitamin K is absorbed through the intestine, again using chilomicrons as transporting vehicles. The liver then places them onto LDLs and they are taken in the blood to various tissues. The only exception to this is with the menaquinones. Having been produced by microflora, they pass from the colon into the lymph system, and then into the liver. If we were to examine cells in bones or other tissues, we would find phyloquinones and menaquinones in the membranes of the cell. Phyloquiniones and menaquinones are excreted in the feces, and metadiones are excreted in the urine. There are a number of reasons that people become vitamin K deficient. We already mentioned the first, that lipid absorption becomes limited because of a lack of fat or other fat-soluble vitamins.

Second, people with chronic intestinal infections may take antibiotics that kill the microflora producing vitamin K. Not only do these antibiotics kill pathogenic bacteria, but also at the same time they kill the organisms needed to supply vitamin K.

HOW VITAMIN K WORKS TO REGULATE
BLOOD CLOTTING AND BONE FORMATION

Vitamin K works in many ways to help the body with many functions. Vitamin K helps to prevent bleeding by aiding in the creation of blood clots. Yet, when the blood clots in the brain or near the heart, the result is very often fatal. The clotting mechanism therefore needs to be activated in the right places and at the right times. An intricate cascade of proteins and chemical reactions regulate the clotting mechanism, and vitamin K plays a crucial role in this. We will not go through all of this, but it is important to know that without coenzymes such as vitamin K, there are certain processes of the body that will not work. Blood clotting is one of them.

Furthermore, strong bones depend on the correct amount and function of vitamin K in our diet. One of the proteins needed in the formation of strong bones is called osteocalcin. Osteocalcin cannot carry calcium unless it is first changed from its inactive state to a state that accommodates the calcium. There are enzymes capable of doing this, but that do not function without the "permission" and binding of vitamin K.

RECENT FINDINGS: VITAMIN K FOR BONE STRENGTH

In order to assess the value of vitamin K intake in the prevention of hip fractures in women, a group began a study in 1984. Hip fractures in elderly women often cause other complications, and if not rehabilitated, can lead to death. The study involved 72,327 women aged thirty-eight to sixty-three who were given a detailed food-frequency questionnaire. Based on their dietary intake, they were placed into different groups, including those who had low intakes of vitamin K and those who had significantly higher intakes. There was a significant drop in relative risk among the women who consumed in their diet the highest amounts of vitamin

K compared to those who consumed the least amounts. The conclusion was that bone health and injury risk was directly correlated to vitamin K intake, lowering the risk by as much as 30 percent.

Another study, done in 1999, compared the bone density of patients diagnosed with glucocorticoid-induced osteoporosis. This is a condition that is caused by prednisolone, a therapeutic hormone for a kidney disease that also unfortunately suppresses bone formation. Because vitamin K was associated with a lowered risk in hip fracture, perhaps it could also suppress the bone damaging effects of prednisolone. Twenty patients who were scheduled for treatments with prednisolone were chosen randomly and divided into two groups of ten. Ten of them were treated with prednisolone alone, and the other ten patients received prednisolone plus 15 mg of menatetreonen, a vitamin K supplement, three times a day. Using x-ray absorptiometry and biochemical markers, they were evaluated before the treatments and ten weeks after to compare the bone densities. Those who received only the prednisolone treatment experienced a significant reduction in their bone material density (BMD). Those who also received the vitamin K did not experience as dramatic a loss in BMD.

RECOMMENDATIONS FOR VITAMIN K

It only takes about one serving of spinach or two servings of broccoli to provide the body with five times the RDA of vitamin K. Yet a recent survey shows that Americans between the ages of eighteen and forty-four are not getting sufficient amounts of this vitamin. Sarah Booth conducted a survey in connection with Proctor and Gamble showing that half of American females get the RDA of vitamin K. Males are consuming even less. Conducting research at the Jean Mayer USDA Human Nutrition Research Center on Aging, she stresses the importance of vitamin K intake.

Vitamin Combinations

Vitamins play an important part in complex chemical reactions in the body. The enzymes needed to orchestrate cellular pathways such as metabolism depend on these vitamins. It is obvious that one enzyme doesn't operate in isolation, but it interacts with many other enzymes to produce a certain end result.

Knowing that enzymes work in concert also teaches us that a

Lack of Power Plants Linked to Esophageal Cancer

A large study published in the December 2000 issue of *Onkologie* states, "Patients with cancer of the esophagus had a nutritional deficit in fresh fruit, vegetables, dietary fiber, and carbohydrates when compared with the other groups."

correct intake of vitamins is crucial not only for individual enzymatic reactions, but for entire pathways. For example, if one enzyme has plenty of a coenzyme to help it do its job, but the enzyme "next door" does not have its corresponding enzyme, the entire pathway is stopped. The point here is that in many cases, vitamins work synergistically. The benefits of their combination are greater than the benefits of each of them added up together.

One of the most convincing studies done to show the synergistic effects of vitamin combinations was done by Katalin Glosonsczy from Maryland. The study was designed to see whether vitamin C enhanced the beneficial effects of vitamin E in preventing heart disease and total mortality. It did. The study's 11,178 elderly subjects (ages 67 to 105) reported all nonprescription drugs, including vitamin C and vitamin E. Multivitamins did not count for using vitamins C or E. In the following nine years, there were 3,490 deaths. Those who were on vitamin E supplements had a 34 percent reduction in risk for total mortality, and a 47 percent decrease in coronary heart disease mortality. This was exciting news for the elderly! However, those individuals who took both vitamin E and vitamin C had a 53 percent less chance to die from heart disease, and 42 percent less chance to die at all in the nine-year period. Evidently, vitamin E is good for a healthy heart and longevity, but combined with vitamin C, it is even better.

What about colon cancer? The University of Washington conducted a study to see if vitamin and mineral supplements would drop the risk for colon cancer. Over a ten-year period, a group of 444 colon cancer patients were compared against 427 people without cancer. The intake of vitamins A, E, C, folic acid and calcium were measured. Also in the study was a group who took some of these and a multivitamin. The group that showed the greatest reduction in colon cancer risk was the group who took a multivitamin supplement along with vitamin E. In fact, the group that took the multivitamin saw a reduction of risk by 51 percent. But those who also took vitamin E had a reduced risk of 57 percent.

Dr. Chung S. Yang, from the Laboratory for Cancer Research in New Jersey, conducted an intervention trial in China for four years. His hypothesis was that because of a very monotonous diet in Linxian, China, there was an especially high incidence of gastroesophageal cancer. After an initial survey, he proposed that the area had the specific deficiency in riboflavin, and vitamins A and C. There were other micronutrients that seemed to be deficient, and so he designed a study to try a variety of different combinations of vitamin and mineral supplements. He involved 29,584 subjects, and tested them on the following four groups of vitamins: 1) retinol and zinc; 2) riboflavin and niacin; 3) vitamin C and molybdenum; 4) vitamin E, beta-carotene and selenium. These nutrients were given in a supplement pill every day. The total mortality rate and the mortality rate caused by gastroesophageal cancer dropped the most in the group that took vitamin E, beta-carotene and selenium.

We mentioned that some of the B vitamins are intricately involved in the breakdown of the homocysteine levels of the body, and thus decreasing the levels of cardiovascular disease. To see if supplements of B-group vitamins would actually lower homocysteine levels in men, Jayne V. Woodside preformed an intervention study. The study involved 101 men all of whom had slightly elevated levels of homocysteine (hyperhomocysteine). Again, Woodside and the other researchers divided the men into different combinations. After eight weeks of either taking B-vitamin supplements (1 mg folic acid, 7.2 mg pyridoxine [B6], and 0.02 mg cyanocobalamin) or the same B vitamins and also various antioxidant vitamins alone (150 mg ascorbic acid, 67 mg RRR-alpha-tocopherol, and 9 mg beta-carotene). Hopefully, these supplements would lower the levels of homocysteine in these men. As it turned out, levels dropped significantly (about 30 percent) in both of these groups. We will discuss homocysteine in further detail later.

References

Backstrom MC, Maki R, Kuusela AL, Sievanen H, Koivisto AM, Ikonen RS, Kouri T, Maki M. Randomised controlled trial of vitamin D supplementation on bone density and biochemical indices in preterm infants. Arch Dis Child Fetal Neonatal Ed. 1999 May; 80(3): F161–6.

Booth SL. Vitamin K: Another Reason To Eat Your Greens. Agricultural Research;

2000 Jan; 16–17.

Feskanich D, Weber P, Willett, WC, Rockett H, Booth SL, Colditz GA. Vitamin K intake and hip fractures in women: a prospective study. Am J Clin Nutr. 1999; 69:74–9.

Losonczy KG, Harris TB, Havlik RJ. Vitamin E and vitamin C supplement use and risk of all-cause and coronary heart disease mortality in older persons: the Established Populations for Epidemiologic Studies of the Elderly. Am J Clin Nutr. 1996; 64:190–196.

Losonczy KG, Harris TB, Havlik RJ. Vitamin E and vitamin C supplement use and risk of all-cause and coronary heart disease mortality in older persons: the Established Populations for Epidemiologic Studies of the Elderly. The American Journal of Clinical Nutrition. 1996; 64:190–196.

Rimm EB, Stampfer MJ, Ascherio A, Giovannucci E, Colditz GA, Willett WC. Vitamin E consumption and the risk of coronary heart disease in men. N Engl J Med. 1993; 328:1450–1456.

Sano M, Ernesto C, Thomas R, Klauber MR, Schafer K, Grundman M, Woodbury P, Growdon J, Cotman CW. Pfeiffer E, Schneider LS, Thal LJ. A controlled trial of selegline, alpha tocopherol, or both as treatment for Alzheimer's disease. N Engl J Med. 1997; 336(17):1216–1222.

Stampfer MJ, Hennekens CH, Manson JE, Colditz GA, Rosner B, Willett WC. Vitamin E consumption and the risk of coronary heart disease in women. N Engl J Med. 1993; 328: 1444–1449.

Tribble DL, PhD. Antioxidant Consumption and Risk of Coronary Heart Disease: Emphasis on Vitamin C, Vitamin E, and Beta-Carotene. American Heart Association. 1999;

Vitamin E supplementation and cardiovascular Events in high-risk patients. N Eng J Med; 342(3):154–160.

Wilkinson RJ, Llewelyn M, Toossi Z, Patel P, Pasvol G, Lalvan A, Wright D, Latif Mohammed L, Davidson R. Influence of vitamin D deficiency and vitamin D receptor polymorphisms on tuberculosis among Gujarati Asians in west London: a case-control study. Lancet. 2000; 355: 618–21.

Woodside JV, Yarnell JW, McMaster D, Yong IS, Harmon DL, McCrum EE, Pattersonm CC, Gey KF, Whitehead AS, Evans A. Effect of B-group vitamins and antioxidant vitamins on hyperhomocysteinemia: a double blind, randomized, factorial-design, controlled trial. American Journal of Clinical Nutrition. 1998 May; 68(3):758.

www.americanheart.org/Scientific/statements/1999

www.who.int

Yang CS. Vitamin nutrition and gastroesophageal cancer. Journal of Nutrition. 2000; 130(2S Suppl): 9338S–339S)

Zamora SA, Rizzoli R, Belli Dominique C, Slosman DO, Bonjour J-P. The Journal of Clinical Endocrinology and Metabolism. 1999; 84(12): 4541–4544.

CHAPTER 9

Fruits and Phytonutrition

There are many different varieties of fruits. In fact, there are literally thousands of different fruit varieties. Though most fruits are good for you, we will limit our discussion to the fruits most commonly available in Western markets. Fruits are a great source of vitamins, minerals, fiber, antioxidants, and phytochemicals. Multiple studies have been conducted on the benefits of fruits. In this section we will identify each fruit, the mythology, folk medicines, and the nutrients they provide for us. Not all fruits have studies on them, but the ones that do are included in this section.

Apple *(Malus domestica)*

Apples belong to the family *Rosaceae*, the same family as the pear, quince, loquat, and medlar. There are countless varieties of apples. There are over 7,000 cultivated apples, but only 100 are grown commercially. Apples were first cultivated in eastern Turkey, southwestern Russia, and regions of Asia Minor, but are native to Europe and Western Asia. Apple growing gradually spread from these areas throughout Europe. Christopher Columbus brought the first apples to the New World.

In Greek, Roman, and Norse mythology, apples were often symbols of immortality and reincarnation. They were the food of the gods and only given to mortals as a reward. The apple was sacred to Aphrodite, the Greek goddess of love, and in history has played a role in courtship and marriage. In the Middle Ages, apples were regarded as symbols of fertility and romantic love. Since apples were connected with gods and magic, many thought they possessed healing or telepathic powers. Some believed a fever could be cured if a holy name was inscribed on apples and eaten three days in a row. We are beginning to recognize that apples really do have the ability to heal.

The saying "an apple a day keeps the doctor away," has a great deal of truth. Apples are cholesterol, fat, and sodium free, and deliver a mere 80 calories per apple (medium sized). Apples are rich in essential minerals like chromium, iron, magnesium, manganese, and potassium. Apples also contain biotin and thiamin (needed to help the brain function) as well as vitamin C. Not all apples are equal in nutritional value. For example, apples can range from being an excellent source to a good source of essential vitamins. One apple contains nearly 20 percent of the fiber we need in our diet to maintain a healthy lifestyle. Apples contain both soluble and insoluble fiber, 80 percent of which is soluble. Insoluble fibers may prevent some cancers. The skin of the apple is dense in fiber, so it is vital you eat the skin when eating an apple.

Not only are apples rich in vitamins, minerals, and fiber, they also contain phytochemicals and antioxidants that are necessary for good health. Flavonoids are found in apples and are recognized for their role in fighting and preventing heart disease. Apples are rich in a class of antioxidants known as polyphenols. These include chlorogenic acid, epicatechin, phloretin glycoside, and quercetin glyocside. As we have discussed before, antioxidants are necessary because they help the body rid itself of free radicals. All these antioxidants and fibers are contained in the skin, so not only will consuming the skin of apples help us stay healthy and strong, it will also reduce our risk of cancer and can even slow the growth of tumor cells.

A study conducted by researchers at St. George's Medical Hospital Medical School in London, UK (Feb 2000) indicated that apples have a strong positive impact on your lungs. Scientists took 2,512 Welshmen aged forty-five to fifty-nine living in Caerphilly and studied them for four years (between 1979 and

1983). The scientists compared the age, height, body mass index (BMI), smoking history, social class, exercise, and total energy intake of these men to see if a correlation existed between the number of apples eaten and the performance of the lungs. The study showed that apples slow deterioration of lung function. That is, those who ate apples regularly had healthier lungs longer than those who did not.

Research indicates that eating two to three apples a day can lower your cholesterol. A study conducted by the University of Paul Sabatier, Institute of Physiology in Toulouse, France, indicated that apples could lower your LDL (low density lipoprotein) cholesterol, while raising your HDL (high density lipoprotein). This could be due to the pectin found in the apple's skin. Pectin has been found to be effective in lowering cholesterol, triglycerides, and blood sugar. Thus whole apples are also good for diabetes. Apples ranked as last on the "glycemic index," which is a measurement of how fast blood sugar rises after eating. In spite of the apple's natural sugar content, it did not raise the blood sugar levels. In actuality, apples can help regulate insulin levels.

Not only are fresh apples good for you, so is their juice. Apple juice contains antioxidants. A study conducted by the Department of Food Science and Technology at the University of California indicates that not only do fresh apples inhibit LDL oxidation, but so do their juices. If you are unable to eat an apple you ought to consider drinking one a day!

Apricot *(Prunus armeniaca)*

Apricots belong to the family *Rosaceae*, the same family as the plum. Apricots originated in northeastern China, near the Russian border. The Chinese began cultivating apricots over 3,000 years ago. Apricots were introduced in Armenia and then into Europe. Many scholars believe that the apricot was the forbidden fruit of Garden of Eden infamy, rather than an apple, because apples were not known in ancient Mesopotamia (the proposed place for the Garden of Eden). The Eastern countries refer to the apricot as the "moon of the faithful" and the ancient Persians believed the apricot to be an aphrodisiac and were called "sun eggs." Apricot pits were used in the early treatment of tumors in 502 A.D. and apricot oil was used to treat tumors and ulcers in the 1600s in England.

Today we can enjoy bigger, brighter and more nutritious apricots as a result of genetic engineering. Apricots can be eaten fresh, canned, and dried. The variety of ways to prepare apricots does not significantly change the nutritional value. Apricots are dense in vitamin A. Dried apricots are very nutritious, but fresh ones are probably your best source as with most plant foods. Roughly 100 grams of apricots will deliver 54 percent of the RDA of vitamin A. Apricots are the third highest source of vitamin A found in commercial fruits. As with other pit fruits, the pit of the apricot is poisonous, so don't eat it! Apricot pits contain a poisonous cyanogenic glucoside known as amygdalin (a two-sugar compound made from benzaldehyde and cyanide). Glucoside is used in the cancer-treating drug Laetrile sold in Canada, Europe, and Mexico. However, according to tests, glucoside does not seem to have any significant effects on cancer. In the United States the pit is used for the amygdalin in medicinal foods.

Avocado *(Persea americana)*

The avocado belongs to the *Lauracea* family as with cinnamon and the laurel. The avocado originated in Central America and Mexico, but then was introduced in the West Indies, where it flourished. Because of its rough skin, the avocado was known as the "alligator pear" and the "avocado pear." The British would take the avocados aboard their ships for the petty officers; hence, avocados came to be known as "midshipman's butter." In the tropics, the avocado was referred to as "poor man's butter."

Many people believe that avocados are fattening and should not be part of a well-balanced diet, but in reality avocados are quite healthy. Avocados contain only 5 grams of fat per serving, while 3 grams of it is monounsaturated fat. Studies have shown that monounsaturated fats can reduce cholesterol levels when they replace saturated fats in the diet. Monounsaturated fats can also benefit people with heart disease and certain kinds of cancer. Avocados contain all the B vitamins (biotin, folic acid, thiamin, and riboflavin) and are also great sources of dietary fiber, folate, potassium, vitamin C, vitamin D (calciferol), vitamin E (alpha-tocopherol), and vitamin K (napthoquinone). They contain no cholesterol and sodium. Avocados are one of nature's most nutrient-dense foods. Avocados are rich in potassium, containing 60 percent more potassium per ounce compared to bananas (UC Berkeley Wellness Letter). Also rich in folate, avocados supply 400 mcg (1/1000 of a gram) per fruit, which is half of the U.S. RDA minimum.

Avocados are also rich in phytochemicals that help prevent chronic diseases. Beta-sitosterol is known as a cholesterol lowering phytosterol, which can help prevent certain types of cancer and heart disease. A study conducted by the California Avocado Commission indicated that a single avocado contains 76 mg of beta-sitosterol per 100 grams. This is four times the amount found in other commonly eaten fruits (apples, bananas, and grapes). Beta-sitosterol is known for its ability to inhibit cholesterol absorption in the intestines, leading to lower blood cholesterol levels. Also phytosterols have been shown to stop the growth of tumor cells. Avocados also contain the antioxidant glutathione, which also reduces and prevents cancer and heart disease. Glutathione neutralizes free radicals that can damage healthy cells during aging, cancer, and heart disease. Avocados contain three times as much glutathione as apples, bananas, cantaloupes, grapes, plums, and cherries.

Banana *(Musa sapientum and Musa paradisica)*

Musa sapientum can be translated to "the fruit of the wise," while *Musa paradisica* means "heavenly fruit." Plantains were also once believed to be the forbidden fruit of the Garden of Eden. Bananas and plantains are part of the family *Musaceae* and the genus *Musa*. These fruits originated in the southeastern part of the world from India to Australia, and then were brought to Hawaii and other tropical islands by the early Filipinos. It took a long time for bananas and plantains to reach Europe. Friar Tomas de Barlanga brought bananas to Europe in 1516. Bananas were not only used as a food staple, they were also grown for the material in the leaves and bark of the tree. This material was used to form everything from strong ropes to tea bags. America's love for the banana grew after the Civil War, when refrigerated transportation made it possible to transport the fruit relatively easily. Bananas were the cheapest fruits in the store and could be purchased year round, making them the number-one consumed fruit in the nation. Apples came in second. In fact, the *Boy Scout*

Handbook of 1915 listed picking up banana peels off of the streets as an example of a good deed.

In South Africa and Panama, the juice of the stem of a banana tree is used to relieve toothaches. In South American folklore, bananas were used to treat peptic and duodenal ulcers. As early as the 1930s, medical literature noted that bananas have healing powers. They were said to cure ulcers, just as Indian folklore insisted. At first, many believed bananas would neutralize stomach acid and soothe irritation, but now we know that bananas actually alleviate ulcers because they strengthen the surface cells of the stomach lining, forming a sturdy barrier against noxious juices.

Bananas aid in digestion because they are rich in fiber. The fiber helps stimulate movement in the intestines. Bananas are good sources of vitamin C, but you would need to eat six bananas in order to fill the U.S. RDA of 60 mg. Bananas are rich in potassium (11 percent of the U.S. RDA). Potassium is a mineral that aids in controlling your body's fluid balance; it is needed for muscle contraction, transmission of nerve impulses and the proper functioning of your body's heart and kidneys. Potassium is also important in regulating water balance and blood pressure. A diet rich in this mineral may reduce the risk of hypertension and stroke.

Bananas also contain vitamin B2 (riboflavin) and vitamin B6 (pyridoxine). Bananas are fat, cholesterol, and sodium free. Bananas also contain all eight essential amino acids. A study conducted by the Cancer Research Laboratory at the University of Auckland indicated that a diet rich in green bananas contained strong antimutagenic properties, thus decreasing the risk of certain cancers.

Blackberry *(Rubus species)*

Blackberries belong to the family *Rosaceae* and belong to the same family as raspberries. Blackberries are native to North and South America, Asia and Europe. There are several varieties according to the differing regions and they vary in color, from dark red to reddish black. Blackberries have been used as foods, medicine, and landscaping hedges for over 2,000 years. In Europe, blackberry juices were used to treat eye and mouth infections until the sixteenth century, and their roots were used to make remedies for dysentery.

Fresh blackberries are an excellent source of vitamin C, containing roughly 21 mg/100 g. Blackberries are also a rich source of folate, providing 10 percent of the RDA. Ranked as the fourth most abundant antioxidant-containing fruit, blackberries are second in preventing oxidation in cells. As in most berries, the antioxidant activity is found in the juicy part of the fruit.

Studies have shown that blackberries have the capability to lower the build-up of LDL (low density lipoprotein) cholesterol. LDL is associated with atherosclerosis, heart disease, and stroke. Blackberries contain the highest LDL inhibitory effect of all berries (see raspberries and strawberries for antioxidant activity).

Blueberry *(Vaccinium angustifolium, V. corymbosum, V. asheii)*

Blueberries belong to the family *Ericaceae*, and are closely related to cranberries, huckleberries, and bilberries. There are about 150 to 450 different species in this family. Blueberries are native to North America. These berries were domesticated in the twentieth century, but were probably collected by the North American Indians and then later by European settlers. Blueberries were once called "star berries," because of the star-shaped calyx on top of each berry. The fruit and root of the bark were used to treat dysentery. Blueberry soup is quite common in European ski resorts to treat colds.

Blueberries are a good source of vitamin C and fiber. A single serving of blueberries (1 cup) delivers 15 percent of the U.S. RDA of vitamin C and 14 percent of the U.S. RDA of fiber. Blueberries are also fat and cholesterol free. Blueberries ranked as number three in their antioxidant richness, but first in their chemical effectiveness in preventing oxidation in cells. Just as with blackberries, the antioxidant activity is in the juicy part of the fruit. Blueberries also reduce the build-up of LDL cholesterol.

A study conducted by the National Institute of Aging (NIA) and the U.S. Department of Agriculture (USDA) at the Human Nutrition Research Center on Aging at Tuft's University in Boston indicated that blueberries could reverse some signs of aging in rats. In this study the rats were given blueberry extract. It appeared that their balance and coordination skills (normal features of aging) were improved. The blueberry extract seemed to reverse the normal deterioration in motor skills associated with aging.

Blueberries ranked as the highest in containing the most oxygen radical absorbance capacity (ORAC) according to the U.S. Department of Agriculture's Center for Aging at Tuft's University. Blueberries are rich in the flavonoid anthocyanin, which gives the blueberry its deep blue coloring. Half a cup of blueberries yields as much antioxidant power as five servings of other fruits and vegetables (apples, broccoli, and carrots).

Cherry *(Prunus avium, Prunus cerasus)*

Cherries belong to the *Rosaceae* family and are found in Asia, Europe, and North America. There are two types of cherries: sweet and sour. The cherry has been associated with virginity from ancient to modern times. The red colored fruit that enclosed a seed symbolized the uterus. According to Buddhist belief, Maya, the mother of Buddha, was offered support and food from a cherry tree when she was pregnant. Cherry stalk was once believed to cure kidney disease and serve as a diuretic. In ancient Greece, cherries were used to treat epilepsy. In the 1920s U.S. physicians prescribed black cherries to cure kidney stones and gall bladder ailments.

Cherries are considered a good source of vitamin C. The amount of vitamin C in cherries, however, changes depending on how the fruit is preserved. Fresh cherries yield 10 mg/100 g of vitamin C, while frozen cherries deliver 5 mg/100 g. Sour cherries have ten times the vitamin A of sweet cherries. Darker cherries also contain more of the phytochemical anthocyanin than lighter cherries. Cherries were listed as the seventh most abundant fruit in antioxidant activity level. Studies suggest that cherries may also reduce the build-up of LDL (low density lipoprotein) cholesterol. Cherries contain about 60 mg to 90 mg/100 grams of the phytochemical polyphenols, which may reduce the risk of cancer.

A study conducted at Forsyth Dental Center indicated that the juice of a black cherry could block 89 percent of the enzyme activity leading to plaque formation and tooth decay.

Cranberry *(Vaccinium macrocarpon)*

Cranberries belong to the family *Ericaceae*, and are the most economically important Vaccinium in the world. Cranberries are closely related to blueberries, rhododendrons (which are poisonous), and azaleas. Cranberries are native to the acid bogs in the northeastern United States and southern Canada. The symbolism and history of cranberries are related to New England history. According to documentation, Native Americans were the first to use cranberries for food. Native Americans appear to have been eating them as early as 1550. There are many historical legends about cranberries and how they came to Massachusetts, where their legend and symbolism is rooted in the first Thanksgiving. American sailors used cranberries to prevent scurvy.

Cranberries are good sources of vitamin C and fiber. Folk remedies claim cranberries can cure urinary tract infections. We continue to use cranberries to treat urinary tract infection. Cranberries acidify the urine by creating hipuric acid, which may be the agent responsible for relieving urinary tract infections. Cranberries are sodium and cholesterol free and contain only 46 calories per 100 grams. Scientists at the Human Nutrition Research Center on Aging at Tuft's University in Boston conducted a study that indicated that cranberry juice was more effective in treating than preventing urinary tract infection (UTI). Cranberries are the only fruit that work in an acidic environment. They do not stimulate the pancreas. To learn more about these berries, see the herb section.

Grape *(Vitis labrusca, Vitis rotundifolia)*

Grapes belong to the family *Vitaceae*, genus Vitis. Grapes can be found in eastern Asia, Europe, and the Middle East between 25 and 50 N latitudes. Cultivation of this fruit began in southwestern Asia over 6,000 years ago and then spread to Greece 3,000 years later. Egyptian hieroglyphics detail the history of grapes as early as 2400 B.C. Phoenicians carried wine varieties to Greece, Rome, and southern France before 600 B.C. The Romans spread grapes throughout Europe. Persian and Indian traders are responsible for spreading grapes to the Far East. Historically, physicians have recommended grapes in cancer therapy; 15 pounds of grapes a day for six weeks was used to cure cancer.

Grapes have been used to make wine since prehistoric times. Dionysus-Bacchus was the Greco-Roman god of wine. On the day of his festival, called "Oschophoria," the Greeks got drunk. They believed the drunken state was symbolic of being a god. It was in this drunken state that the gods could see the future. In several religions, wine is symbolic of the blood of life. Traditionally grapes were considered good for all dyspeptic conditions, febrile conditions, liver and kidney troubles, tuberculosis (lungs and bones), hemorrhoids, varicose veins, osteomyelitis, gangrene, cancer, and other malignant diseases.

Grapes provide 18 percent of the U.S. RDA of vitamin C. Grapes have always been known as a "health food," because of their antioxidant and phytochemical content. It is assumed that the darker grapes contain more phytochemicals than lighter grapes. The phenolic (polyphenols protect the brain and connective tissues from aging) compound resveratol is the best-known protective agent found in grape skins. This compound can inhibit tumor formation in four ways:

- Stops DNA damage
- Enhances DNA repair capacity
- Slows/Inhibits cell transformation from normal to cancerous
- Slows tumor growth

Resveratol also contains anti-inflammatory properties that can be very useful for the prevention of colon cancer. Raisins, dark grapes, and wine all contain this protective Resveratol. However, the alcohol in wine enhances certain chronic diseases, so consuming fresh or dried grapes and grape juice is much more beneficial than wine.

Red grapes ranked sixth in comparison with other fruits in their antioxidant effectiveness against damaging free radicals. In a scientific study raisins ranked second to other fruits in the amount of antioxidant content. In a study conducted by the Cardiology Section of the Department of Medicine at the University of Wisconsin in Madison, WI, scientist found that polyphenolic compounds including flavonoids found in red wines and grapes can reduce platelet aggregation and lower rates of cardiovascular disease.

Grape seeds have also been known for their protective value, but will not be discussed in this section. To find out more about their beneficial powers, see the herb section in Appendix C.

Grapefruit *(Citrus paradisica)*

The grapefruit belongs to the family *Rutaceae,* and is part of the genus Citrus. The grapefruit first appeared in the 1700s. No one seems to know anything of its origin, though many now speculate that it is a hybrid of other citrus fruits. Some believe it is a hybrid of the "forbidden fruit" of the Caribbean.

Grapefruit are excellent sources of vitamin C. An average serving delivers a whopping two-thirds of an adult's daily minimum requirement. Grapefruit juice contains citrus flavonoid compounds not in other citrus juices. The most prevalent flavonoid is naringin, which is responsible for the characteristic bitter taste of grapefruit juice. Grapefruit has phytochemicals called monoterpenes in its skin. In experiments involving laboratory mice, monoterpenes appear to protect against cancer cells.

Grapefruit is an amazing food for the heart. It contains compounds that lower blood cholesterol, clean out plaque (arterial debris) and might even reverse atherosclerosis. These powerful compounds are mainly found in the fruit's pectin (skin). A study in Japan indicated that grapefruit stopped tumor growth and even caused remission of malignancy. Other studies in Japan indicate that the grapefruit rind contains antimutagenic properties. This is believed to be a result of the high vitamin C content in grapefruit. The rinds of citrus fruits are high in vitamin content and cancer fighting properties, so it would not be a bad idea to eat the rinds, too.

Guava *(Psidium guajava)*

Guavas belong to the family *Myrtaceae* and are known as the "apple of the tropic." Guavas are native to the tropical Americas, from Peru to Mexico. European colonizers took guava back to Europe and to their African and Southeast Asia colonies.

Guavas are rich in vitamin C, containing 165 mg of vitamin C per fruit. That is twice the amount of vitamin C in kiwi, making guava one of the top-ranking fruits in vitamin C density. Guavas also contain niacin (vitamin B3), and vitamin A. They are also high in potassium and dietary fiber. Guavas can lower triglyceride levels in blood, and decrease hypertension, while also increasing high density lipoprotein (HDL), the good cholesterol levels.

A study conducted by the Heart Research Laboratory Medical Hospital and Research Center in Moradabad, India indicated that eating one guava before meals would decrease the absorption of fat, particularly saturated fat. This leads to a decrease in total cholesterol, triglycerides, and blood pressure. Guavas are also high in fiber.

A study conducted by the Department of Botany, Guru Nanak Dev University in Amritsar, India (June 93) indicated that guavas contain antimutagenic properties and can inactivate mutagens, thus helping to prevent cancer.

Kiwifruit (Actinidia deliciosa)

Kiwis belong to the *Actinidiacea* family; the kiwi was first called the *Actinidia chinensis*, but was changed to its present name in the 1980s. The kiwi was first named the Chinese gooseberry, but was later changed to "kiwi." The name was then replaced in the 1960s by the first Americans to import the fruit from New Zealand. The kiwi was named after the brown, round, flightless bird that is native to New Zealand, because they resemble each other. The French call this fruit "souris vegetale" translated as "vegetable mouse."

The kiwi is native to south and central China, but commercial cultivation began in New Zealand in the 1930s. Kiwi is an extremely nutrient-dense food. They contain high concentrations of vitamins and minerals per calorie compared with other fruits. For example, kiwis are an exceptional source of vitamin C. A single fruit delivers 115 percent of the U.S. RDA. Kiwis are also rich in iron, folate, and potassium. Kiwis are also a good source of fiber.

Lemon (Citrus limon)

Lemons belong to the family *Rutaceae* and are related to all the other citrus fruits. Lemons probably developed in Southeast Asia. Lemons were first mentioned in Sanskrit writings in 800 B.C. Lemons moved from the Mediterranean to Asia and northern Africa in the Middle Ages. Then they were brought to South America and the Caribbeans by Spanish and Portuguese colonizers. Lemons were used to treat and cure scurvy as early as the sixteenth century. In the third century, the Romans believed lemon was an antidote for all poisons.

Lemons contain the phytochemicals monoterpenes. These phytochemicals generate protective enzymes, which can interfere with the action of carcinogens, thus helping prevent cancer. We discussed terpenes in chapter 5. They also act as an anti-ulcer remedy and can prevent dental decay (see grapefruit and vitamin C).

Lime *(Citrus aurantifolia)*

The lime belongs to the family *Rutaceae* and is related to the other citrus fruits (oranges, lemons, and grapefruits). To prevent "limey" (scurvy), English sailors used limes. As with other citrus fruits, limes contain monoterpenes. For more information on monoterpenes, see chapter 5.

Mango *(Mangifera indica)*

The mango belongs to the family *Anacardiaceae* and is related to the cashew and pistachio. Mangos were first cultivated in Southeast Asia and India, and then spread to England and Europe, when England occupied India in the 1800s. They were then brought to Brazil and the West Indies in the 1700s. They were later taken to Florida in the nineteenth century.

According to folklore, mangoes had a variety of uses. Remedies for bronchitis, internal hemorrhage, and toothaches were made with the twigs and leaves of the fruit.

Mangoes contain amino acids, carbohydrates, fatty acids, minerals, protein and vitamins. Mangoes are rich in vitamin C (one fruit equals U.S. RDA) and have the highest fruit concentration of vitamin A. The darker the flesh, the more vitamin A it contains.

Melon, Cantaloupe *(Cucumis melo)*

The cantaloupe melon is native to the sub-Saharan eastern tropical part of Africa, but was actually naturalized in India. From India, the fruit spread to Greece, Italy and the rest of the Mediterranean world.

According to Chinese folklore, cantaloupes were used to treat hepatitis. In Guatemala the seeds are crushed and eaten to expel worms. In the Philippines, cantaloupe is used to treat cancer and in India it is used as a diuretic.

Like mangoes, cantaloupes are high in potassium and rich in vitamin A. Half of the U.S. RDA of potassium and vitamin A can be filled with a single serving of this melon. Some studies suggest that cantaloupe also has cancer-fighting properties.

Orange (Citrus sinensis)

The orange belongs to the same family as the other citrus fruits, *Rutaceae*. Oranges were first mentioned in Chinese literature in 2400 B.C, where they first originated. Through trade over the land and sea, oranges were spread to Europe and the greater part of the Mediterranean area. Oranges spread to the Caribbeans and South America by the Spanish and Portuguese explorers in the early fifteenth and sixteenth centuries. Florida began growing oranges as early as the eighteenth century. In folklore, oranges played a big role in marriage. The orange tree produces white flowers, which symbolized virginity, while the fruit themselves represented fertility.

A single orange can meet about 20 percent of the U.S. RDA of folate. They are also a great source of vitamin C, with one orange supplying all the required U.S. RDA. Oranges contain the phytochemical monoterpenes in their skin. One such phytochemical called "d-limonene" compromises more than 90 percent of the oil found in the orange peel.

Papaya (Carica papaya)

The family *Caricaceae* only has two fruits: the papaya and the passion fruit. They are native to southern Mexico and Central America. They spread to the South with the Indians. It was then spread to the Caribbean, Europe and the Pacific Islands by the Spanish explorers. In Samoa, the papaya's inner tree bark was used to relieve toothache. Columbus noted that the natives were able to consume large qualities of meat and fish without getting indigestion. This was due to the fact that the Indians consumed an unripe papaya after meals. The papaya fruit pulp is used in a number of cosmetic products (facial creams and shampoos).

A single serving of papaya can meet 20 percent of the U.S. RDA of folate and provides 75 percent of the U.S. RDA of vitamin C. The papaya ranked second to the mango as the best source of carotene. The papaya contains a proteolytic enzyme found in the latex called papain. Papain retains proteolytic activity over a wide pH range. Because of this, papain is used during surgical procedures to dissolve ruptured spinal discs. Papain is known as "nature's scalpel" because it degrades dead tissues.

Peach *(Prunus persica)*

The peach belongs to the family *Rosaceae* along with other stone fruits. Peaches were first cultivated in China, before histories were written. In China the peach was a symbol of life and immortality. From China, peaches were distributed to Persia and then to Europe. The Spanish explorers brought peaches to the New World. In Roman mythology, the peach was the fruit of the goddess Venus (goddess of love). People believed they were an aphrodisiac. Peaches are also associated with sincerity or truth. In ancient Egypt, the Egyptians used peaches as offerings to the God of Tranquility. In the West, the peach is associated with sensuality. In folk medicine, peach bark was used as an herbal remedy for a wide variety of ailments, from bladder inflammation to urinary tract problems. Peaches were used as a natural laxative.

A 100-gram peach will supply 5 percent of the U.S. RDA of the vitamin niacin (B3). Both canned and fresh peaches are rich in vitamin A. Peaches are also a good source of vitamin C; a single peach can yield 10 percent of the vitamin C our bodies need every day for good health. These fruits are also rich in potassium.

Pear *(Pyrus communis)*

The pear belongs to the family *Rosaceae* and originally came from in eastern Europe and Asia Minor. The pear can now be found in Europe, northern Africa, and the Americas, as well. Homer referred to the pear as "the gift of gods." The pear dates back thousands of years ago and spread throughout North

America by the French Jesuit missionaries. Pears are believed to promote healthier hair and a healthier complexion.

Fresh pears are a great source of dietary fiber. The fiber found in pears is mostly in the form of pectin. Pears are rich in potassium, and vitamin A, B, and C. They are cholesterol and sodium free. Pears contain a little fat, but they are unsaturated fats, which are essential in a healthy diet. Pears also contain natural alcohol.

Pineapple *(Ananus communis)*

The pineapple belongs to the family *Bromeliaceae*. The pineapple is native to Paraguay and southern Brazil. Indians distributed it to other countries in Central and South America. The Spanish and English explorers brought the fruit to Europe. The first pineapple was very seedy, containing about 3,000 seeds per fruit. The pineapple we now enjoy is seedless. In 1885, the first commercial plantation was established in Oahu, Hawaii. Pineapples are used for a variety of other things beside food. They are used to tenderize meat, stabilize latex paint, and to make threads and course textiles.

Pineapples are 80 to 85 percent water and 12 to 15 percent sugars. Most pineapples are a good source of vitamin A and C, containing about 20 percent of the U.S. RDA of vitamin C in a single serving. Though we enjoy canned pineapples, they lose about a third of their vitamin C content when processed. However, even canned, pineapples are still a good source of vitamin C. Pineapples contain the enzyme bromelain. Some claim bromelain combats arthritis, heart disease, and other chronic illnesses. Bromelain tablets can be bought in health food stores.

Plum *(Prunus domestica)*

The plum belongs to the *Rosaceae* family. There are countless varieties of plums, but they are all the result of the crossing of three species: the European plum, *Prunus domestica*; the Japanese plum, *Prunus salicina*; and the American plum, *Prunus americana*. The European plum probably developed in ancient Rome and has been cultivated in Europe for over 2,000 years. The European plum is probably the most important commercial plum. Japanese plums originated in China, where they have been cultivated for thousands of years. Two hundred to four hundred years after the Chinese began growing plums they were brought to Japan and then spread throughout the world.

Plums are rich in riboflavin (B2). Two (66 gram-sized) plums provide about a sixteenth of the U.S. RDA. Plums are also good sources of vitamin C. Dried prune plums (prunes) are the most antioxidant rich of all fruits and vegetables. Studies have shown that fresh plums have the fourth highest chemical effectiveness in preventing oxidation in cells in comparison to other commercial fruits. Most of the chemicals responsible for this antioxidant activity are in the juice. Dried plums (prunes), like dried figs, contribute a useful amount of calcium toward meeting the recommended daily requirement of 800 mg. Plums are also rich in carotenoids and a good source of potassium, sodium, calcium, magnesium, iron, and zinc. Prunes and their juices are known for their laxative properties. Prune juice can reduce the plasma low density lipoprotein cholesterol.

Raspberry *(Rubus idaeus, Rubus strigagus)*

Raspberries belong to the family *Rosaceae* and are related to the blackberry. The species *Rubus idaeus* is the wild European raspberry, while *Rubus strigagus* is the red raspberry found in North America. Raspberries travel well, as plants or seeds. Traders and soldiers brought them to Europe. The Romans were also active in spreading raspberries.

The British improved the fruit in the Middle Ages, sent them to its colonies, including America in the late eighteenth century . The red raspberry was already present in America however. A variety of the Southwest Asian raspberry, *Rubus idaeus* variety strigosus, is indigenous to eastern North America. The black raspberry *Rubus occidentalis* is found only in North America, and wasn't domesticated until the 1800s.

Laboratory tests suggest some berries may reduce the build-up of LDL (low density lipoprotein) cholesterol, a contributor to heart disease, stroke and atherosclerosis. Raspberries were tested as having the second highest LDL inhibitory effect.

As with other berries, raspberries contain bioflavonoids that give the berries their bright colors. Bioflavonoids can also maintain health and promote longevity. Bioflavonoids are helpers of the antioxidant vitamin C. Thus bioflavonoids are important in the neutralization of free radicals, and in the building and strengthening of the collagen matrix of your gums, bones, and skin. Bioflavonoids can also protect the body against cancer, heart diseases, reduced memory, and other chronic degenerative diseases.

Studies indicate that red and black raspberries have antiradical activity. They also indicat that the extract of these berries inhibit the activity of xanthine oxidase, which is an enzyme that initiates free-radical formation at a cellular level. The antioxidant properties of these berries can also have a beneficial effect against chronic degenerative diseases that are associated with free radicals.

Strawberry *(Fragaria virginiana)*

Strawberries belong to the family *Rosaceae*. The strawberries we eat now have only been cultivated in North America for about 200 years. North American Indians sent seeds to Europe in the sixteenth century where modern production began. The Chilean Indians domesticated another species of the strawberry, *Fragaria chiloensis*. The Spanish are responsible for spreading it to the rest of South America. A French intelligence officer, Frezier, introduced the plants to France in 1714.

Strawberry juice was used in England as glue for loose teeth, and as a cure for mouth ulcers. Teas were brewed from the leaves and used as an antidiarrheal by the Indians in western Washington. Strawberries were used as a mild laxative, diuretic and astringent. In Western folk medicine, strawberries were used to cure acne, ringworm, and chronic ulceration. In the Middle Ages, a blend of strawberries was used as a general panacea. Strawberries have been used in cosmetics to condition the skin and to whiten the teeth. As with most fruits, the strawberry is a symbol of fertility.

Strawberries are one of the few fruits containing pantothenic acid. Six strawberries can deliver roughly a third of the U.S. RDA. Strawberries are also rich in vitamin C, delivering 131 percent per 100 grams of the U.S. RDA. Strawberries have a fairly high quantity of ellagic acid, which may aid in preventing cancer. Ellagic acid can inhibit cancer or the mutations caused by cancerous elements, such as benzopyrene or aflotoxin in human, rat, and mice tissue.

Scientists think the acid neutralizes active cancer-causing agents by stimulating specific enzymes that combat cancer.

In one study, strawberry consumption seemed to reduce the risk of prostate cancer. Strawberries may also inhibit the absorption of HIV into cells, and the HIV enzyme activity in DNA. A study conducted by Konowalchuk and Speirs published in *The Journal of Food Science* indicated that strawberry extract can reduce subsequent infections with viruses. Strawberries are also rich in the fiber pectin, which can reduce blood cholesterol.

Ranked as the sixth most antioxidant-rich fruit and vegetable, strawberries are an amazing fruit. Studies suggest that some berries may decrease the build-up of LDL (low density lipoprotein) cholesterol. Strawberries were tested as having the fifth highest LDL inhibitory effect of all the berries investigated, while further studies have shown that strawberries are third in fighting free radicals found in the body. Strawberries, as with raspberries, contain a protective antioxidant called "anthocyanin." As strawberries ripen, their antioxidant power also increases.

Not only do strawberries contain protective phytochemicals and antioxidants, they are also fat free.

Watermelon (Citrullus lanatus)

Watermelons belong to the family *Curcurbitacae*. Though watermelons are melons, they belong to a different botanical family than the cantaloupe, *Cumis melo*. Watermelons are 92 percent water and are related to cucumbers and squash. They are native to the Kalahari desert of southern Africa. In Kalahari, tribesmen grind the seed for bread, dry the flesh, and eat the young fruit as a vegetable. Watermelons were cultivated by the ancient Egyptians and were then spread throughout the world. Watermelons are often associated with summer, and are one of America's favorite fruits. Mark Twain described it in his novel *Pudd'n Head* as the food angels eat.

Lycopene is found in high levels in watermelon, which is an antioxidant that is known to reduce the risk of cancer and other diseases. The American Heart Association recognized watermelon as being a heart-healthy food because of its nutritional properties.

Lycopene is responsible for the bright red color found in watermelons. It is part of a larger class of phytochemicals called carotenoids (discussed in more detail in chapter 3). Carotenoids neutralize compounds that are created during photosynthesis, such as hydrogen peroxide or single oxygen atoms that attack and destroy cell membranes and damage the cell (free radicals). Out of all the carotenoids, lycopene is the most effective oxygen neutralizer. One lycopene molecule can neutralize several oxygen radicals. A study conducted by Harvard University indicated that men who ate diets rich in lycopene (tomatoes, tomato products, and watermelon) had a much lower risk of developing certain cancers, especially prostate cancer. Watermelons contain 14 to 15 mg of lycopene per 2-cup serving.

Watermelons are a good source of the B6 vitamin pyridoxine. Pyridoxine helps your body break down and generate amino acids and create new cells. These new cells specialize in producing hemoglobin (used in the immune system to fight disease). One cup of watermelon delivers 0.23 mg of pyridoxine.

Watermelon is a very good source of vitamin C, with a typical serving supplying an adult with one half their daily vitamin C requirement. Watermelons are also fat and cholesterol free. Watermelon is also an excellent source of potassium (116 mg/100 g) and vitamin A (366 IU/100 g).

References

Annie Lise Roberts. Cornucopia: The Lore of Fruits and Vegetables. Knickerbocker Press 1998.

Apple: BB Lala Kaushal and PC Sharma. Dr YS Parmar University of Horticulture and Forestry, Nauni, Solan, Himachal Pradesh, India

Apple-Malus domestica Borkh. http://www.uga.edu/hortcrop/rieger/apple.htm 5/30/00

Apricot Producers of California. http://www.apricotproducers.com

Apricot: VM Ghorpade and Milford A Hanna–University of Nebraska, Lincoln, Nebraska. SS Kadam–Mahtama Phule Agricultural University, Rahuri, Maharashtra, India.

Apricots-Prunus armeniaca http://www.uga.edu/hortcrop/rieger/apricot.htm 5/30/00

Avocado: SS Kadam, Mahtama Phule Agricultural University, Rahuri, Maharashtra, India. DK Salunkhe–Utah State University, Logan, Utah

b+pubmed&list_uids=10822289&dopt=abstract

Banana and Plantain. http://www.uga.edu/hortcrop/rieger/apple.htm 5/30/00

Barbara Martin-Worley. Best Dietary Supplement: Fruits and Vegetables. Colorado State University Cooperative Extension, Denver County. December 18, 1998.

Berries: PM Kotecha–Mahtama Phule Agricultural University, Rahuri, Maharashtra, India. DL Madhavi–University of Illinois, Urbana, Illinois.

Blackberries and Raspberries-Rubus spp. . http://www.uga.edu/hortcrop/rieger/apple.htm 5/30/00

Blueberries and Eyesight,Food Style 21, Vol. 3 No. 3, March 1999.

Blueberries-Vaccinium spp. http://www.uga.edu/hortcrop/rieger/blueberry.htm 5/30/00

Butland BK, Fehily AM, Elwood PC. Diet, Lung Function, and Lung Function Decline in a cohort of 2512 Middle Aged Men. Department of Public Health Sciences, St. George's Hospital Medical School, Cranmer Terrace London, UK.

California Apricot Council. http://www.califapricot.com

Casalini-C; Lodovici-M; Briani-C; Paganelli-G; Remy-S; Cheynier-V; Dolara-P. Effect of Complex Polyphenols and Tannins from Red Wine (WCPT) on Chemically Induced Oxidative DNA Damage in the Rat. Eur-J-Nutr. 1999 Aug; 38(4): 190–5.

Cool Stuff about Apples-Nutrition. 5/12/00

Copyright 1997 Washington Apple Commission

Curtis J Mettlin and Kunio Aoki. Recent Progress In Research On Nutrition And Cancer. Wiley-Liss, New York 1990.

David Scofield Wilson and Angus Kress Gillespie. Rooted in America: Foodlore of Popular Fruits and Vegetables. The University of Tennessee Press, Knoxville 1999.

DK Salunkhe and SS Kadam. Marcel Dekker. Handbook of Fruit Science and Technology: Production, Composition, Storage, and Processing. Marcel Dekker, Inc. 1995.

FA Tom?s-Barber?n and RJ Robins. Phytochemistry of Fruits and Vegetables. Oxford Science Publications 1997.

Getty T Ambau. The Importance of Good Nutrition, Herbs and Phytochemicals For YourHealth, Good Looks, and Longevity. Falcon Press International, CA 1997.

Heart Disease and Cancer January 10, 2000. Santa Ana, Calif. http://www.avoca-do.org

http://www1.epicurious.com/e_eating/e02_summering/summerfruits/apricot.html

Jean Carper. Food Pharmacy: Dramatic New Evidence That Food is Your Best Medicine. Bantam Books 1988.

Jozef V. Joossens, Michael J Hill, and Jef Geboers. Diet and Human Carcinogenesis. Excerpta Medica, Amsterdam 1985.

Julia Daly. Antioxidant Activity of Apples is high, says Cornell Scientists February 5, 1999.

K Tazawa, Hideo Ohkami, Iwao Yamashita, YasuharuOhnishi, tomohiro Saito, Masahiro Okamoto, Kiichi Masuyama, Kazumaro Yamazaki, Shigeru Takemori, Mitukazu Saito, and Hedikik Arai–Anticarcinogenic and/or antimetastatic Action of Apple Pectin in Experimental Rat Colon Carcinogenesis and on Hepatic Metastasis Rat Model. School of Nursing and Second Department of Surgery, Toyama Medical and Pharmaceutical University, Toyama, Japan.

Kedar N Prasad and Frank L Meyskens, Jr. Nutrients and Cancer Prevention. Humana Press–New Jersey 1990.

Keevil-JG; Osman-HE; Reed-JD; Folts-JD. Grape Juice, But Not Orange Juice or Grapefruit Juice, Inhibits Human Platelet Aggregation. J-Nutr. 2000 Jan; 130(1): 53–6.

Kneckt P, Isotupo S, Rissanen H, Heliovaara M, Jarvinen R, Hakkinen S, Aromaa A, Reunanen A–Quercetin Intake and the Incidence of Cerebrovascular Disease. National Public Health Institute, European Journal of Clinical Nutrition. May 2000; 54 (5): 415–417. http://www.ncbi.nlm.nih.gov:80/entrez/que....

Miyagi-Y; Miwa-K; Inoue-H. Inhibition of Human Low-Density Lipoprotein Oxidation by Flavonoids in Red Wine and Grape Juice. Am-J-Cardiol. 1997 Dec 15; 80(12): 1627–31.

National Watermelon Promotion Board: Fun Facts. http://www.watermelon.org

National Watermelon Promotion Board: Health and Wellness. http://www.watermel-on.org

National Watermelon Promotion Board: What is Lycopene. http://www.watermel-on.org

Pat Kendall, Ph.D., R.D. Nutritional Benefits of Fruits and Wines. Food Science and Human Nutrition Specialist Colorado State University Cooperative Extension. June 4,1997.

Pearson DA, Tan CH, German JB, Davis PA, Gershwin ME. Apple Juice inhibits low density lipoprotein oxidation. Department of Food Science and Technology, University of California, Davis USA.

Stein-JH; Keevil-JG; Wiebe-DA; Aeschlimann-S; Folts-JD. Purple Grape Juice Improves Endothelial Function and Reduces the Susceptibility of LDL Cholesterol to Oxidation in Patients with Coronary Artery Disease. Circulation. 1999 Sep 7; 100(10): 1050–5.

Takayuki Shibamoto, Junji terao, and Toshihiko Osawa. Functional Foods For Disease Prevention I: Fruits, Vegetables, and Teas. Oxford Universtiy Press 1998.

Takayuki Shibamoto, Junji Terao, and Toshihiko Osawa. Functional Foods for Disease Prevention II–Medicinal Plants and Other Foods. American Chemical Society, Washington DC 1997.

The California Avocado Commission. http://www.avocado.org

The California Avocado Commission. Phytochemicals Found in Avocados May Help Fight

The Natural Food Hub –Natural Food-Fruit. www.naturalhub.com

The Natural Food Hub –Natural food-Vegetables. www.naturalhub.com

U. S. FDA/Center for Food Safety and Applied Nutrition HHS, USDA Report 1995 Nutrition and Your Health: Dietary Guidelines for Americans.

Vincenzo Zappia, Fulvio Della Ragione, Alfonso Barbarisi, Gian Luigi Russo, and Rossano Della Iacovo. Advances in Nutrition and Cancer 2. Kluwer Academic/Plenum Publishers, New York 1999.

Wang H, Cao G, Prior RL.1996. 'Total antioxidant capacity of fruits'. J Agric Food Chem 1996; 44:701–5. Joseph, J.A., Shukitt-Hale B., Denisova, N.A. Bielinski D., Martin, A., McEwen, J.J., & Bickford, P.C. 1999 "Reversal of age-related declines in the neuronal signal transduction, cognitive, and motor behavioral deficits with blueberry, spinach, or strawberry dietary supplementation." Journal of Neuroscience, September 15, 1999, Vol. 19, No. 18. pages 8114–8121.

Vinson, J. A., Hao, Y., and Zubik, L. 1998 'Phenol antioxidant quantity and quality in foods: vegetables.' J. Agric. Food Chem. 46:3630, l998. (includes analysis of commercially dried/treated figs).

www.naturalhub.com

CHAPTER 10

Vegetables: Finding the Power Plants

Vegetables are the major source of dietary fiber, minerals, and vitamins of a healthy diet. Vegetables are also a rich source of phytochemicals needed in the body for proper health. Vegetables also supply proteins, fats, and carbohydrates in a human diet. Vegetables are a good source of folic acid, niacin, pantothenic acid, riboflavin, thiamin, vitamin A, and vitamin C. Vegetables provide the minerals calcium, iron, magnesium, and phosphorus. Each vegetable provides a different amount and type of vitamins, minerals, and phytochemicals. Consuming a variety will ensure proper nutrition.

Also as an overall rule of thumb, remember that it's better to consume fresh vegetables rather than cooked; cooking vegetables tends to dilute the chemical potency of the plant.

Artichoke *(Cynara scolymus)*

The artichoke belongs to the family *Compositae*, which is part of the daisy family. The artichoke is closely related to the thistle. There are many types of artichokes, but the most familiar type is the globe artichoke. The globe artichoke is small, green and cabbage like. The part of the globe artichoke we eat is the immature flower bud, which is actually the less healthy part of the plant. However, the rest of the artichoke is very bitter. Other types of artichokes are consumed whole. Artichokes are native to the western and central Mediterranean regions, where they have been eaten for over 2,500 years. The artichoke has been cultivated since the fifteenth century, making it one of the world's oldest cultivated vegetables.

In the beginning, artichokes were only used for medicinal purposes. In France, for example, artichokes were used for those suffering from depression. The globe artichoke has long been known as a diuretic and an aid to digestion. For centuries, artichokes have been used to treat specific liver and gallbladder diseases and as a remedy for snakebites. Artichokes were thought to be an aphrodisiac for centuries. They were known for their nutty flavor and the fact that they can be a tasty fingerfood. The artichoke heart is also difficult to obtain, and getting to it is a labor of love for artichoke lovers.

The artichoke is rich in vitamins A, B, C and the minerals calcium, iron and potassium. These vitamins and minerals are known for their cholesterol-fighting properties. The artichoke contains the compound cynarian, which helps protect human arteries from hardening and also keeps serum triglyceride levels low. Often foods will taste sweeter after eating artichoke because cynarian stimulates the taste buds that detect sweetness. Cynarian seems to help with the production and flow of bile. Cynarian may be a cholagogue, increasing the production of bile in the liver; a choleretic, increasing the flow of bile from the gall bladder; and a choliokinetic, increasing the contractive power of the bile duct. Artichoke leaves also contain some pharmacologically active properties that may help the functioning of the brain and parts of the central nervous system. The artichoke also contains acids that can activate liver function. Artichokes can help with atherosclerosis, liver problems, memory loss, and triglyceride levels.

Asparagus (Asparagus officinais)

The asparagus is part of the Lily family. Though there is little known about the origin of the asparagus, it is native to the eastern part of the Mediterranean. The Egyptians often offered bundles of asparagus to their gods. The ancient Greeks collected the wild asparagus, but it was the Romans who first cultivated it in 2000 B.C. The Greeks and Romans were the first to use it in medical ways. Asparagus now grow in central Europe, North America, western and central Asia, and northern Africa.

This vegetable was used medicinally around the world. The underground stems of the plants were used to make remedies to alleviate bee stings, toothaches, and venereal disease. Syrups from the plant have been used to make potions to cure heart palpitations and increase urine production. Asparagus was also used to remove blackheads and pimples.

Asparagus are rich in potassium, folate, and vitamin A. One cup of asparagus, which is equivalent to 134 g, delivers 365.8 mg of potassium, 171 mcg of folate, and 781.2 IU of vitamin A. The vitamin A content in asparagus varies according to the color of the plant. Dark green asparagus contains more vitamin A than white or blanched asparagus. Asparagus are cholesterol and nearly sodium and fat free. They contain phytosterols that contain anticancer properties. Asparagus also contains rutin that can help prevent small blood vessels from rupturing.

Beans *(Leguminosae)*

Beans belong to the family *Leguminosae*. The bean has been a dietary staple for many countries. They are an excellent source of protein, nitrates, iron, and phosphates. In some countries, beans replace meat entirely. There are hundreds of bean variations and subvariations. The bean can be eaten at any point of its life cycle, from sprouted seeds, to pods, to mature seeds. It can be eaten fresh, dried, frozen, and canned.

The Greeks and the Romans avoided beans because they were rumored to induce insanity and nightmares. The oracles of ancient times also avoided them because it was thought that they would lose the right to divine revelation. In England, beans were often placed on graves to ward off ghosts and were even used in the exorcism of evil spirits. Though there are hundreds of bean species, we will only discuss a few that have played an exceptional part in history.

The American haricot, *Phaseolus vulgaris*, is also known as the "common bean." This bean is native to southwestern Mexico and was first cultivated over 7,000 years ago. There are over 500 different species of common bean, including the black, black-eyed pea, marrow, navy, pigeon, pinto, string bean, and yellow eye. The haricot bean is also known as the "French bean." The haricot is rich in protein, vitamin A, vitamin C, calcium, and phosphorus.

The lima bean, *Phaseolus lunatus*, is named after the capital of Peru. The lima bean is native to tropical America. This bean predates the haricot. The lima bean is also a great source of vitamin A, phosphorus, protein, fiber, and amino acids.

The broad bean, *Vicia faba*, is also known as the "fava bean" in the United States. This bean has been the staple of Europe since the Bronze Age.

Lentils, *Vicia lens*, are the oldest cultivated beans in the world. Lentils originated in the Near East and have been cultivated since 7000 B.C.

The chickpea, *Cicer arietinum*, is also referred to as the garbanzo, gram, or Egyptian pea. This bean originated in the Mediterranean and is popular in Indian and Middle Eastern cuisine. It has been cultivated for over 5,000 years. The chickpea is an excellent source of calcium, phosphorus, ascorbic acid, and iron.

The Asian soybean, *Glycine maxo*, is not only used as a food staple, but it is also used to make many different commercial products. For instance, soy is used to make fertilizer and paint. Soy is very high in protein and is often used as a meat substitute. The soybean is originally from China. For more information about soy, please see chapter 3.

Beans are great for the cardiovascular system. Beans are an excellent source of both soluble and insoluble fiber. Beans can lower your LDL cholesterol and are great regulators of insulin. Beans, rich in protease inhibitors, act as anticancer agents.

Beet *(Beta vularis)*

This vegetable belongs to the *Chenopodiaceae* family and was thought to have originated in the Mediterranean. Beets are a good source of sugar and are added to dishes for flavor and color. Beets are rich in potassium, folate, calcium, magnesium, sulfur, and vitamin C.

Broccoli *(Brassica oleracea italica)*

Broccoli is a member of the *Cruciferae* family with the cabbage, brussel sprouts, and cauliflower. Broccoli originated in Italy. We have placed studies conducted about the *Cruciferae* family in the cabbage section. In a survey conducted in the United States, broccoli and cauliflower were called America's favorite vegetables. Interestingly enough, more women indicated broccoli was their favorite vegetable compared to men.

Broccoli is rich in chlorophyll, which has demonstrated some ability to block cell mutations, which is the cause of cancer. Broccoli is also rich in carotenoids, which is a leading anticancer agent. Broccoli is rich in potassium, folate and vitamins A and C. Broccoli contains sulphoraphane, which is also known for its anti-cancer causing elements. Sulphoraphane does not suppress cancer cells, but actually blocks them. It stimulates the production of enzymes in the liver that destroy cancer-causing chemicals. When this happens, it stimulates the body's own natural detoxification system known as Phase II enzymes.

Since the early 1950s tests have been conducted on the nutritional benefit of broccoli. Those who consume even the smallest amounts of broccoli reduce their risk of cancer significantly. Broccoli can prevent colon, esophageal, larynx, lung, pharynx, prostate, oral cavity, and stomach cancers.

Brussels Sprouts *(Brassica oleracea gemmifera)*

Brussels sprouts are also part of the *Cruciferae* family. Brussels sprouts are rich in sulfur, as their broccoli cousin. Brussels sprouts have been grown in the vicinity of Brussels, Belgium, for hundreds of years, hence the name.

Brussels sprouts are rich in chlorophyll, indoles, dithiolthiones, carotenoids, and glucosinolates, which are all active cancer-fighting chemicals. Glucosinolates are responsible for the bitter taste and smell of Brussels sprouts and broccoli. Brussels sprouts contain the chemical sinigrin, which can restrain the growth of cancerous cells. Another chemical that is found in Brussels sprouts is allyl isothiocyanate, which is a breakdown product of sinigrin. This chemical works by making cancerous cells go through apoptosis, or self-destruction. See cabbage for studies.

Cabbage *(Brassica oleracea)*

The cabbage belongs to the *Cruciferae* family as well. It is believed that the cabbage originated in northern Europe and then spread throughout the Mediterranean. The cabbage is known to be one of the world's oldest cultivated vegetables. Cabbage has been used for medicinal purposes since the time of the ancient Greeks and Romans. It was believed that it could cure almost every disease, from wounds to cancer. It was even recommended by the Native folk healers in America to cure yeast infections of the feet, hands, head, and skin.

Cabbage contains the chemical anthocyanin, which gives the cabbage its range of color, from greens to purples. Cabbage contains a vast array of chemicals that are beneficial to our bodies. Two are sulfur and histidine, both of which inhibit tumor growth and can prevent colon and rectum cancer. Other chemicals found in cabbage include: chlorophyll, dithiolthiones, flavonoids, indoles, isothiolthiones, phenols (caffeic and ferulic acids), vitamin C, and vitamin E. All of these chemicals have cancer-fighting properties. Cabbage can also lower your LDL (bad cholesterol) cholesterol and raise your HDL (good cholesterol) cholesterol.

A study conducted by the Brassica Chemoprotection Laboratory and Department of Pharmacology and Molecular Sciences at John Hopkins University's Medical School, found that Brassicas (cabbage, cauliflower, Brussels sprouts, and broccoli) are rich in Phase II enzymes, which inactivate major carcinogens in the body by destroying their reactive centers. It was also found that Brassicas contain sulphuraphane, which has anticarcinogenic properties. In another study conducted by the Department of Chronic Diseases and Environment Epidemiology, at the National Institute of Public Health and Environmental Protection in the Netherlands indicated that over 100 glucosinolates were identified in the *Brassica* family. Glucosinolates are responsible for inhibiting the growth of cancer cells. They are also antifungal and antibacterial.

Carrot *(Daucus sativus)*

The carrot belongs to the family *Umbelliferae*, which is the parsley family. Carrots are native to Afganistan, but were not cultivated until they spread to the Mediterranean. At first carrots were only used for medicinal purposes and not as a food. The ancient Greeks used the carrot plant to relieve stomachaches and to increase virility. In the 1800s, Iranian men believed that the carrot held aphrodisiac properties.

Carrots come in all different shapes and sizes, ranging from white, orange, to purple. The Dutch first introduced the orange carrots that we eat today. Carrots are rich in beta-carotene, which helps fight cancer. Beta-carotene is converted into vitamin A in the liver and controls cell differentiation. Carrots are high in sugar and are also rich in vitamins B and C, calcium, phosphorus, iron, and magnesium.

Cauliflower *(Brassica oleracea botrytis)*

The cauliflower belongs to the *Cruciferae* family. It contains all the same chemicals found in the *Brassica* genus and has all of the same benefits. Cauliflower can reduce the risk of colon, rectum, stomach, and possibly prostate and bladder cancers. Unlike its cousins broccoli, cabbage, and Brussels sprouts, the cauliflower does not contain high amounts of chlorophyll or carotenes (see cabbage).

Celery *(Apium graveolens)*

The celery belongs to the family *Apiaceae* and is one of the oldest recorded vegetables in history. This vegetable is native to the Mediterranean region. Ancient Greeks crowned winning athletes with celery leaves and stems. Celery belongs to the parsley family with the carrot. Celery contains phthalide, which is a natural sedative. In China, celery juice is used to reduce hypertension.

One hundred grams of celery delivers roughly 6.3 grams of protein, 2.1 grams of minerals, 1.4 grams of fiber, and 1.6 grams of carbohydrates. Celery also contains calcium, phosphorus, iron, carotene, thiamin, vitamin C, niacin, riboflavin, and vitamin A.

Cucumber *(Cucumis sativus)*

The cucumber belongs to the family *Cucurbitaceae*. Native to southwestern Asia, the cucumber has been cultivated for over

12,000 years. The cucumber is a symbol of fertility in many cultures. Cucumbers are also mentioned in the Bible (Numbers 11:4–5). They were cultivated by the Hebrew slaves during their imprisonment in Egypt. The Romans made wine out of cucumbers and also used them for cosmetic purposes.

Cucumbers are related to the melon family and are almost 96 percent water. Cucumbers contain no cholesterol, fat, fiber, or sodium and contain small amounts of vitamins and minerals. Cucumbers are used in a wide array of cosmetic purposes ranging from whitening teeth to softening the skin. They are also used medicinally to purify the blood and alleviate coughs.

Eggplant (Solanum melongena)

The eggplant belongs to the family *Solanaceae*, which is also known as the deadly nightshade family. The eggplant is technically a fruit, but is not eaten as one. This plant originated in tropical Asia and has been cultivated for over 4,000 years. It was first cultivated in India and then was introduced to the Arabs, who brought it to Spain where it was grown by the Moors. In the sixteenth century, the eggplant was known as the "apple of love" and believed to be an aphrodisiac by the Spaniards. In the northern part of Europe, the eggplant was not eaten but used as decoration. They were known as the "mad apple" in northern Europe because it was thought to inflict insanity, fever, and epilepsy on those who consumed them.

Eggplants are not very nutritious, but contain large contents of calcium and potassium. In Japan, the eggplant is used to whiten teeth, but there are other benefits that come with the consumption of this fruit. The eggplant can lower cholesterol in the blood. It contains substances that bind cholesterol in the intestines and carry it out of the body so it will not be absorbed. Eggplants are rich in protease inhibitors. In Nigeria, eggplants are regarded as a contraceptive, an antirheumatic agent and anticonvulsant. In traditional Korean medicine, the eggplant is used to treat pain, measles, stomach cancer, alcoholism, and used externally to cure burns. Today the eggplant is known for its cancer-fighting properties and cleansing the arteries of fatty plaques.

Hot Pepper *(Capsicum)*

Hot (chili) peppers are related to the deadly nightshade family *Solanaceae*, as well as the tomato, potato, eggplant, and tobacco. The Incas, Mayas, and Aztecs commonly used chili peppers. It was Christopher Columbus who introduced the chili pepper to Europe. He mistook it for the coveted peppercorn, but the Europeans nonetheless were thrilled to have chili peppers.

Hot peppers are rich in vitamin C (nine times that of an orange), potassium, fiber, folic acid, and vitamins B6 and E. These peppers also contain the chemical capaicin, which is responsible for the heat and burn of the vegetable. In Mexico, the vegetable is used to cure stomach problems. Chili peppers also aid in arthritis, bronchitis, epilepsy, malaria, parasitic infections, and toothaches.

Lettuce *(Lactuca)*

There are many types of lettuce belonging to the *Compositae* family. The four types are: head (capitata), cutting or leaf (crispa), cos or romaine (longifolia), and asparagus or stem (asparagina). There are also two known variations of head lettuce known as crisp head and butter head.

All lettuces are not equal in nutritional value: the darker and leafier the lettuce, the more nutrients it contains. Lettuce is a good source of vitamin A, calcium, and iron. Lettuce also contains some proteins, carbohydrates, and vitamin C. When lettuce is cooked, the vitamin C content decreases significantly. Lettuce is often associated with diet. Those who are watching their weight often consume salads. In the United States, iceberg lettuce is the most consumed variation of lettuce, but it has little nutritional value. Try to go for the greener and leafier lettuce to get more nutrients in your salad.

Mushroom *(Agaricaceae)*

The mushroom belongs to the family *Agaricaceae*. All mushrooms are fungi, but only half of the 100,000 species of fungi are mushrooms. The emperor Nero proclaimed mushrooms to be the "food of the gods." Mushrooms were used by Native Americans and during Viking rituals because of their intoxicating and hallucinogenic properties. In Mexico, the mushroom symbolizes knowledge and enlightenment, while in China it is a symbol of leadership. The mushroom is symbolic of fertility because of the rapid growth and reproduction of the vegetables.

Mushrooms contain no sugars, few carbohydrates, but many vitamins, minerals, and protein. Mushrooms are particularly dense in phosphorus and calcium. The mushroom is technically not a vegetable because it does not produce chlorophyll, seeds, flowers, or roots. Oriental mushrooms can stimulate the immune system, inhibit blood clotting, and slow down the development of certain cancers. Some mushrooms contain antitumor powers (shiitake, oyster, enoki, and tree ear). Shiitake mushrooms may even lower blood cholesterols.

Onion *(Allium cepa)*

The onion belongs to the Lily family. The skin of the onion can range from white, to yellow, to red. Onions have been cultivated for over 5,000 years. Though they also grow wild throughout the world, they are one of the oldest cultivated vegetable crops known to man. To the ancient Egyptians, the onions were a symbol of the universe. Onions were often offerings to the gods. In Rome and Eastern Europe, the onion was recognized as a symbol of eternity.

Historically onions were eaten and used for medicinal purposes. The warmer the climate, the sweeter and milder onions are in taste. They were often eaten raw like apples. Onions were used as an antiseptic agent and applied to bee stings and burns. Onions also induce perspiration and were used to treat congestion and colds.

Onions are rich in vitamin C, sulfur, and mineral salts. They lower blood sugar levels. Onions also lower LDL (bad) cholesterol, and raise HDL (good) cholesterol.

Pea *(Pisum sativum)*

There are hundreds of pea varieties, but only two types are cultivated: field and garden. The pea is one of the world's oldest vegetables. Carbonized pea seeds have been found in western Asia and in Europe, dating back to 7000 B.C. The Chinese first began using the pea for food in 2000 B.C. The green pea wasn't popularly eaten in the West until the French royalty demanded them on their table. It was the common garden pea that Gregor Mendel used for his genetic experiments. Customarily, unwed females lucky enough to find a nine-pea pod, would hang the pod on their doors. The first eligible male to walk through the door was to become her spouse. Ironically, the pea has also been used as an antifertility agent.

Peas are rich in proteins and soluble fiber. One cup of peas provides 8 grams of protein, which is equivalent to 1 oz of cooked lean meat. The fiber can lower your LDL cholesterol and control blood sugar. Green peas contain a substantial amount of vitamin A and C. They are rich in calcium, potassium, phosphorus, and iron. Fresh peas are low in sodium. Not all peas are equal in nutritional value. Frozen peas actually lose about 50 to 70 percent of their vitamin C when thawed. Peas also contain concentrated sources of protease inhibitors that kill the activation of certain viruses and chemical carcinogens.

Potato *(Solanum tuberosum)*

The potato belongs to the family *Solanaceae*, the nightshade family. The potato stands next to wheat, rice, and maize as the fourth major food crop in the world. The potato originated in the Peruvian Andes and was cultivated there for centuries. This vegetable was introduced by the Spanish explorers to Europe in the sixteenth century. The potato was first feared because it belonged to the nightshade family. Potatoes provide more nourishment per acre than grain and will also grow in poor soil. England and Ireland readily accepted this new vegetable.

Potatoes were believed to fight rheumatism and purify blood. Potatoes also aid in digestion, and have anticancer agents and antiviral agents. Potatoes contain high concentrations of a protease inhibitor, which can neutralize certain viruses and carcinogens. Potatoes and their skin are rich in chlorogenic acid, a polyphenol that prevents cell mutations, a precursor of cancer.

Potatoes are a rich source of carbohydrates, but also provide significant amounts of other nutrients. Potatoes contain proteins, iron, the vitamin B-complex, and vitamin C.

Spinach *(Spinacia oleracea)*

Spinach belongs to the family *Chenopodiaceae*. Spinach is probably native to Southwest Asia, but it can be found throughout the world. Spinach was first cultivated by the Arabs and then brought to Spain by the Moors.

Spinach is rich in iron and calcium. But because of the oxalic acid found in spinach, calcium absorption is minimal. Spinach is also rich in potassium and contains some magnesium and phosphorus. Spinach is rich in vitamin A and K, and also contains significant amounts of folate.

According to new research conducted by Harvard University, eating cooked spinach at least twice a week can cut the risk of cataracts in men by half. The National Eye Institute also states that incorporating at least two servings of spinach weekly in your diet can cut the risk of macular degeneration (leading cause of blindness) in half as well.

Spinach is high in vitamin K, which is used to build strong bones. Spinach can lower the risk of hip fracture from osteoporosis as much as 30 percent according to a joint study conducted by Harvard University and Tufts University. Spinach also contains alpha and beta-carotene, lutein, zeaxanthin, and the minerals potassium and magnesium. As stated above, spinach is an excellent source of vitamin K, but is also the richest plant source of folic acid. One half-cup serving of spinach provides two-thirds of the daily-recommended value of folic acid.

Spinach can lower the risk of stroke, colon and rectal cancer, macular degeneration, cataracts, heart disease, osteoporosis, memory loss, Alzheimer's disease, depression, and birth defects.

Squash *(Cucurbita)*

Squash belongs to the *Cucurbita* family. Squash are unique to America and have been cultivated for over 9,000 years. The squash is part of the Native American triad with corn and beans, also known as the "inseparable sisters." Squash is a generic term used in America that includes squash, gourds, and pumpkins. The squash is divided into two different types: winter and summer squash. Pumpkins are a type of winter squash popular for have been noted for their cancer-fighting properties. They are also rich in vitamin A.

Winter squash is characterized with an outer tough skin, irregular shape, and orange pulp and seeds. The seeds and pulp are eaten separately. These squash include pumpkins, acorn, butternut and Hubbard. Summer squash has a mild taste and is quite tender. It is most often eaten whole. Summer squash includes yellow straightneck squash and zucchini. Summer squash is low in energy value in comparison to the winter squashes.

Tomatoes *(Lycopersicon esculenta)*

Tomatoes belong to *Solanaceae*, the nightshade family. The tomato is native to the Andes and was spread throughout Central America by the Spanish Conquistadors. Europeans first avoided tomatoes because they belonged to the deadly nightshade family. The tomato was surrounded by superstition: many believed tomatoes caused cancer and gout. The tomato's Latin name can be translated into "wolf peach," but the French refer to it as pomme d'amour: the "love apple." The tomato is a native of North America and may have been cultivated by the Aztecs as early as 700 A.D. Tomatoes are actually berries and are therefore fruits. However, they are most often thought of as vegetables because they are usually prepared in similar ways with other vegetables. In fact, the U.S. Supreme Court actually officially declared that tomatoes were vegetables in the late 1800s. Tomatoes are the third most popular vegetable eaten by Americans.

The nutritional value of tomatoes varies according to where it is grown. One medium tomato has only 35 calories and provides 40 percent of the RDA of vitamin C. Tomatoes are also a good source of vitamin A, providing 20 percent of the RDA. Concentrated tomato products such as tomato sauce or paste provide even higher concentrations of tomato nutrients.

Tomatoes have also recently been spotlighted for their potential in fighting cancer. A 1995 study found that men who ate large amounts of tomatoes had a lower incidence of prostate cancer. Furthermore, a very small recent study using lycopene supplements (a natural antioxidant) made from tomatoes showed promise in slowing the growth of prostate cancer in men who had already developed the disease. Participants receive 15 mg of lycopene. A half-cup of tomato sauce contains almost 22 mg.

Lycopene, which is an antioxidant that is known to reduce the risk of cancer and other diseases, is found in high levels in tomatoes, but more in tomato products. Lycopene is responsible for the bright red color found in watermelons. It is part of a larger class of phytochemicals called carotenoids (discussed in more detail in chapter 3). Carotenoids neutralize compounds that are created during photosynthesis, such as hydrogen peroxide or single oxygen atoms that attack and destroy cell membranes and damage the cell (free radicals). Out of all the carotenoids, lycopene is the most effective oxygen neutralizer. One lycopene molecule can neutralize several oxygen radicals. A study conducted by Harvard University indicated that men who ate diets rich in lycopene (tomatoes, tomato products, and watermelon) had a much lower risk of developing certain cancers, especially prostate cancer.

References

Annie Lise Roberts. Cornucopia: The Lore of Fruits and Vegetables. Knickerboxer Press, New York 1998.

Artichoke (Cynara scolymus).6/13/00
http://members.xoom.com/_XMCM/mangey/artichoke.htm

Artichoke, Globe. Botanical.com A Modern Herbal Mrs. Grieve. http://www.botanical.com/botanical/msgmh/a/artic066.html

DK Salunkhe and SS Kadam. Marcel Dekker. Handbook of Vegetable Science and Technology: Production, Composition, Storage, and Processing. Marcel Dekker, Inc. 1998.

FA Tom?s-Barber?n and RJ Robins. Phytochemistry of Fruits and Vegetables. Oxford Science Publications 1997.

Food Pharmacy.

Getty T Ambau. The Importance of Good Nutrition, Herbs and Phytochemicals For YourHealth, Good Looks, and Longevity. Falcon Press International, CA 1997.

Globe Artichoke. http://extension-horticulture.tamu.edu/PLANTanswers/vegetables/globeart.html 6/9/00.

Jean Carper. Food Pharmacy: Dramatic New Evidence That Food is Your Best Medicine. Bantam Books 1988. Curtis J Mettlin and Kunio Aoki. Recent Progress In Research On Nutrition And Cancer. Wiley-Liss, New York 1990.

Jed W. Fahey, Katherine K. Stephenson, and Paul Talalay. Gluconsinolates, Myrosinase, and Isothiocyanates: Three Reasons for Eating Brassica Vegetables. Brassica Chemoprotection Laboratory and Department of Pharmacology and Molecular Sciences, School of Medicine, John Hopkins University. Baltimore MD 1998.

John Heinerman. Heinerman's New Encyclopedia of Fruits and Vegetables: Revised and Expanded.Parker Publishing Company. New York 1995.

Jozef V. Joossens, Michael J Hill, and Jef Geboers. Diet and Human Carcinogenesis. Excerpta Medica, Amsterdam 1985.

Kedar N Prasad and Frank L Meyskens, Jr. Nutrients and Cancer Prevention. Humana Press—New Jersey 1990.

Michael G.L. Hertog, Geert van Poppel, and Dorette Verhoeven. Potentially Anticarcinogenic Secondary Metabloites from Fruits and Vegetables. Department of Chronic Diseases and Environmental Epidemiology, National Institute of Public Health and Environmental Protection, the Netherlnads 1997.

Takayuki Shibamoto, Junji terao, and Toshihiko Osawa. Functional Foods For Disease Prevention I: Fruits, Vegetables, and Teas. Oxford Universtiy Press 1998.

Takayuki Shibamoto, Junji Terao, and Toshihiko Osawa. Functional Foods for Disease Prevention II–Medicinal Plants and Other Foods. American Chemical Society, Washington DC 1997.

Vincenzo Zappia, Fulvio Della Ragione, Alfonso Barbarisi, Gian Luigi Russo, and Rossano Della Iacovo. Advances in Nutrition and Cancer 2. Kluwer Academic/ Plenum Publishers, New York 1999.

Why Your Best Friend could be a Brassica. 5/17/00.

CHAPTER 11

Using Herbal Treatments for Health Problems

The use of herbs to treat health problems is an ancient practice experiencing a modern-day revival. Many herbs have pointed the way for the discovery of life-saving drugs and have eventually lead to the creation of today's pharmaceutical industry. In the surge to find more "natural" medicines, many have gone back to the roots of the modern pharmacy. People are returning to herbs.

Herbs are almost indistinguishable from vegetables. We use a pretty flexible principle in naming some plants "herbs" and others vegetables. In the end, the only difference between an herb and vegetables is that we tend to eat herbs in small quantities in comparison to vegetables. Herbs are often used for their inessential chemicals to promote health, aid in overcoming diseases, treat a deficiency or flavor foods. Most often herbs are plants that have a history or tradition of use that goes back hundreds or thousands of years for medicinal purposes.

The herbal remedy industry has boomed in recent years, filling the shelves of health-food stores, and promising to cure just about any disorder or disease you can think of. People rush to stores and sites on the Internet to purchase herbs in order to treat or prevent a great variety of problems. An impressive number of companies are now touting their ware's superiority and effectiveness.

Generally, herbs are safer to use and have fewer side effects than many modern medicines. This is often because they are milder in their doses compared to prescription medicines. A mild herbal treatment may be all that is required in treating many of the minor conditions people experience.

Despite the fact that herbs are generally milder than prescription medicines, it is still important to be aware of the chemicals in any herbal remedy before taking it. Herbal treatments are also commonly used for problems for which a doctor's visit is not necessary, and are thus often self-prescribed. We hope to provide some basic reliable information on some of the most prominent herbs on the market today.

We will also try to clarify some oft-repeated terms to help you feel comfortable in the intense marketing arena of herbal remedies. Lets start with the perception of what an herb is and what it does, whether good or bad.

Herbs Are Undeveloped Drugs

Some plants contain chemicals that can change or influence the function of the body. Herbs are often used to treat and, in some cases, prevent illness. Though herbal substances are milder and have fewer side effects than modern prescription drugs, they should not be used carelessly. It is important to know some basic things about the plants from which an herbal remedy is made as well as something about the process of making an herbal supplement before taking an herbal remedy.

First, it would be wise to know what part of the plant is being used to make a supplement. The chemical composition can vary greatly for each part of an herb. It is important to know what part of a plant is supposed to be used for medicinal purposes. While one part of a plant may be completely safe and edible, it may not be true for the whole plant. For example, the rhubarb plant's stalks may be eaten raw while the leaves are poisonous.

Chemicals "naturally" created in plants can be just as toxic as "unnatural" chemicals produced in laboratories. On the other hand, these same chemicals may be therapeutic under the right conditions. Make sure you know what to expect by learning about an herb before taking it. Many herbs have undesirable side-affects, while others seem to have none. In the end, however, it is important to take responsibility for learning about an herb before eating it. This is particularly true when it comes to herbal remedies.

Herbs as Medicine

Legally, in the United States, herbs are to be used strictly as supplements and cannot be used as medications. However, the fact is, most herbs are used to treat physical conditions, and are thus used medicinally. When herbs are used as medicine the intent is to change something about how the body is working. This is the same intent in taking over the counter medications. There are some noteworthy differences between herbs and drugs, however, that prevent herbal supplements from legally standing toe to toe with drugs. Herbs generally lack the dosage accuracy and information that most developed drugs have. Herbal remedies are thus less consistent and dependable than prescription drugs.

How to Choose Your Supplements

Start by reading the label. It is important to know what to look for because you can often tell the difference between conscientious companies and unscrupulous suppliers by the information provided on the label. Often it is not so much what is on the label as it is what is left out. The quality of the information that the supplier is willing to give you can be indicative of the quality of the herb inside.

Herbal supplement labels should clearly indicate six important things: what part of the plant was used, what the herb's Latin name is, whether the chemicals in the supplements were carefully monitored or standardized, dosage information, side effects associated with the herb, and an expiration date.

Different parts of the plant contain different chemicals. If the root is therapeutic, don't buy a supplement that is made from the leaves. This information ought to be readily available on the label. The company should be specific about the variety of herb they are selling. Some herbs share the same common name but are completely different species and differ in chemical composition.

Not only do different parts of plants contain different chemicals, but different plants of the same species, depending on their individual genetics and where and under what conditions they were grown and harvested, can have variable chemical concentrations. It is important that the chemical concentrations are monitored to assure both the potential effectiveness and safety of the herb. Some herbs have different effects on the body in different concentrations.

Check to see if the concentration of the herb is standardized. This means that a certain amount of various substances are guaranteed to be in the bottle, or in the case of negatively influencing compounds, guaranteed not to be in the bottle in appreciable amounts. Standardization is the best way to ensure consistent results. Dose numbers should be presented in weight, grams, and/or percentages of total weight. Do not be impressed by labels that only mention ratios of one substance in comparison to another because these are not measures of amounts and don't tell you anything about how much of a chemical is actually there.

Unfortunately standardization does not solve all of the potential problems associated with dosage inaccuracy in herbal supplements. There has not been enough attention in rigorous scientific circles yet to promote extensive testing and research of herbs. As a result, we are relatively unsure of how many of the chemicals in herbs affect the body. In fact, we have yet to identify the active chemicals in many herbal remedies. Thus it is possible that the chemicals believed to be therapeutic in an herb may not be all that helpful. In such cases it is possible that sometimes the wrong chemical compounds are standardized while truly helpful ones are ignored. Despite this, standardization is still considered the best way to gauge quality and safety.

The bottle should indicate how often and how much of the herb should be taken. For example: One tablet of this herb should be taken twice a day, after meals. Dosages can also be an effective way to calculate costs. A less concentrated herbal supplement may require you to take two or three tablets while another only requires you to take one in order to get the same effect. If both bottles have the same number of pills, and cost the same, the most cost effective choice is the herb that is concentrated and can be used more.

Because the active constituents and their modes of action are not determined and total effectiveness may include the activities of more than a single element, it is usually a better idea to buy supplements which contain the whole herb, though standardized to certain constituents. If you buy the constituents alone they may not have all the ingredients making the herb most effective.

Look for bottles that have expiration dates. Herbs are going to be most effective and predictable when fresh. Different herbs can keep for different lengths of time. A sample that is several months or even years old may have changed in chemical composition and may have stronger or weaker effects.

Herbal companies usually make some claims as to what the herb is used for on the bottle. Often web sites and accompanying literature can be filled with claims and testimonials of an herb's effectiveness. Testimonials, however appealing, are not good sources of evidence to base a decision on taking an herbal remedy on. Often testimonial evidence is little more than modern folklore. In addition, in cases where the testimony is based in truth, so little is known about the effects of herbs that it is likely that there are many other factors involved in successful treatment that are not due to the herb itself. In order for claims to be credible they ought to be grounded on well-designed and supported scientific experiments. We will talk more about this in chapter 17.

Many herbs will have side effects. Pregnant and nursing mothers should be particularly cautious in taking herbs. Again, we are still learning about the effects of herbs. Despite the fact that herbs have been used for thousands of years, we are still relatively uninformed about the potential effects of an herb on the body. Adding any herb that is not a normal part of the diet could make large changes in the physical and chemical behaviors of the body. On the other hand, herbal remedies may have no effect at all. While some herbs are incredibly safe and effective others have the potential to cause problems, and may be poisonous.

Some herbs contain potent drugs. Some of these herbs were used before the advent of modern medicine to treat equally serious health problems. Even when administered by knowledgeable authorities, the inaccuracy of the composition of chemicals in these herbs makes it difficult to manage doses. As a result, sometimes people experienced serious side effects and even died. The isolation and artificial manufacture of the effective chemicals within these herbs meant precision dosage was possible. Some dangerous herbs are being offered on the market today. Some have been connected to serious problems and even death. In the end, we simply urge you to be informed of all an herb's effects before taking it. Search out information especially on safety and side effects.

Wild Crafted Herbs

Some herbs are wild crafted, meaning they were collected from a natural source growing without the aid of man. Some herbs are now rare in the wild because of a high demand in the herbal market. Many states have begun restricting the harvesting of some herbs on state and federal lands in order to protect species from becoming extinct.

The effects of the chemicals in an herb are the same whether grown wild or cultivated. Protect wild plants by not purchasing rare or threatened varieties of wild herbs.

Misleading Claims

There are many herbal companies. Some are careful to make honest and informed representations of their products and others are not so careful. Beware of companies that make claims for their herbs that sound more like miracle cures. A good rule to follow is an old one: if something sounds too good to be true—it probably is.

If you are surfing the internet or going shopping in a health food store and run across a company claiming an herb or product they sell will cure or otherwise treat cancer, AIDS, diabetes, or any other serious, life-threatening condition, don't be inclined to believe them. Not only is it illegal for them to make these claims, but also such claims are almost certainly untrue. It would be unwise to make purchases from a company that makes illegal claims. If they are willing to risk making illegal claims they may also be taking other risks in areas such as manufacturing.

In the United States the Dietary Supplement Health and Education Act of 1994 was passed making it illegal for an herbal supplier to market their herb as a cure, prevention, treatment or diagnosis of any disease. According to Section 6 of the Act, herbal suppliers cannot make any statements about the herb that claim therapeutic results. Herbal sellers can only make statements claiming how an herb affects the structure and/or function of the body as nutritional support.

Allowed claims include: health maintenance (people are already healthy), nondisease claims (calm stomach, help sleep), and claims for minor symptoms associated with normal life stages (hot flashes, PMS).

Just what constitutes a serious health condition is continually in the process of definition as the industry and the FDA face new problems and concerns. According to the FDA: "Serious conditions associated with aging, pregnancy, menopause, and adolescence, such as toxemia of pregnancy, and osteoporosis, will continue to be treated as diseases." Herbal companies cannot claim to be therapeutic for any serious health condition until they are proven safe and effective and approved for such uses.

This doesn't mean that all herbal companies follow such guidance. The FDA warns hundreds of herbal companies every year, and even litigates against some for making claims for products that are either unsubstantiated or untruthful. Some companies are particularly creative in making claims for their products. They attempt to support their claims with research papers and expert testimonials. However, often research is fabricated or misrepresented while expert testimony comes from doctors on the payroll.

Not all situations are as negative as these. Many companies are respectable and honest with consumers. The herbal remedy market is confusing and intimidating; the key is to do your research so you can distinguish between substance and hype. In the end we urge you to take the time and effort to learn something about an herb and the distributor before purchasing and taking it.

If You Have a Serious Health Problem

If you have a real or serious medical problem such as diabetes, heart disease, asthma, etc. it is important for you to know that herbs should not replace conventional and proven medical therapies. Please continue taking your prescribed medications as directed by your physician. Always consult your physician before using herbs at the same time as your medications because some medications react negatively with herbs.

Allergies

Herbs contain many molecules just about any of which could generate an allergic reaction. If you experience rashes or other discomfort after taking an herb discontinue its use. If you already know you have allergies to certain plants it would be a good idea to do some research to see if the herbs you intend on taking are related to something you are allergic to. Plants that are related to one another tend to contain some of the same chemicals.

Making Your Own Supplements

Some herbs are toxic in nature if not handled and processed correctly. Sometimes toxic plants can be misidentified as herbs. You should not attempt making your own supplements without the direction of an expert, as the results could be very negative.

CHAPTER 12

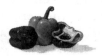

Using Herbs as Part of Your Diet

D irectly following are some descriptions of some of the most commonly used herbs on the market today. This represents a brief review of only a small sample of the herbs available for purchase. The reviews and statements made in the following section are meant to be informative and are not meant to diagnose, cure, prevent or treat any serious condition or disease. The information is accurate according to the best knowledge of the authors.

A great place to look for updated advice concerning herbs and herbal supplements is the *Nutrition Action Health* letter, which is funded by a nonprofit organization called the Center for Science in the Public Interest (www.cspnet.org). They publish a booklet on supplements that reviews current scientific information and products in a straightforward, easy to understand manner. And since they aren't actually trying to sell you anything but are just trying to inform you, they can be trusted more than most other sources.

Spice up Your Life

Many herbs that you find in your every day spice cabinets are not only flavorful, but they also have many health benefits. These herbs are normally used in very small amounts, just to add flavor to the food you eat. This is the exact same way that you can get the benefits from them. Larger amounts of some of these herbs may prove to be irritating. So, use those herbs, spice up your life with the many helpful phytochemicals from a large variety of flavorful plants.

Here is a list of some of the herbs that you might have in your cabinet and the benefits that may be associated with them (garlic, ginger and turmeric are studied in greater detail in the dietary herb section and the herbal glossary in Appendix C).

Allspice *(Calycanthus floridus/occidentali)*

Allspice contains a compound called pimentol that is an antioxidant comparable in power to vitamin E. It also contains chemicals that inhibit the growth of fungi.

Anise *(Illicium spp.)*

Anise also has been shown to inhibit the growth of fungi. Anise has also been shown to have antimicrobial effects, acting as a preservative, when used in other foods. Anise contains a substance called anisatin, which is an antagonist of receptors in the brain and has the potential to be toxic if enough is consumed. It also contains a molecule called safrole that is both toxic and mutagenic, but is destroyed during processing and cooking of the herb. Anise is related to basil.

Basil *(Ocimum gratissimum)*

Basil has been shown to have antimicrobial properties against several different strains of microbes.

Black Pepper *(Piper nigrum)*

Black pepper may have a protective effect on the colon against the development of cancers. It is able to decrease the activity of an enzyme called beta-glucuronidase, which is usually activated by carcinogens.

Black pepper contains compounds that can be irritating when inhaled to the point of potential serious health risk if inhaled in large amounts. Most people naturally sneeze to remove it from their airways. If it is able to penetrate in large amounts it causes edema in the tissues of the lung that may make it difficult to breathe. It can also irritate the lining of the stomach by removing the protective mucus lining and activating pain receptors. This is a good reason for consuming only moderate amounts of this herb. The chemical in black pepper that causes the burning sensation is called piperine and is able to produce partial desensitization, or lack of feeling.

It also contains a molecule called safrole that is both toxic and mutagenic, but is destroyed during processing and cooking of the herb. Raw black pepper has been shown to cause sister chromatid exchanges, so cooking it might be better.

Cayenne Pepper
(Capsicum annuum var. annum, group longum)

Cayenne pepper has been shown to effect cells in the intestine. Research has shown that it increases the permeability of membranes for ions and some sugars. Researchers suggest that it may be connected with food allergies. It also activates slow adapting chemoreceptors in the intestine.

Celery
(Apium australe, Apium filiforme, Apium graveolens)

Celery itself is more of a food, and can be consumed in greater amounts, celery seed is an herb consumed in smaller amounts. Celery contains a substance called lutein, which was shown in a very large study to be associated with decreased odds for developing colon cancer. Lutein is also found in spinach, broccoli, lettuce, tomatoes, oranges, carrots and other greens as well as celery. Rats that drank celery juice for eight weeks showed a decrease in serum cholesterol levels and an increase in bile acid secretion.

Chili Pepper/Red Pepper
(Capsicum annum L., Solanaceae)

Red pepper is able to decrease the activity of an enzyme called beta-glucuronidase, which is usually activated by carcinogens. This may have a protective effect on the colon against the development of cancers. A good reason for only consuming moderate amounts of this herb is that if you eat a lot it can also irritate the lining of the stomach by removing the protective mucus lining and activating pain receptors. The chemical that causes the burning sensation that is experienced by ingestion of red pepper is called capsaicin. The effects this chemical has on the nerves in your mouth can change how you experience other substances. The chemical causes almost complete desensitization or loss of feeling with the rapid application of a series of small doses.

Chives
(Allium ramosum, Allium schoenoprasum, Allium tuberosum)

This herb is closely related to garlic and onions. Along with garlic and onions, ingestion of this herb is associated with a decreased risk for esophageal and stomach cancers. It also seems to have weak antimutagenic properties. Chives and other green vegetables have been linked to a decreased risk for colon cancer.

Cinnamon *(Cinnamomum verum)*

Cinnamon contains a substance that may directly inhibit LPS bacterial endotoxin. Its antibacterial and anti aflatoxin properties have also been demonstrated.

Cloves *(Syzygium aromaticum L)*

Cloves have been shown to inhibit the growth of fungi. Cloves contain a molecule known as biflorin that is a good antioxidant. Cloves also contain a substance called eugenol, which has been shown to reduce oxidative damage in the liver caused by iron. It has also been indicated to reduce lipid peroxidation possibly by inhibiting the production of hydroxyl radicals and superoxide anion. Both eugenol and acetyl eugenol, another chemical in cloves, have been indicated to have blood-thinning capabilities that may be even more potent than aspirin. Eugenol has also been shown to reduce the mutation inducing oxidative damage caused by tobacco on *in vitro* cell lines. In human beings the oil of cloves was historically used as a local anesthetic. It is possible to overdose on clove oil, and the consequences can be serious resulting in coma, fits, clotting problems and liver damage. Eugenol given intravenously in larger concentrations has been indicated as a possible cause of noncardiogenic pulmonary edema in rats.

Coriander *(Coriandrum sativum)*

Coriander may have antibacterial activity against some food borne pathogens. It has also been indicated to decrease tissue cholesterol and triglycerides, decrease LDL and VLDL, increase HDL and increase the synthesis of bile acids in the liver. It appears to have the ability to promote the secretion of insulin and the incorporation of glucose into glycogen for energy storage. This indicates possible use in diabetics after further safety and efficacy tests are undertaken.

Cumin *(Cuminum cyminum)*

Cumin may protect against colon cancers. It is able to decrease the activity of an enzyme called beta-glucuronidase, which is usually activated by carcinogens. It also contains a molecule called safrole that is both toxic and mutagenic, but is destroyed during processing and cooking of the herb.

Fennel *(Foeniculum vulgare)*

Fennel has been indicated to inhibit pathogenic bacterial growth. Fennel has a drug interaction. It interferes with the plasma concentration, bioavailablity and urinary recovery of the antibiotic ciprofloxacin. These effects are possibly due to the rich metal cations present in fennel. The essential oils of fennel, rosemary and sage are able to cause convulsions if over used.

Fennel is a member of the Apiaceae family that also includes anise, celery, coriander and cumin. Allergies to one of these makes allergy to any of the others more likely.

Marjoram *(Origanum majorana)*

Marjoram contrasts from many other spices as it may possibly stimulate the growth of bacteria.

Nutmeg *(Myristica fragrans)*

Nutmeg has been repeatedly shown to be antibacterial. The substance in nutmeg that has this effect is called malabaricon C. The volatile oil in nutmeg is called myristicin and it can be present in toxic doses in about 5 grams of nutmeg. Tests have been done on rats, but rats aren't nearly as sensitive to the oil as humans are. This oil has the ability to weakly bind to DNA. Eating nutmeg in this large of an amount in a normal diet is highly improbable since it is usually used in very small and dilute amounts.

Oregano *(Origanum vulgare)*

Oregano and mint are both very effective antifungal agents in foods. Oregano is also an effective antibacterial agent. Thyme has been shown to be more effective. Both Oregano and Thyme contain a substance called carvacrol, an essential oil that kills bacteria by changing cell wall permeability for cations. The loss of cations leads to the bacteria cells death.

Oregano has also been indicated to have antioxidant and anticarcinogenic properties.

Paprika *(Capsicum annuum var. annuum)*

Paprika is rich in carotenoids, such as canthaxanthin, which are great antioxidants. Paprika contains a substance called capaicin that can cause bradycardia, or slow heart beats, a good reason why to use it as a spice and not a food.

Parsley *(Petroselinum crispum)*

This herb belongs to the Apiaceae family and is rich in flavonoids, cumarines and vitamin C, which may give it antioxidant properties when ingested.

Pimento *(Capsicum annuum var. annum, group grossum)*

Pimento was also shown to have antibiotic abilities against food borne pathogenic bacteria in experiments.

Rosemary *(Rosemarinus officinalis L.)*

Rosemary contains antioxidants that may have a antimutagenic, hepatoprotective effect according to a study that used rats as subjects. One of the antioxidants is called rosmarinic acid. This antioxidative ability has been shown in another study that showed that rosemary produced lower phospholipid hydroperoxides in red blood cells compared to that in control fed mice. Research done thus far indicates that rosemary does not help cell-mediated immunity. Ingestion of concentrated rosemary oil, which contains some very reactive substances, has the potential to lead to convulsions and other ill effects. It takes a lot of herb to make oil. It should be used as a flavoring herb, not as a food.

Sage *(Salvia officinalis)*

Sage contains a substance called rosmarinic acid, a polyphenol that may have protective antioxidant abilities.

Thyme *(Thymus vulgaris)*

Thyme was found to be by far the most effective herb against both gram-positive and gram-negative bacteria of all the herbs tested in a recent study.

Dietary and Common Herbs

Some herbs have a few Latin names that identify them specifically and are used more or less by different sectors of the world. Following sections contain more recent knowledge about the herb, it's functionality and efficacy, and the negative aspects and side effects associated with the use of the herb. Attention was given to the quality of research available for each of the supplements. These herbs and the medicinal herb section have more detailed information available in Appendix C. References are also available in the Appendix C.

Aloe Vera *(Aloe Barbadensis)*

Aloe vera is a succulent member of the lily family and has quite a few common names. It is known as Aloe, Barbados Aloe, Burn plant, Curacao aloe, Medicine plant, Mediterranean aloe, Saqal, and True Aloe.

Aloe vera is useful in treating minor burns and sunburns. It has two functions in the treatment of burns. First, it provides evaporative cooling and soothes the burn. Second, it helps to stimulate your body to begin the process of healing. Aloe vera seems helpful as an additive in many lotions, cosmetics and various skin products for various skin conditions including psoriasis. It is not helpful in the case of radiation therapy-induced skin discomfort.

Aloe vera should not be used on serious burns or on any cuts. It has not been shown to have strong antibiotic abilities. Also, ingestion of Aloe vera is not recommended. Although aloe vera has been shown to work effectively when ingested as a laxative, there is also a significant risk of kidney damage with long-term use. The outer portions of the plant tend to cause allergic reactions. Use of the plant should be restricted to the clear inner gel.

Chamomile

(Matricaria chamomilla/ Chamomilla recutita, Anthemis nobelis, Chamaemelum nobile)

Chamomile has several common names including: anthemis, garden chamomile, german chamomile, ground apple, matricary, pinheads, roman chamomile, and sweet false chamomile. Both species, German and English, are supposed to have the same effects.

Chamomile is usually used to help settle the stomach and relieve gastrointestinal discomfort. It is often used as an herbal tea. The scent is relaxing to some people. The plant may have mildly anti-inflammatory properties when applied topically. It may also help in healing wounds. It is a mild and safe herb. To date, there are no known side effects or contraindications, despite hundreds of years of use. Allergies to this plant occur and it is recommended that if you are allergic to members of the same family of plants you may wish to avoid using chamomile. Related plants include asters, chrysanthemum, dog fennel, may weed, pineapple weed and ragweed. If you experience any ill effects you should stop using the herb.

Cranberry *(Vaccinium macrocarpon)*

The cranberry has a few common names including: Bear berry, Bounce Berry, and Crane berry. Cranberry is thought to be a shortened version of the name Crane berry. Cranberries are very high in vitamin C.

Cranberries contain substances that make it more difficult for bacteria to stick to the wall of the bladder. Ingestion of cranberry products can help prevent and treat bladder infections when used in combination with antibiotics and other modern therapies. The berries do not have any known side effects and are often used as a food product in many different kinds of beverages, breads, cereals, jams, jellies, and sauces. As is true with any fruit, consumption of large amounts of cranberries can lead to diarrhea and intestinal discomfort. Cranberries are only used in a prevention or facilitative capacity. Urinary infections can lead to very serious problems if left untreated. People who have urinary infections should see a doctor.

Cranberries don't seem to work in a preventative manner for people suffering from bladder infections related to the condition of neurogenic bladder.

Blue berries and some other berries that are close relatives of cranberries have been shown to have the same helpful properties as cranberries.

Garlic (Allium Sativum)

Garlic is a member of the lily family. It is commonly used in many cultures as a seasoning or spice. Garlic seems to lower cholesterol levels and blood pressure, thus it may be helpful in preventing atherosclerosis. Unfortunately, as more interest has been focused on garlic in recent years, these claims have not yet been substantiated. Many claim garlic has mild antifungal and antimicrobial effects. Garlic may also serve to thin the blood. Early investigations have begun to determine if garlic may inhibit cancer cell growth but a lot more research remains. Garlic is a rich source of sulfur, an essential micromineral that is used in many of the systems of the body.

Eating garlic may also help prevent bug bites. Studies have shown that garlic applied topically works as an insect repellent. Most people probably wouldn't actually do this because of the smell but, interestingly, if you eat garlic the chemicals enter your body and eventually some will exit through sweat glands in your skin. This would, of course, make your skin taste like garlic and may make it less appetizing to bugs. Mother's milk also takes on the flavor of garlic consumed in the diet.

If your garlic supplement doesn't have the characteristic odor, it probably lacks allicin, the effective element of garlic, and is of questionable value. People who are taking blood thinners like aspirin or warfarin should avoid using large amounts of garlic as it may have an additive effect leading to bleeding disorders. Garlic oil can be irritating to mucus membranes. Keep this in mind when cooking with garlic.

Ginger (Zingiber Officinalis)

Common ginger is known by a few other names: Asian ginger, Canton ginger and culinary ginger. Ginger may lower cholesterol levels when used in combination with garlic. The combined effect of garlic and ginger is supposed to be greater than garlic alone. It also seems to act as a blood thinner. However, as with garlic, further research is needed to substantiate some of these claims.

Ginger does appear to be useful in reducing the severity of nausea caused by seasickness. It also appears to be able to speed up the motility of the digestive system when it has been slowed down chemically. Whether faster gastric motility is generated in a normal system and whether faster movement would be good or not is disputable.

Ginger contains some compounds that are strong antioxidants. It also appears to be an anti-inflammatory. Ginger is a safe herb and is often used as a food item. Many oriental and western dishes contain ginger, from sweet and sour pork to ginger snaps and pumpkin pie. People taking anticoagulants, pregnant women, and people with gallbladder disease should avoid taking high concentrations of ginger.

Tea *(Camellia Sinensis/Thea sinensis/Camellia thea)*

This is the same tea that the Chinese have been drinking for thousands of years. It has become quite popular with the rest of the world in the last few hundred of years. As a beverage it is second only to water in consumption around the world. It apparently has some great health benefits associated with it. Tea has been shown to contain powerful antioxidants that may prove useful in controlling inflammation, atherosclerosis and heart disease. Huge observational studies have indicated that regular consumption of tea is connected to a reduced risk of stroke, cancer and heart disease. These are observations and the actual results could have something to do with other habits of tea drinkers as well as the tea itself.

Tea has been mentioned as a source of dietary fluoride, but it really doesn't contain enough to be useful. It would take over 30 cups of tea to supply a 133-pound adult female with enough fluoride to meet her RDA.

Tea that is not decaffeinated contains appreciable amounts of caffeine, though not as much as coffee. Caffeine can become addicting, and has even been a drug of abuse on occasions.

Caffeine has been shown to interfere with natural sleep in children, reducing the amount of time they spend in bed. Caffeine is a stimulant that causes the heart to beat harder. Caffeine together with tannins, other chemicals in tea that have vasoconstricting effects, result in a brief rise in blood pressure after tea consumption. People with high blood pressure may be better off avoiding caffeine consumption.

Caffeine can also interfere with the function of other drugs. This has been demonstrated for some psychological drugs. Pregnant women should not consume caffeine, or women planning on becoming pregnant who are also using the antiepileptic drug Phenobarbital. When the two substances are used together the result is an increased risk for serious congenital birth defects. Nursing mothers should also avoid consuming caffeine.

Caffeine alone seems to be detrimental to fetal development and infant health in controlled animal experiments. Older people should also avoid caffeine consumption as caffeine may also contribute to fragile bones in the elderly. You should always consult your doctor or pharmacist before consuming caffeine containing foods or drinks with medications. It would be a better idea to drink decaffeinated tea products to avoid these negative effects.

People who drink tea at high temperatures are at higher risk for esophageal cancer. In order to avoid this problem tea drinkers should drink their tea warm or iced instead of hot.

Turmeric *(Curcuma longa)*

Turmeric is a commonly used spice that is native to India. It is an ingredient in many food dishes. Turmeric contains a chemical with strong antioxidant abilities called curcumin, which has been indicated to have anticarcinogenic properties as well. It seems to be able to induce apoptosis, or programmed cell death, in many different cancer cell lines. More research remains to be done to verify these results.

The antioxidant effects may also function to protect the liver from damage. Turmeric appears to be completely safe when eaten in reasonable amounts. Excess amounts may have undesirable effects.

Medicinal and Exotic Herbs

Black Cohosh *(Cimicafuga racemosa or Actaea racemosa)*

Black cohosh has many common names including: Actaea, baneberry, bugbane, black snakeroot, bugwort, Cimicifuga, cohosh, rattle root, rattle weed, and squawroot. Cimicifuga means "to drive away", and is related to the name bugbane, which refers to the plants use as a bug repellant. The plant is often wild crafted and may face pressure in the wild due to difficulties in domestic cultivation.

Black cohosh contains phytoestrogens, plant derived chemicals that resemble human estrogens in structure or function. These phytoestrogens have been shown to bind to estrogen receptors. Black cohosh is useful in the treatment of the hot flashes of menopause, working in some of the same fashions as estrogen therapy. It is unknown if it has some of the other benefits and/or drawbacks of estrogen therapy, but research has been promising.

Premenopausal women and pregnant or nursing mothers should not take black cohosh. It may interfere with the menstrual cycle and normal development. Unlike other herbs, there is evidence that black cohosh could be a factor in some reproductive problems. Never take Black cohosh if you think you might be pregnant.

Side effects of Black cohosh include abdominal pain, changed heart rate, dizziness, nausea, seizure, and headache. There are other possible side effects and this herb is thought to have a sedative effect. It should not be taken for long continuous periods of time.

Chaste Tree Berry *(Vitex agnus castus)*

The chaste tree berry has several common names including Abraham's balm, agnus castus, chaste tree, hemp tree, monk's pepper tree, monk's tree, and safe tree.Chaste tree berry may be useful in the treatment of premenstrual syndromes due to its ability to reduce PMS symptoms. Studies have indicated that it has an influence on the receptors for dopamine resulting in an increase of two reproductive hormones, LH and FSH. Studies have also indicated that use of this herb results in the reduction of premenstrual syndrome symptoms.

Side effects include abdominal discomfort and headache. Allergic rashes are not entirely uncommon. If allergies or negative effects occur, stop taking this herb immediately.

One study has connected chaste tree berry with abnormal ovulations, but such a connection has not been proven conclusively. It is probably wise to avoid or at least be cautious in the use of this herb if you are pregnant or planning to become pregnant because the true effects of chaste tree in these situations are not yet known. Also use caution with this herb if you are on hormone therapy.

Echinacea *(Echinacea angustifolia/purpurea/pallida)*

Echinacea also goes by other names: black sampson, indian head, narleaf purple, purple cone, red sunflower, or snake root.

This herb is often used as an immunostimulant. It is supposed to help in the treatment of colds and flues. There are few good efficacy studies done on this herb. One thing appears fairly certain: echinacea will not prevent either a cold or flu. Studies indicate the herb may be helpful when taken at the onset of symptoms in reducing the length and severity of illness. People who used echinacea beginning at the onset of symptoms recovered faster and did not feel as sick as those who did not take it. Studies on this herb are encouraging; however, more research is needed to solidify its worth. We also know little about this herb's long-term effects, so it's still a good idea to be careful how you use it.

Long-term use of echinacea has also been connected to liver damage. People with liver damage should avoid using echinacea. This is an herb that should only be used for a short term.

Echinacea side effects occur rarely and include fever, nausea and vomiting. Consult your physician before taking this herb in conjunction with any medications. Also, pregnant or nursing mothers and small children should use caution with echinacea because science still has some to learn.

Feverfew
(Tanacetum Parthnium, Chrysanthemum parthenium)

Feverfew is also known by a few common names: manzanilla, featherfew, featherfoil, and febrifuge plant.

Feverfew has gained popularity in the treatment and prevention of migrane headaches. Feverfew contains substances that act as cyclo-oxygenase inhibitors. An example of a cyclo-oxygenase inhibitor is aspirin. These chemicals probably use the same pathways to reduce headache pain. Feverfew also contains a flavonoid named tanetin or santin that seems to have anti-inflammatory effects. This substance in combination with the cyclo-oxygenase may make feverfew helpful for painful inflammatory conditions such as arthritis.

Feverfew has a few side effects. It may cause drowsiness. If the raw herb is ingested, it may irritate mucus membranes in the mouth leading to oral ulcers and mouth sores. Allergies to feverfew are also not uncommon. As always, we advise caution to pregnant and breastfeeding mothers using this herb. Unborn and newborn children are very sensitive and should be handled with care when it comes to herbs.

Ginkgo Biloba

This giant among herbs is also known as the maidenhair tree. It is a full sized deciduous tree that is beginning to be common in landscaping. *Ginkgo biloba* contains substances that thin the blood and improve circulation. It apparently does this by interfering with clotting factors. *Ginkgo biloba* seems to be helpful for people suffering from circulation abnormalities. Research indicates that gingko may be helpful in treating Alzheimer's disease, stroke, and depression caused by cerebral blood flow insufficiencies. The gingko leaves contain a powerful antioxidant.

The leaves are the part of the plant used as an herb. The fruit flesh contains a toxin that resembles vitamin B6 and interferes with the real vitamin's functions. It causes symptoms of vitamin deficiency. The main symptom of intoxication is convulsions, though it can cause death. Do not consume seed flesh. The nut within the fruit is often roasted and eaten.

Side effects are rare though it has been reported to cause mild gastrointestinal discomfort, headache, dizziness, rashes, burning eyes, breathlessness, nausea, and vomiting when taken in high doses. The most serious side effect is spontaneous bleeding. There have been several cases of bleeding connected with combinations of *Ginkgo biloba* and other prescription or over the counter blood thinners such as warfarin or aspirin. Ginkgo should never be taken with other blood thinning drugs or herbs.

Ginseng, American *(Panax quinquefolius)*

American ginseng may increase endurance and energy. Some research has been done but much more remains to be done to test these claims. Some claim American ginseng helps curtail stress. As with other claims, there is an absence of current, significant research on American ginseng's effect on stress, if it has one.

American ginseng contains a powerful antioxidant that may be helpful in controlling oxidation. It also contains a molecule that appears to have antifungal properties. The same molecule seems to have the ability to inhibit an enzyme called reverse transcriptase, an enzyme that is specific to retroviruses such as HIV. All of these effects were demonstrated outside of living systems. In order to see if it is safe in living systems, it needs to be tested further to see if it is effective.

There are no known side effects linked to American ginseng. So far research has not found any evidence that excessive doses are toxic, but science has not done enough research to say they are. In normal doses, this herb should be safe for regular consumption.

This herb is often wild crafted and is experiencing a great deal of pressure in the wild. Ginseng is protected by law in some states. In North Carolina, digging up someone else's ginseng from a fenced bed is a felony offense. It has been successfully cultivated and need not be harvested in the wild. Again, we urge you not to support decimation of wild herbs by purchasing products from companies that do not threaten wild populations.

Ginseng, Korean *(Panax ginseng)*

This is the original ginseng used in oriental medicine for thousands of years. This herb is supposed to help increase endurance and energy while reducing stress. Research done so far has not substantiated these claims. In fact, current research has indicated that ginseng may not be as effective as once thought in increasing the ability of muscles to perform work.

There have been a few experiments looking at the psychological effects of ginseng on animals. Ginseng tends to reduce aggression in mice. More recently, researchers have found that when ginseng components are separated, some tend to calm animals while others tend to increase excitability and aggression. When test animals were placed under stress they tended to react abnormally after eating ginseng. Ginseng supplemented animals tend to "freeze up" and be less inquisitive about their environment.

Upon scientific study, long-term ginseng supplementation seems to have no influence on life span or weight. Korean ginseng also appears to have little on cholesterol or lipid levels in the blood and may not reduce the risk of atherosclerosis. Ginseng apparently contains a very potent antioxidant that may help prevent oxidative damage occurring as a result of physical stress. It also contains compounds that may have anticarcinogenic properties. It may have an ability to reduce blood sugar levels. It might also cause vascular relaxation, and blood thinning: possibly resulting in decreased blood pressure. Researchers hope to find a chemical in ginseng that may prove to be helpful in treating impotence.

Side effects are few and include headache and changes in blood pressure when taken in large doses. Because of its effect on blood pressure, you should use caution in taking Korean ginseng with other blood thinning agents, or by people who have problems with blood pressure, blood clotting, heart problems, hypoglycemia, or insulin-dependant diabetes. Avoid taking ginseng for longer than three months. Pregnant women should avoid taking ginseng because it has been linked to a three-fold increased risk in developing gestational diabetes. Nursing mothers and small children should also avoid ginseng.

Ginseng, Siberian
(Eleutherococcus senticosus, Acanthopanax senticosis)

This plant is distantly related to the true ginsengs mentioned above. It is not a true ginseng. It is known by several common names including: ciwujia, devil's bush, touch-me-not (do not confuse with impatiens), and Ussurian thorny pepperbush.

There is very little information available on the function of this herb. What research has been done is fairly inconclusive. So far it appears to be ineffective in increasing physical or psychological performance.

It appears to have side effects including stomach irritation and diarrhea. It also should not be taken with the prescription drug digoxin. Always consult your physician or pharmacist about taking this herb with medications.

Goldenseal *(Hydrastis canadensis)*

Goldenseal belongs to the buttercup family and has several common names including: eye balm, eye root, ground raspberry, hydrastis, indian plant, jaundice root, orange root, turmeric root, yellow eye, yellow indian paint, yellow paint, yellow puccon, yellow root and wild turmeric.

Externally and internally, goldenseal may have antibiotic or bacteriostatic abilities. This may be due to a substance called berberine. However, berberine occurs in highly variable amounts, making it very important that this herb is standardized. It also appears to have anti-inflammatory abilities and possibly anticarcinogenic abilities. In a single study, goldenseal seemed to have a stimulating effect on the immune response. Much more research is necessary to substantiate these effects.

Some herbal companies claim that goldenseal can help lessen the symptoms of diabetes. Research has shown that goldenseal cannot modify the main causes of diabetes: low functional insulin levels and high blood glucose. It is not legal to make this claim, which is a disease claim, without FDA approval. Nonetheless, you may find some companies making the claim. Diabetes is a serious disease, and herbal supplementation cannot take the place of conventional and proven therapies.

Unfortunately, berberine seems to be an inhibitor of an enzyme called NADH oxidase, which functions in the electron transport system making energy. Even very small concentrations of goldenseal were inhibitory. This pathway of inhibition is not unlike the effect of the chemical arsenic, a commonly recognized poison. Goldenseal has also been connected to reports of damaged internal organs. It should never be taken for long periods of time if one chooses to take it internally at all. Ingestion of the raw herb may cause irritation of the mucus membranes. Pregnant women should avoid it because it has been connected to miscarriages and other negative results. It should not be given to nursing women or children.

It appears to work as a depressant and has been connected to hypertension, convulsions, cardiovascular malfunction, and CNS damage. Some of these negative effects are backed up by science, and some are not. However, the negative effects that are backed up by science are serious enough to doubt the wisdom in using the plant for purposes that have yet to be substantiated in scientific research.

Goldenseal is harvested mostly from wild crafted sources and is protected as a threatened or endangered species in some areas. In fact, harvesting goldenseal in some states could cost harvesters a heavy fine or even jail time. Some herbal companies have begun to cultivate this herb in an effort to preserve wild stock. If you do decide to buy it, check and see if the company you buy from can certify that the herbal extract they sell is not from diminishing wild populations.

Hawthorn *(Crataegus spp.)*

Hawthorn also goes by several other common names including: bread and cheese tree, gazels, hagthorn, halves, haw, hazels, hedgethorn, holy thorn, ladies meat, may tree, mayblossom, quickset, thorn, and whitethorn.

The hawthorn fruit is rich in vitamins and pigments. Hawthorn seems to modify cardiac output, or heart rate and the amount of blood pumped, but varying studies contradict one another, preventing any strong claims from being substantiated. Some experiments claim hawthorn extracts cause an increase in heart muscle contractility and heart rate, resulting in increased cardiac output. Other experiments claim hawthorn caused increased contractility, but decreased heart rate, leading to decreased cardiac output. Until some clear information becomes available we cannot recommend it as a supplement, especially to people who suffer from a disease as serious as heart disease.

Side effects are rare and may include: abdominal discomfort, facial pain and tachycardia or increased heart rate.

Milk Thistle *(Silybum marianum)*

This prickly plant has become most famous for a purported ability to protect and detoxify the kidney and liver. Milk thistle contains several substances that are collectively called silymarin. Some of these substances are powerful antioxidants and have been shown to have protective effects for the kidney, liver and pancreas when they are exposed to various toxins. Chemically induced damage, such as from alcohol, is reduced in animals that are supplemented with milk thistle. Other studies have also shown that, although it reduces damage, it cannot overcome or prevent damage to organs that are constantly accosted with toxins. The toxins retain the overriding effect. People shouldn't count on milk thistle's antioxidants to save them from the consequences of an alcoholic or otherwise abusive substance lifestyle.

These same antioxidant chemicals in milk thistle have anticarcinogenic properties just as many other antioxidants. They may reduce the incidence of chemically induced prostate, breast, and cervical cancers. They can also reduce the chance of developing skin cancers when applied topically.

As is true with all plants, milk thistle can cause allergic reactions in some people. If you experience rashes, nausea, tight throat or any other negative symptom, it may be best to stop taking the herb. Milk thistle may cause diarrhea, gas and upset stomach. It should only be taken in recommended amounts.

Saw Palmetto
(Serenoa serrulata, Serenoa repens, Sabal serulta)

Saw Palmetto is known by a few other common names including: dwarf palmetto, fan palm, palmetto scrub, and sabal.

Saw palmetto has gained renown in the world for its apparent effect on benign prostatic hyperplasia (BPH), also known as enlargement of the prostate gland. Saw palmetto apparently stops the prostate from enlarging and improves urinary parameters. It has not been shown to cause any actual regression of prostatic growth except for in a transition epithelial area. In the research done this far saw palmetto has out-performed placebos consistently. This herb has begun to generate a great deal of excitement in the urinary pathology field. Scientific support is growing for its use. More studies are on the way.

The berries are used for medicinal purposes. Most saw palmetto in the market today is wild crafted though it can't exactly be called rare. Until recently it was considered a pest plant. Cultivation of the plants has been attempted several times, without tremendous success. The plants often grow but are not near as productive as wild growing strands, if producing fruit at all. The pressure on wild populations is becoming intense. More research is being conducted to try to find ways to cultivate productive plants.

The only known side effect, gastrointestinal discomfort, occurs rarely. If you think you have enlargement of the prostate gland and experience discomfort, consult a doctor immediately. Although saw palmetto may help, BPH is a serious condition that should be monitored by a physician. BPH can be life threatening if it worsens enough to interfere with proper urine flow, leading to irreversible kidney damage.

Saw palmetto is an herb that is specifically for the use of men. There is no data showing any benefits to women. Although it is an herb with low side effects and low toxicity, women, whom don't have prostate glands, seem to have no need for it. Women who could be or are pregnant or nursing should avoid ingesting saw palmetto. It is unknown what effect it could have on fetal development or infant growth.

St. John's Wort *(Hypericum perforatum)*

St. John's wort is known by a few common names: hard hay, hypericum, klamath weed, and St. Johnny's wort.

St. John's wort has been heavily researched and used in Germany. Rigorous tests indicate that St. John's wort seems to be effective in treating symptoms of mild depression. Please note that to date it has only been used to treat mild depression. Its effectiveness has not been determined in serious depression. Serious depression is considered life threatening. If you experience symptoms of serious depression consult a qualified professional.

St. John's wort may have antibacterial abilities when applied externally. However, it is not effective against all bacteria and care should be taken because it may cause an allergic rash.

St. John's wort contains a chemical that seemed promising in inactivating the HIV virus. This chemical is a photodynamic pigment named hypericin. The chemical requires light in order to inactivate the virus. Unfortunately light reactions cause changes in the chemical structure that can inflict damage to healthy living tissue. Researchers hoped to balance this negative effect by balancing dosage and viral kill with cytotoxicity. Many different doses have been tested. Even large doses, which made subjects extremely sick, did not induce a detectable change in viral load. Thus far, researchers have concluded that the molecule is too toxic to be used in the amounts necessary to inactivate the virus in living systems.

238 / POWER PLANTS

Research has also attempted to use hypericin to inactivate HIV in donated blood. If a way could be found to use hypericin to inactivate HIV in blood, then remove the hypericin before the blood is transfused so it wouldn't be toxic to the recipient, it would be easier to provide virus free blood transfusions. Unfortunately the HIV virus required such large concentrations of hypericin to destroy the virus that it also destroyed the blood cells, making the blood useless. Hypericin was more promising in treating more susceptible animal viruses such as bovine viral diarrhea virus, which is similar to human hepatitis C.

Current research is ongoing about whether hypericin may be used to make cancer cells more susceptible to radiation therapy and/or help induce apoptosis of cancer cells. This enters the field of medicinal and medical drug use. It may prove useful in this area, not as an herb, but as a refined drug. Precise dosage and professional monitoring will accompany this research that may also have associated dangers.

When used in recommended amounts, side effects are fairly rare and include: allergic reactions, dry mouth, confusion, dizziness, fatique, gastrointestinal discomfort, nervousness, and sensitivity to light.

There are quite a few drugs that St. John's wort should not be taken with. In fact St. John's wort is one of the only herbs on which the FDA has published a public health advisory about the problem of drug interactions. St. John's wort has been shown to interfere with the effectiveness of the anti-HIV drug indinavir. Other drugs operating along the same pathways may be influenced. These include: oral contraceptives, heart medications, antidepressants, antiseizure medications, cancer medications, and the medication cyclosporine (which is used to prevent organ transplant rejection). St. John's wort may make these drugs less effective and should not be used in conjunction with them. This is definitely enough reason to consult your physician or pharmacist about drug interactions before taking this herb with any current medications.

Large doses of this herb can lead to photosensitivity, a response that was noted among the human subjects in the HIV study mentioned above. Using large amounts of the herb is not advisable without qualified medical counsel. Doses should not exceed 900 mg/day.

Valerian *(Valeriana officinalis)*

Valerian is also known by several common names including: American valerian, all-heal, Capon's tail, common valerian, English valerian, fragrant valerian, garden heliotrope, phu, setewale, stink root, St. George's herb, and vandal root.

Valerian has come to be used as a sedative. There really isn't a lot of research on valerian but what is out there indicates that it does have a sedative effect and may help some people sleep. More research is definitely warranted.

Valerian may have cytotoxic effects, causing liver damage if used for long periods of time. If you have liver disease you should avoid taking valerian. Valerian is believed to be a hypnotic drug and should not be used for long periods of time so as to avoid dependence and withdrawal problems. Be aware that due to the sedative nature of this herb it may increase reaction time and should not be taken before driving or operating heavy equipment.

Chinese Herbs

The Chinese have paid more attention to herbal uses over the course of time than any other culture. With thousands of years of documented medicinal herb use, the Chinese now have a very large collection of plants with ascribed medicinal purposes. In fact some of the herbs mentioned in the herbal section of this book are of Chinese origin (ginseng, ginkgo etc.). These and other plants have been used for medicinal purposes for hundreds or even thousands of years in some cases. Some of them may be valuable medical tools. Some are probably more dangerous than helpful. Some of them are probably prime examples of how long herbs can continue being used when they are nothing more than fancy placebos.

There are literally hundreds of Chinese herbs, and they are often used in combinations. Very little information is available to us at this time to ascertain the safety or efficacy of most of these herbs.

There is danger in the use of many Chinese herbal preparations because the ingredients are often of unknown origin, quality, and function. There have been many problems associated with misidentification of one herb for another due to name confusion or other errors. The herbs that are best known are often those that have negative effects. Following are a few of the best-studied

Chinese herbs outside of those in the herbal section. It is wise to know what these herbs are so if you see them on a label you can know to use caution in using them.

Ephedra *(Ma Huang, Ephedra sinica, Ephedra antisyphilitica)*

This short evergreen shrub from northern china is an herb that has been the topic of much discussion in the herbal and legal world recently. There has been considerable debate and controversy over ephedra in recent years. The chemical in this herb is known as ephedrine. Ephedrine has been used as an over the counter bronchodialator in the past. A bronchodialator is a type of drug used to widen the airways for asthmatics. In fact this is the same purpose for which this herb was used for a long period of time in Chinese medicine. It is a legitimate medicinal use, though whether or not it should be available with out a prescription has been an argument for some time.

The first current hot topic concerning Chinese ephedra is it's relatively modern use for increasing energy, performance, and helping with weight loss. This is not known to be a traditional use of the herb. Because of the numerous and eager clientele that can be accumulated in the weight loss industry, there has been a drastic increase in the use and misuse of this herb, though the scientific evidence for its efficacy is lacking. Even when this herb was being used as a bronchodialator there were reports of severe side effects and even deaths in people who used the herb frequently or excessively. Even more concern has been generated over uses of ephedra and the health of consumers who are taking it.

The drug ephedrine has powerful effects on the body as a stimulant. It is said to have similar effects to the common and dangerous street drug methamphetamine, also known simply as meth. In fact, more concentrated versions of this herb have been chosen by many thrill seekers as a legal drug of abuse in substitution for illegal drugs. It may be combined with other stimulants to increase its effects. This tendency to use ephedra for psychostimulation and abuse is reflected in some of the product names under which Ephedra products are being marketed. Such names include Herbal Ecstasy and Ulitmate Xphoria.

Use and abuse of ephedra and ephedrine products have been tightly linked to many deaths. It is also often mixed with other drugs and stimulants, such as caffeine (kola nut), in efforts to get more intense stimulatory results. This often serves to worsen the situation and intensify the risk. Because of the capacity for abuse, accidental overuse, and dangerous side effects, many states have begun regulating ephedra. Until recently, even warning labels were not required or included on many products containing ephedra. Some still do not carry warning labels. The regulations on this herb were still largely undecided at the writing of this book.

Ephedra's side effects are serious and not altogether uncommon. In the state of Texas alone the health department reported over 1,400 adverse effects and injuries relating to ephedra and ephedrine associated products between 1993 and 1999. One ephedra/kola nut product generated over one hundred reports of adverse effects in a single year.

The side effects cover an alarming range with the mildest effects being nausea, headache, tremor, psychosis, and irregular heartbeats. More serious side effects including hepatitis, heart attack, high blood pressure, stroke, seizures, and even death. Different people have highly variable sensitivities to the herb. Oddly enough, one side effect mentioned was fatigue. People coming down from ephedra highs often feel tired as the herb's effects wear off. References to this herb as being equal to weight loss drugs or, presumably, any other drugs, are considered drug claims by the FDA and are not legal.

In response to serious illnesses and injuries, including multiple deaths, associated with the use of dietary supplement products that contain ephedrine alkaloids" the FDA recommends the following guidelines:

- Doses as high as 8 mg in a six-hour period or 24 mg of ephedrine alkaloids in a twenty-four-hour period should be avoided.
- Don't use ephedrine containing products for longer than seven days.
- Don't use ephedrine products with other stimulants such as caffeine or yohimbe.
- Our recommendations would be to avoid using this product without consulting a qualified physician first for direction.

Dong Quai
(Angelica sinensis; aka Dang Gui, Angelica Root)

Dong quai is usually used to relieve menopausal symptoms. It is said to contain phytoestrogens. Very little scientific information has been collected on the efficacy of this herb, but the studies that do exist are generally negative. Given the current information it is unlikely that this herb is useful for this purpose.

In a well-designed, double-blind, randomized, placebo controlled trial, seventy-one post menopausal women were treated with Dong quai or a placebo for twenty-four weeks. Using standard measures of uterine, vaginal and menopausal symptoms the researchers concluded that Dong quai did not have estrogen like responses in tissue and did not help relieve menopausal symptoms.

The second study reported that Dong quai was phototoxic, carcinogenic, and antiarrhythmic. It is also anticlotting and has been implicated in interactions with the blood thinning drug warfarin.

Dong quai should not be taken with blood thinning medications as bleeding disorders may result. Pregnant women or small children should not take dong quai.

Guang Fang Ji
(aka snakeroot, guaco, aristolochia fangchi, aristolochia spp.)

These herbs are often used for weight loss, and seem to be going the same direction as many of the recent diet fads: a dangerous one. Aristolochia fangchi has been connected to over one hundred cases of kidney damage and at least 18 cancers of the urinary tract from a single incident of herbal misidentification that took place in a Belgium weight loss clinic in 1992–3. Patients were accidentally given Aristolochia fangchi instead of another herb named Stephania tetrandra. Since then several other incidences of organ damage have been connected with this herb in England and France.

Many members of the Aristolochia family contain a substance called aristolochic acid. Aristolochic acid leads to a particular type of kidney damage in humans. Oddly enough it doesn't appear to have this effect in rats. The herb causes fibrosis, or the accumulation of connective tissue, in the cortex of the kidneys. This kind of fibrotic kidney damage only occurs as a result of taking these herbs and has been named Chinese-herb nephropathy. It is a serious problem, many of the above-mentioned cases required kidney transplants in order to prevent death.

Aristolochic acid is also a potent carcinogen. In a study published by *The New England Journal of Medicine* the urinary tracts of patient's whom were being seen for Chinese-herb nephropathy were checked for cancer. Of the thirty-nine who underwent surgery, eighteen, or forty-six percent, had cancer in the epithelium of their urinary tract. Another study of patients with Chinese-herb nephropathy found cancer in 40 percent of participants. Most of the remaining patients had abnormal epithelium that was not yet cancerous. Aristolochic acid is a potent carcinogen in mice as well as humans. In rats renal lesions developed in response to aristolochic acid within three days of a single dose. It appears to cause carcinogenesis through activation by cytochrome P450 producing carcinogenic byproducts.

Spice References

Adlova GP, et al. The Development of Bacterial Growth Stimulants from Plants. Zh Mikrobiol Epidemiol Immunobiol. Jan-Feb 1998. (1): 13–7.

al-Sereiti MR, Abu-Amer KM, Sen P. Pharmacology of Rosemary (Rosmarinus officinalis Linn.) and its Therapeutic Potentials. Indian-J-Exp-Biol. 1999 Feb; 37(2): 124–30.

Azumi S, Tanimura A, Tanamoto K. A Novel Inhibitor of Bacterial Endotoxin Derived from Cinnamon Bark. Biochem Biophys Res Commun. 1997. 234(2): 506–10.

Babu US, Wiesenfeld PL, Jenkins MT. Effect of Dietary Rosemary on Cell-Mediated Immunity of Young Rats. Plant Foods Hum Nutr. 1999. 53(2): 169–74.

Bartine H, Tantaoui-Elaraki EA. 1997. Growth and Toxigenesis of Aspergillus flavus Isolates on Selected Spices. J Environ Pathol Toxicol Oncol. 16(1): 61–5.

Basilico MZ, Basilico JC. Inhibitory Effects of Some Spice Essential Oils on Aspergillus Ochraceus NRRL 3174 Growth and Ochratoxin A Production. Lett Appl Microbiol. 1999. 29(4): 238–41.

Burkhard PR, Burkhardt K, Haenggeli CA, Landis T. Plant-Induced Seizures: Reappearance of an Old Problem. J Neurol. 1999. 246(8): 667–70.

Chithra V, Leelamma S. Hypolipidemic Effect of Coriander Seeds (Coriandrum sativum): Mechanism of Action. Plant Foods Hum Nutr. 1997. 51(2): 167–72.

Clarke GD, Davison JS. Mucosal Receptors in the Gastric Antrum and Small Intestine of the Rat with Afferent Fibres in the Cervical Vagus. J Physiol Lind. 1978. 284:55–67.

Dessirier JM, O'Mahony M, Carstens E. Oral Irritant Effects of Nicotine. Psychophysical Evidence for Decreased Sensation Following Repeated Application of and Lack of Cross-Desensitization to Capsaicin. Ann N Y Acad Sci. 1998. 855:828–30.

Dorman HJD, Deans SG. Antimicrobial Agents From Plants: Antibacterial Activity of Plant Volatile Oils. Journal of Applied Microbiology. 2000. 88:308–16.

Ejechi BC, Souzey JA, Akpomedaye DE. Microbial Stability of Mango (Mangifera indica L.) Juice Preserved by Combined Application of Mild Heast and Extracts of Two Tropical Spices. J Food Prot. 1998. 61(6): 725–7.

Fahim FA, Esmat AY, Fadel HM, Hassan KF. Allied Studies on the Effect of Rosmarinus Officinalis L. on Experimental Hepatotoxicity and Mutagenesis. Int J Food Sci Nutr. 1999. 50(6):413–27.

Farag SD, Abo-Zeid M. Degradation of the Natural Mutagenic Compound Safrole in Spices By Cooking and Irradiation. Nahrung. 1997. 41(6): 359–61.

Fejes S, et al. Investigation of the in Vitro Antioxidant Effect of Petroselinum Crispum (Mill) Nym. Ex A.W. Hill. Acta Pharm Hung. 1998. 68(3):150–6.

Fyfe L, Armstrong F, Stewart J. Inhibition of Listeria Monocytogenes and Salmonella Enteriditis By Combinations of Plant Oils and Derivatives of Benzoic Acid: The Development of Synergistic Antimicrobial Combinations. Int J Antimicrob Agents. 1997. 9(3): 195–9.

Gao CM, et al. Protective Effect of Allium Vegetables Against Both Esophageal and Stomach Cancer: A Simultaneous Case-Referent Study of a High-Epidemic Area in Jiangsu Province, China. Jpn J Cancer Res. 1999. 90(6): 614–21.

Gonzalez de Mejia E, Loarca PG, Ramos GM. Antimutagenicity of Xanthophylls Present in Aztec Marigold (Tagetes erecta) Against 1-Nitropyrene. Mutat Res. 1997. 389(2–3): 219–26.

Gray AM, Flatt PR. Insulin-Releasing and Insulin-like Activity of the Traditional Anti-Diabetic Plant Coriandrum Sativum (coriander). Br J Nutr. 1999. 81(3): 203–9.

Gulbransen G, Esernio-Jenssen D. Aspiration of Black Mustard. J Toxicol Clin Toxicol. 1998. 36(6): 591–3.

Hallstrom H, Thuvander A. Toxicological Evaluation of Myristicin. Nat Toxins. 1997. 5(5): 186–92.

Hammer KA, Carson CF, Riley TV. Antimicrobial Activity of Essential Oils and Other Plant Extracts. J Appl Microbiol. 1999. 86(6): 985–90.

Hao YY, Brackett RE, Doyle MP. Inhibition of Listeria Monocytogenes and Aeromonas Hydrophila by Plant Extracts in Refrigerated Cooked Beef. J Food Prot. 1998. 61(3): 307–12.

Hartnoll G, Moore D, Douek D. Near Fatal Ingestion of Oil of Cloves. Arch Dis Child. 1993. 69(3): 392–3.

Hitokoto H, et al. Inhibitory Effects of Spices on Growth and Toxin Production of Toxigenic fungi. Appl Environ Microbiol. 1980. 39(4): 818–22.

Hu JF, et al. Diet and Cancer of the Colon and Rectum: A Case-Control Study in China. Int J Epidemiol. 1991. 20(2): 362–7.

Ilori M, et al. Antidiarrhoeal Activities of Ocimum Gratissium (Lamiaceae). J Diarrhoeal Dis Res. 1996. 14(4): 283–5.

Jensen JE, et al. Hot Spices Influence Permeability of Human Intestinal Epithelial Monolayers. J Nutr. 1998. 128(3): 577–81.

Kakemoto E, et al. Interaction of Anisatin with Rat Brain Gamma-Aminobutyric AcidA Receptors: Allosteric Modulation by Competitive Antagonists. Biochem Pharmacol. 1999. 58(4): 617–21.

Kawaguchi AT, et al. Afferent Reinnervation After Lung Transplantation in the Rat. J Heart Lung Transplant. 1998. 17(4): 341–8.

Lachowicz KJ, et al. The Synergistic Preservative Effects of the Essential Oils of Sweet Basil (Ocimum basilicum L.) Against Acid-Tolerant Food Microflora. Lett Appl Microbiol. 1998. 26(3): 209–14.

Lagouri V, Boskou D. Nutrient Antioxidants in Oregano. Int J Food Sci Nutr. 1996. 47(6): 493–7.

Lichtenberger LM, et al. Effect of Pepper and Bismuth Subsalicylate on Gastric Pain and Surface Hydrophobicity in the Rat. Aliment Pharmacol Ther. 1998. 12(5): 483–90.

Liu L, Simon SA. Similarities and Differences in the Currents Activated by Capsaicin, Piperine, and Zingerone in Rat Trigeminal Ganglion Cells. J Neurophysiol. 1996. 76(3): 1858–69.

Madrigal BE, et al. Sister Chromatid Exchanges Induced In Vitro and In Vivo by an Extract of Black Pepper. Food Chem Toxicol. 1997. 35(6): 567–71.

Nalini N, Sabitha K, Viswanathan P, Menon VP. Influence of Spices on the Bacterial (Enzyme) Activity in Experimental Colon Cancer. J Ethnopharmacol. 1998. 62(1): 15–24.

Ono H, et al. 6-Methylsulfinylhexyl Isothiocyanate and Its Homologues as Food-Originated Compounds with Antibacterial Activity Against Escherichia coli and Staphylococcus aureus. Biosci Biotechnol Biochem. 1998. 62(2): 363–5.

Ouattara B, et al. Antibacterial Activity of Selected Fatty Acids and Essential Oils Against Six Meat Spoilage Organisms. Int J Microbiol. 1997. 37(2–3): 155–62.

Oya T, Osawa T and Kawakishi S. Spice Constituents Scavenging Free Radicals and Inhibiting Pentosidine Formation in a Model System. Biosci Biotechnol Biochem. 1997. 61(2): 263–6.

Plouxek CA, Ciolino HP, Clarke R, Yeh GC. Inhibition of P-Glycoprotein Activity and Reversal of Multidrug Resistance In Vitro by Rosemary Extract. Eur J Cancer. 1999. 35(10): 1541–5.

Reddy AC, Lokesh BR. Effect of Curcumin and Eugenol on Iron-Induced Hepatic Toxicity in Rats. Toxicology. 1996. 107(1): 39–45.

Reddy AC, Lokesh BR. Studies on the Inhibitory Effects of Curcumin and Eugenol on the Formation of Reactive Oxygen Species and the Oxidation of Ferrous Iron. Mole Cell Biochem. 1994. 137(1): 1–8.

Shinohara C et al. Arg-Ginipain Inhibition and Anti-Bacterial Activity Selective for Porphyromonas Gingivalis by Malabaricone C. Biosci Biotechnol Biochem. 1999. 63(8): 1475–7.

Slattery ML, et al. Carotenoids and Colon Cancer. Am J Clin Nutr. 2000. 71(2): 575–82.

Srivastava KC. Antiplatelet Principles from a Food Spice Clove (Syzygium aromaticum L). Prostaglandins Leukot Essent Fatty Acids. 1993. 48(5): 363–72.

Stager J, Wuthrich B, Johansson SG. Spice Allergy in Celery-Sensitive Patients. Allergy. 1991. 46(6): 475–8.

Sukamaran K, Kuttan R. Inhibition of Tobacco-Induced Mutagenesis by Eugenol and Plant Extracts. Mutat Res. 1995. 343(1): 25–30.

Tang X, Edenharder R. Inhibition of the Mutagenicity of 2-Nitrofluorene, 3-Nitrofluoranthene and 1-Nitropyrene by Vitamins, Porphyrins and Related Compounds, and Vegetable and Fruit Juices and Solvent Extracts. Food Chem Toxicol. 1997. 35(3–4); 373–8.

Then M, et al. Plant Anatomical and Phytochemical Evalutation of Salvia Species. Acta Pharm Hung. 1998. 68(3): 163–74.

Tsi D, Tan BK. The Mechanism Underlying the Hypocholesterolaemic Activity of Aqueous Celery Extract, its Butanol and Aqueous Fractions in Genetically Hypercholesterolaemic Rats. Life Sci. 2000. 66(8): 755–67.

Ultee A, Kets EP, Smid EJ. 1999. Mechanisms of Action of Carvacrol on the Food-Borne Pathogen Bacillus Cereus. Appl Environ Microbiol. 65(10): 4606–10.

Wan J, Wilcock A, Coventry MJ. The Effect of Essential Oils of Basil on the Growth of Aeromonas Hydrophila and Pseudomonas Fluorescens. J Appl Microbiol. 1998. 84(2):152–8.

Wicker P. Local Anaesthesia in the Operating Theatre. Nurs Times. 1994. 90(46): 34–5.

Wright SE, Baran DA, Heffner JE. Intravenous Eugenol Causes Hemorrhagic Lung Edema in Rats: Proposed Oxidant Mechanisms. J Lab Clin Med. 1995. 125(2): 257–64.

Yang B, et al. Purification, Cloning, and Characterization of the CEL I Nuclease.

Biochemistry. 2000. 39(13): 3533–41.

Zhu M, Wong PY, Li RC. Effect of Oral Administration of Fennel (Foeniculum vulgare) on Ciprofloxacin Adsorption and Disposition in the Rat. J Pharm Pharmacol. 1999. 51(12): 1391–6.

Chinese Herbs References

Ephedra:

Cupp. 1999. Herbal Remedies: Adverse Effects and Drug Interactions. Am Fam Physician 59(5): 1239–45.

FDA WARNS AGAINST DRUG PROMOTION OF HERBAL FEN-PHEN

FDA/CFSAN Federal Register 62 FR 30677 June 4, 1997 Dietary Supplements Containing Ephedrine Alkaloids Proposed Rule, http://vm.cfsan.fda.gov/~lrd/fr97064a.html (6-23-00)

Gorey, Wahlqvist, and Boyce. 1992. Adverse Reaction to a Chinese Herbal Remedy. Med J Aust. 157(7): 484–6.

Gurley et al. 1998. Ephedrine Pharmakinetics After the Ingestion of Nutritional Supplements Containing Ephedra Sinica (Ma Huang). Ther Drug Monit. 20(4): 439–45.

http://reporternews.com/1999/texas/ephed0226.html

http://vm.cfsan.fda.gov/~lrd/form1.html

http://www.fda.gov/bbs/topics/ANSWERS/ANS00832.html

Nadir, Agrawal, King and Marshal. 1996. Acute Hepatitis Associated with the Use of a Chinese Herbal Product, Ma-huang. Am J Gastroeterol. 91(7): 1436–8.

Powell, Hsu, Turk and Hruska. 1998. Ma-huang Strikes Again: Ephedrine Nephrolithiasis. Am J Kidney Dis. 32(1): 153–9.

White et al. 1997. Pharmacokinetics and Cardiovascular Effects of Ma-huang (Ephedra sinica) in Normotensive Adults. J Clin Pharmacol. 37(2): 116–22.

Zaacks et al. 1999. Hypersensitivity Myocarditis Associated with Ephedra Use. J Toxicol Clin Toxicol. 37(4): 485–9.

Zahn, Li, and Purssell. 1999. Cardiovascular Toxicity After Ingestion of "Herbal Ecstasy". J Emerg Med. 17(2): 289–91.

Dong quai:
Hirata, Swiertz, Zell, Small and Ettinger. 1997. Does Dong Quai have Estrogenic Effects in Postmenopausal Women? A Double Blind, Placebo Controlled Study. Fertil Steril. 68(6): 981–6.

Page and Lawrence. 1999. Potentiation of Warfarin by Dong Quai. Pharmacotherapy. 19(7): 870–6.

Aristolochia fangchi:

Cosyns et al. 1998. Chinese Herbs Nephropathy-Associated Slimming Regimen Induces Tumors in the Forestomach but no Interstital Nephropathy in Rats. Arch Toxicol. 72(11): 738–43.

Cosyns et al. 1999. Urothelial Lesions in Chinese-Herb Nephropathy. Am J Kidney Dis. 33(6):1011–7.

http://www9.cnn.com/2000/HEALTH/alternative/06/08/herbal.dangers/index.html

Lord et al. 1999. Nephropathy Caused by Chinese Herbs in the UK. Lancet. 354(9177):481–2.

Mengs and Stotzem. 1993. Renal Toxicity of Aristolochic Acid in Rats as an Example of Nephrotoxicity Testing in Routine Toxicology. Arch Toxicol. 67(5): 307–11.

Stengel. 1998. End-Stage Renal Insufficiency Associated with Chinese Herbal Consumption in France. Nephrologie. 19(1): 15–20.

Stiborova et al. 1999. Aristolactam I a Metabolite of Aristolochic Acid I upon Activation from an Adduct Found in DNA of Patients with Chinese Herbs Nephropathy. Exp Toxicol Pathol. 51(4–5):421–7.

CHAPTER 13

Phytonutrition and the Prevention of Cardiovascular Disease

D isease of the heart and blood vessels, also known as cardio-vascular disease (CVD) is America's number one killer. Almost sixty million people are afflicted with one or more forms of CVD in the nation today. Nearly one million people die from CVD each year accounting for 41 percent of all deaths in the United States and claiming more lives than the next seven causes combined. Somebody dies from some form of CVD about every thirty-three seconds. Many believe that CVD is a disease that afflicts primarily men. This is false. Counting total deaths, more women have died annually from CVD than men since 1984. More than half a million women die a year from CVD, more than the next fourteen causes of death in women combined! This disease is as serious for women as it is for men. We hear about coronary artery disease, heart attack, high blood pressure, and stroke almost every day, but what are they and what causes them?

Hypertension

One of the most common heart conditions threatening the health of many is high blood pressure or hypertension. Hypertension affects one in four adult Americans. Over 50 percent of those sixty and above have high blood pressure, a level rising to over 65 percent in individuals over age seventy. In the American Heart Association's 2000 Heart and Stroke Statistical Update hypertension was listed as a primary or contributing cause of about 210,000 deaths.

Blood pressure is the force blood exerts on blood vessel walls as the heart pushes it through the body. As blood circulates through the body, it does not move in a steady stream, but in short spurts. When the heart beats, it forces blood quickly through the blood vessels, causing a momentary rise in blood pressure. As the heart relaxes between beats blood moves more slowly through the blood vessels, and blood pressure returns to its resting state. Blood pressure thus rises and falls with each heartbeat. Blood pressure is thus given in two numbers. The first number is called the systolic blood pressure, or the pressure of the blood as the heart beats. The second number is called the diastolic blood pressure, or the pressure of the blood as the heart is resting between beats.

A healthy individual will have a systolic blood pressure below 130 and a diastolic blood pressure below 85. A person at risk for hypertension will have a systolic blood pressure between 130 and 139 and a diastolic blood pressure between 85 and 89. A person is diagnosed with hypertension when their blood pressure goes above 140/90.

Hypertension does not manifest any symptoms of its own, but promotes the development of other, more serious heart conditions. High blood pressure is called the silent killer because most people with high blood pressure do not know they have it. For an individual to know whether or not they have hypertension they need to have their blood pressure tested.

High blood pressure is the number one risk factor for strokes. Hypertension contributes to the hardening of blood vessels. Individuals with hypertension are three times more likely to have coronary artery disease, often leading to heart attacks. Because of the increased pressure of the blood, the heart must work harder to push blood through the blood vessels. This causes the heart to tire more rapidly and weaken over time, making hypertension a major contributor to congestive heart failure. Extra pressure on the blood vessel walls can weaken them, potentially causing bulges or ruptures. When blood vessel walls bulge, it is called an aneurysm. When they rupture, it is called a hemorrhage. Blood vessels in the brain and kidneys are especially sensitive to aneurysms and hemorrhages caused by hypertension. Hemorrhages in the brain can lead to strokes while those in the kidneys may cause kidney failure.

Atherosclerosis

Arteriosclerosis and atherosclerosis are two prominent diseases of the circulatory system. These conditions are frequently observed together and often lead to many other heart problems. Arteriosclerosis is the progressive hardening and thickening of the arteries. Tough fibrous tissues replace the elastic tissues of the arteries and cause them to stiffen and become rigid. In time calcium deposits can build up in the artery walls, making them inflexible, almost like a bony tube.

Atherosclerosis is slightly different. Atherosclerosis is the progressive narrowing of the arteries. Fatty plaques accumulate inside blood vessels. Though we do not yet know how atherosclerosis initiates, we do understand many different problems associated with it. Cholesterols from LDLs, the bad kind of cholesterol, begin to accumulate on the inside of blood vessel walls. This process is aided by free radicals. Free radicals in the blood can oxidize LDLs and make them stickier than normal LDLs. Oxidized LDLs build up along the blood vessel walls speeding up the progression of atherosclerosis. As we have discussed earlier, smoking not only chars the lungs, but also introduces large quantities of free radicals into the blood, substantially increasing the risk of atherosclerosis for smokers.

As cholesterol builds up in arteries, the smooth muscle cells that form part of the blood vessel wall begin to grow and multiply. Both smooth muscle cells of the artery and white blood cells from our immune system start ingesting great quantities of cholesterol. They eventually become large foam cells, further adding to the deposits along the arterial walls. Eventually these plaques can completely stop all blood flow.

Atherosclerosis is often accompanied by arteriosclerosis. Thus the arteries usually become rigid with fibrous tissue and calcium deposits as fatty plaques grow. The deposition of cholesterol and the great increase in the number of cells in the area of the plaque causes a rough bulge to form on the inside of the blood vessel. This can cause three major problems. First, the increased pressure associated with such bulging can cause brittle arteries to burst, leading to internal bleeding and massive hemorrhages. Second, the bulge can completely block blood flow within the vessel. Third, the rough surface of the plaque can initiate the formation of a blood clot.

Blood clots can also block the normal flow of blood. A stationary blood clot is known as a thrombus, while a moving blood clot is called an embolus. Both kinds are extremely dangerous. When atherosclerosis and arteriosclerosis occur in blood vessels carrying blood to the heart, the condition is called coronary artery disease. Coronary artery disease is the most significant indicator of heart attack risk. Because the blood vessels are already partially blocked by atherosclerotic plaques, it is much easier for them to be completely closed by tiny blood clots. The blockage of blood flow in the coronary arteries results in a heart attack.

Atherosclerosis is caused by several related factors. Principle among them is high LDL and low HDL levels in the blood. Stress, genetics, high blood pressure, diabetes, smoking, and insufficient exercise contribute significantly to atherosclerosis.

Stress causes high blood pressure and the narrowing of the arteries because the body releases chemicals that cause the muscles in our arteries to contract when stressed. This contraction of the arteries decreases their diameter, making blockage more likely. The same chemicals that tell the arteries to contract also cause the heart to pump harder and faster. This increased strain on the heart increases the risk of heart failure, among other problems.

Genes are another factor in the likelihood of developing atherosclerosis. Though still little understood, researchers know that heredity plays a big role in atherosclerosis. A history of atherosclerosis in the family is usually an accurate indicator that a person has a greater disposition to get it than others without a similar family history.

Despite the role that genes play in the development of atherosclerosis, dietary factors play a huge part in determining an individual's risk of acquiring this disease. A great many studies have shown that a healthy diet with lots of fruit and vegetables is one of the most important ways to avoid atherosclerosis and the other heart diseases that come about as a result of it. One of the principle reasons for this effect is that fruit and vegetables are high in antioxidants and compounds such as vitamins A, C, and E and the carotenoids and flavonoids. These substances protect the body from atherosclerosis because they prevent the oxidation of the

LDL particles that circulate in our blood. If LDLs are not oxidized, they do not contribute substantially to the formation of the fatty plaques that block the blood flow in atherosclerotic vessels.

People who eat large amounts of fruit and vegetables have higher plasma antioxidant capacity than those who don't. This means that the antioxidant defense systems in the blood can neutralize more free radicals in those individuals. The LDLs of people who increase their diets with more fruits and vegetables have been shown to demonstrate greater resistance to oxidation from free radicals.

The quintessential antioxidant vitamin is vitamin E. Very many studies have shown the effectiveness of this dietary component in preventing LDL oxidation. In three major studies dietary supplementation with vitamin E dramatically decreased the risk for heart disease. The first study reported the results of the U.S. Nurses' Health Study, which included over 87,000 women, and found that women taking dietary vitamin E supplements had a 34 percent decrease in risk for cardiovascular disease. The U.S. Health Professional's Follow-up Study, which had nearly 40,000 male participants, found a decrease of 39 percent in men taking vitamin E supplements. The Iowa Women's Health Study, which included over 34,000 participants, found a 47 percent reduction in mortality from cardiac disease in women who ate foods high in vitamin E as opposed to those who didn't. Researchers also found in the Cambridge Heart Antioxidant Study that nonfatal heart attacks decreased by 47 percent in patients given vitamin E supplements.

Not all studies though, corroborate the beneficial effects of vitamin E supplementation. The results of the recently released HOPE study showed no significant effect of vitamin E supplementation on the prevalence of cardiac disease. This study involved nearly 10,000 patients at high-risk for cardiovascular events such as heart attacks and strokes. These patients already had some form of cardiovascular disease, diabetes, or some other significant risk factor. The likely reason that vitamin E had no effect on the outcome of disease in these patients is because vitamin E has preventative functions instead ex post facto antiatherogenic activity. Vitamin E prevents the oxidation of LDLs in the blood stream and in that manner inhibits build-up of atherosclerotic plaques. If those fatty build-ups already exist, there is little that vitamin E can do.

Coronary Artery Disease

Coronary artery disease, also known as CAD, is essentially atherosclerosis of the arteries that supply blood to the heart. They are essential to the appropriate function of the heart, supplying oxygen and nutrients to the heart muscles. Without these nutrients, the heart would stop beating. When coronary arteries are partially blocked, the blood flow to the heart is decreased and the heart cannot function at peak performance.

The most frequent symptom of CAD is angina, also called angina pectoris. Angina is usually described as a squeezing or crushing pain in the chest that sometimes spreads to the abdomen, neck, shoulders, and down the arms. The pain frequently spreads to the left side of the body. Sometimes the pain is described as a burning sensation and may be mistaken for heartburn or indigestion. There are two principle types of angina: stable and unstable.

Stable angina is a less serious, more predictable pain that usually occurs after physical exertion, emotional stress, exposure to extreme temperatures, smoking, or eating a large meal. The pain of stable angina usually lasts for one to five minutes and goes away after a few minutes of rest. In the case of unstable angina, the symptoms are more irregular, more frequent, and more severe. Much smaller exertions or none at all can set them off and they can occur multiple times a day. Unstable angina is a strong indicator of an imminent heart attack. Other symptoms of CAD include sweating, lightheadedness, breathlessness, and heart palpitations, all of which are also associated with heart attacks. In fact, CAD is the greatest risk factor for heart attack.

Even though CAD can cause angina, it is frequently asymptomatic, or in other words, it manifests no symptoms. This makes this disease especially dangerous because an individual can have a strong predisposition for heart attacks and not know it. Doctors can tell if you have CAD (even if you don't ever experience angina) by conducting an exercise stress test. During an exercise stress test, an electrocardiogram (frequently called an ECG or EKG) is taken to measure the flow of electricity around the heart during exercise. Even though an individual with CAD will show normal ECG patterns at rest, when they begin exercising, usually on a treadmill, the patterns will change. As the person begins to exercise the heart pumps faster and harder and requires more blood. Because the arteries are partially blocked, they cannot supply sufficient blood to the heart and the muscle begins starving for oxygen. This causes enough change in the ECG patterns that a physician can diagnose CAD. Doctors can also detect CAD with a test called a coronary angiogram. Dye is injected into the coronary arteries and a series of x-rays are taken to observe the blood flow through the blood vessels of the heart. In this manner, blood vessel blockage can be directly visualized.

Because CAD is essentially atherosclerosis and arteriosclerosis of the coronary arteries, the two diseases have the same causes. As with most other heart diseases that we will be discussing here, eating more fruits and vegetables can decrease the risk of developing them. To briefly mention one study, researchers found in a survey of over 11,000 men and women, that individuals with high carotenoid intakes experienced angina pectoris much less frequently than others whose carotenoid intake was not as high. Because angina is one of the few symptoms of CAD, it is likely that carotenoids play a preventative role in this disease.

Heart Attack

A myocardial infarction, or heart attack, is caused by the complete blockage of the coronary arteries. The blockage of blood flow to a tissue is called ischemia. Without its normal blood supply the heart cannot function correctly and frequently stops working altogether, a condition known as cardiac arrest. The restoration of blood flow, called reperfusion in medical terms, must occur within minutes, or the heart tissue will begin to die because of lack of oxygen. If blood flow is not restored to the heart soon enough, irreparable heart damage will occur even if the heart attack victim survives. A great deal of heart attack damage is a direct result of the lack of oxygen to the muscle tissues of the heart. However, free radicals also do a lot of damage to the heart when blood flow resumes. This is called ischemia-reperfusion injury.

Free radical damage associated with myocardial infarction does not occur during ischemia, but during reperfusion. Or, in other words, the heart suffers oxidation damage when the heart again receives oxygen rich blood after recovering from a heart attack. Enzymes in the heart create reactive oxygen species following a heart attack. The lack of oxygen during ischemia causes a few normally helpful enzymes to lose their cofactors. When oxygen is reintroduced to the tissues during reperfusion those modified enzymes begin producing free radicals because they are not able to function normally due to the loss of their cofactors.

In addition, the tissue damaged by the lack of oxygen releases chemicals attracting white blood cells. These white blood cells, in turn, produce free radicals. This huge production of reactive species overwhelms the heart tissue's antioxidant defenses. These free radicals then kill many more heart cells. Heart muscle cannot replace dead cells. Thus, a loss of heart tissue can weaken the heart's ability to pump blood forever. In addition, the destruction of many heart cells can create weak spots in the heart structure, leading to heart failure.

A diet high in fruit and vegetables is one of the best ways to avoid heart attacks and the problems that they cause. A study published in the *American Journal of Clinical Nutrition* in 1999 reported a strong inverse correlation between the consumption of fruits and vegetables and heart attacks. The study group included over 34,000 Seventh-Day Adventists and showed that people with high intakes of fruit, vegetables, nuts, and grains were at a significantly decreased risk for heart attacks and various forms of cancer. Specifically, male vegetarians experienced heart attacks at a rate 37 percent less than their nonvegetarian counterparts. These powerful health effects were not solely attributable to the lack of meat.

An Italian study with nearly 47,000 participants also found a strong relationship between a high consumption of vegetables and many chronic diseases. Those who ate a large amount of vegetables had a decreased chance for heart attacks and angina.

Another important benefit of eating many fruits and vegetables that relates directly to heart attacks is that those foods provide much needed fiber to our diets. Fiber is known to help protect against heart attacks. One study conducted on vegetable, fruit, and cereal fiber intake with nearly 44,000 participants showed that those who had a higher fiber intake experienced much fewer heart attacks. The correlation was even stronger in people who died of heart attacks.

Stroke

A stroke is very similar to a heart attack. It is caused in similar ways and demonstrates the same basic pattern of damage. The only difference is that the blood flow is blocked on its way to the brain rather than the heart. It has often been called a "brain attack." Like a heart attack, a stroke is most frequently caused by the blockage of an artery narrowed by atherosclerosis. A ruptured artery can also cause a stroke if the artery that is broken open fails to bring oxygen to the brain as a result of the rupture. This type of stroke is called a hemorrhagic stroke. When blood does not reach a part of the brain for either of these two reasons, the brain tissues begin to die because they do not receive the oxygen they need. Nerve cells are especially sensitive to oxygen depravation. They will die quickly if blood flow is denied for even short periods of time.

Ischemia-reperfusion injury occurs also in the brain as it does in the heart. A great deal of oxidative damage occurs to the brain tissue by free radicals. When a stroke occurs, blood flow is usually cut off to only a part of the brain and not the whole brain itself. Because different physical and mental functions are located in different parts of the brain, damage done to specific areas causes the loss of the physical and mental abilities associated with the damaged regions. Again, like the muscle cells of the heart, nerve cells do not regenerate. Thus, damage done to the brain by stroke is more or less permanent unless other parts of the brain compensate for the dead tissue.

A branch of the U.S. Nurses' Health Study investigated specifically the effect that diet had on the incidence of stroke in women. They found that women who ate a diet high in fruits and vegetables had strokes much less frequently than those whose fruit and vegetable intake was not as high. The foods that were most notable for their healthy contribution were cruciferous vegetables, green leafy vegetables, and citrus fruit including fruit juices. This report continues to show the beneficial effects that dietary fruits and vegetables can have on our health.

Exercise is also a significant factor in preventing stroke. A study published in the *Journal of the American Medical Association* found that thirty minutes a day of some sort of physical activity can decrease risk of stroke by as much as 30 percent. These benefits can be derived from vigorous activities like jogging, bicycling, and racquet sports, but even a brisk walk will do the trick. The study reported no difference in the benefits derived at different ages so it doesn't matter if you start to exercise at age eighteen or eighty, you will still get the benefits.

Congestive Heart Failure

Congestive heart failure sounds like something sudden and traumatic, but it is not. Congestive heart failure is a chronic disorder that occurs when the heart weakens to the point that the amount of blood it pumps is insufficient to serve the body's needs. The weakened heart is unable to effectively push blood through the arteries and veins of the body. Because of this, blood frequently accumulates in two principle places: the veins leading from the lungs to the heart, and the veins that carry blood from the rest of the body to the heart.

Excess blood in the veins leaving the lungs causes the lungs to fill with fluid. Consequently, people with congestive heart failure often experience shortness of breath and chronic coughing or wheezing. Excess blood in the veins that drain from the rest of the body into the heart causes swelling of neighboring tissues. This swelling is observed most frequently in the lower extremities. Sufferers of congestive heart failure also experience tiredness and fatigue. Because the heart can't pump enough blood for the whole body, the body redirects the majority of the blood to the most essential organs. This leaves only a small supply of blood for the muscles, which makes them tire easily. The body also directs blood away from the digestive tract causing loss of appetite, nausea, and digestive problems. Some individuals with congestive heart failure experience rapid heart rates and heart palpitations because the heart is trying to pump faster to make up for its inability to pump effectively.

There are several causes of congestive heart failure. Many of the controllable factors include: hypertension, CAD, heart attack, obesity, and alcohol or drug abuse. High blood pressure can make the heart work harder and cause it to weaken over time. CAD can limit blood flow to the muscle tissue, preventing it from working at peak efficiency. A heart attack can damage and even kill parts of the heart, forcing the remaining muscle to work harder than possible. Obesity forces the heart to work harder than normal. Excessive use of alcohol and drugs damages the heart significantly.

Other factors, outside of our control, can also play a considerable role. Congenital heart defects and heart valve disorders caused by the malformation of the heart in development can lead to a weakened heart. Disease of the heart muscle caused by viral or bacterial infection can also weaken the heart.

Risk Factors and Prevention

All of the heart diseases share the same general risk factors. Some factors such as heredity, age, and gender cannot be controlled, but our decisions about how we live our lives determine the majority of our risk. As we have discussed, eating a diet high in fats and cholesterol and low in fruits and vegetables is one of the principle ways people place themselves at risk for heart disease. Extra fat and cholesterol in a diet contributes to atherosclerotic plaques in the blood vessels. On the other hand, fruit and vegetables provide us with chemicals that can help ward off heart problems.

Fiber actually reduces the amount of cholesterol absorbed by the bloodstream from the digestive system. Eating fiber rich foods causes a fiber mesh to form in the intestines. This mesh traps fats, cholesterol, and bile acids, partially preventing them from entering the bloodstream. The rate by which fat and cholesterol is absorbed is decreased, causing more of the fat we eat to be excreted rather than being absorbed into the blood stream. Of course, lower levels of fat and cholesterol in the blood, decrease the risk of diseases such as atherosclerosis and coronary heart disease.

The Scottish Heart Health Study, using over 11,000 participants, demonstrated a strong inverse correlation between dietary fiber intake and the risk of heart disease. As individuals ate a diet with more fruits and vegetables to give them the necessary fiber, they experienced less heart problems. Other studies corroborate this relationship as well.

The simple carbohydrates in fruits and vegetables provide the body with an optimal fuel source. Fruits and vegetables also con-

Other Ways to Prevent Coronary Heart Disease

A recent study published in the February 2002 issue of *Medizinische Klinik* examined the possibilities of preventing coronary heart disease through nonpharmacological therapy. Scientists conluded that "Life-style factors such as a healthy eating pattern, nonsmoking and regular physical activity call contribute to an enormous health benefit in the general population and save money for the public social systems. Therefore the promotion of this healthy life-style should be a major aim of the health policy."

tain many vitamins and phytochemicals that ward off heart disease. A study published in the *European Journal of Clinical Nutrition* reviewed many other studies dealing with fruit and vegetables and the risk of heart disease. They found that people who eat diets high in fruits and vegetables, even without further dietary supplements, enjoy a 15 percent reduction in heart disease.

Obesity, sedentary lifestyle, smoking, and excessive alcoholic intake all contribute significantly to the development of heart disease. Studies show that when individuals eat an appropriate diet, exercise regularly, do not smoke and avoid excessive use of alcohol, their chances from acquiring heart disease drop significantly.

Homocysteine

Homocysteine has recently received attention from medical researchers and the media for its role in heart disease. Homocysteine is an amino acid that is involved in the synthesis and degradation of two other amino acids: methionine and cysteine. Recent studies have linked high levels of homocysteine in the blood to atherosclerosis and coronary artery disease.

Dr. Kilmer McCully first made the connection between homocysteine and heart disease over thirty years ago. Dr. McCully noticed some interesting recurring symptoms in children with a rare genetic disorder called homocystinuria. These children lacked an enzyme required in the degradation of homocysteine. As a result, they had excessive concentrations of homocysteine in their blood. In order to rid themselves of the excess homocysteine, they excreted large amounts of it in the urine. Thus, the disease was coined "homocystinuria". Children with homocystinuria usually have mild mental retardation, light-colored hair, ruddy complexion, and dislocated lenses in the eyes. The symptoms interesting Dr. McCully, however, were the atherosclerotic plaques in their blood vessels and the fact that the children also suffered from arteriosclerosis. These children frequently died from heart attacks, strokes, and kidney failures caused by blood clots developing in the arteries.

HOMOCYSTEINE AND CARDIOVASCULAR DAMAGE
Although older people suffer regularly from cardiovascular disease, the fact that these children demonstrated the same conditions was highly irregular. The only reasonable explanation was the high level of homocysteine in the blood. Dr. McCully set to

work to see how the two were linked and published his first paper on the subject in 1969. Since then many studies, several of them large, have confirmed exactly what Dr. McCully suspected: high levels of homocysteine in the blood is strongly related to cardiovascular disease.

In 1992 a ten-year study with nearly 15,000 participants was released dealing with the relationship of homocysteine levels in the blood and heart attack rates. The study showed that there is a significant correlation between moderately high levels of plasma homocysteine and heart attacks. Another study with over 1,000 participants showed that people with high levels of homocysteine also demonstrated greater levels of arterial blockage by atherosclerotic plaques. Literally dozens of other studies corroborate these findings.

Scientists are beginning to move from determining that a relationship exists between homocysteine levels in the blood and the risk of cardiovascular disease to discovering why this relationship exists. Homocysteine promotes the progress of ateriosclerosis and atherosclerosis.

Research indicates that homocysteine may damage arterial walls, beginning the processes of both these diseases. One of the ways that homocysteine might damage the cells that line the vessel walls, known as endothelial cells, is by production of free radicals. Free radicals produced in the blood plasma can have two deleterious effects. First, they can directly attack the cells of the blood vessel wall causing an inflammatory response ultimately leading to atherosclerosis. The inflammation attracts white blood cells, which contribute to plaque formation by becoming foam cells. The second way that free radicals produced by homocysteine contribute to atherosclerosis is by oxidizing LDLs. We have discussed this aspect of free-radical damage previously.

There is a lot of evidence linking homocysteine to the production of free radicals. First, the free radical, superoxide ion, is produced when the concentration of homocysteine increases. Second, antioxidant enzymes of people who have high levels of homocysteine in their blood demonstrate greater activity than people with low levels of homocysteine in their blood. This increased enzymatic activity indicates an increased oxidative stress in the blood, against which the body is trying to defend itself. Third, when antioxidants are placed into test systems, damage to the cells of blood vessel walls is decreased.

The second way homocysteine does damage to arterial walls is by attaching itself to proteins. This is called homocysteinylation. Though it is not uncommon for molecules to attach to proteins in a healthy body, often homocysteinylation alters the function of important proteins working within arteries. This promotes damage to arterial walls.

Another factor that contributes to the development of atherosclerotic plaques is the growth of smooth muscle cells comprising a layer of the blood vessel walls. When these cells divide at greater rates than normal smooth muscles cells, atheroscelerosis is a common result. Homocysteine has been shown to cause these smooth muscle cells to proliferate while inhibiting the growth of the endothelial cells that line the inside of the blood vessel and are in immediate contact with the blood. The mechanisms of this action is still unclear, but it appears that homocysteine interferes with the signal pathways that regulate cell growth. It also seems that the effects of that interference differ between types of cells.

HOMOCYSTEINE AND ENDOTHELIAL CELLS

Homocysteine seems to interfere with endothelial cells, which are important cells that line arterial walls. Endothelial cells play an important function in several aspects of vascular control. One such function is called vasodilation, or the dilation, or relaxation, of arteries. The speed blood travels through blood vessels is dependant on blood pressure. When blood pressure is high, the blood moves very quickly. The endothelial cells help regulate the speed of blood by releasing nitric oxide. Nitric oxide causes the muscle cells surrounding arteries to relax, increasing the diameter of the artery and lowering the pressure (and thus slowing the speed) of blood. Homocysteine damages the endothelial cells, so they do not produce nitric oxide in response to increased blood velocity. This dysfunction can cause high blood pressure.

When Homocysteine interferes with the ability of endothelial cells to dilate blood vessels there is also an increased risk for atherosclerosis. This is because blood vessels remain narrow, a condition exacerbated by arterial plaques. The narrower the blood vessel, the easier it is for a blood clot to block it. A blood clot generated by an atherosclerotic plaque can quickly block a narrow artery causing a heart attack, stroke, or some other physiologic problem.

Homocysteine also contributes directly to the formation of blood clots by interfering with the body's natural defenses against blood clot formation. Endothelial cells produce proteins called annexins. These proteins assist in the activation of enzymes that break up spontaneous blood clots. Homocysteine attaches to the part of the annexin protein that would normally bind to the enzyme, preventing the break up of blood clots. Because the homocysteine molecule blocks the activation of the anticlotting enzymes, many clots are not dissolved before they form large blockages.

HOW TO LOWER YOUR HOMOCYSTEINE LEVELS

Homocysteine is obviously a damaging molecule. However, there are ways to lower the levels of homocysteine in your blood and protect yourself from health problems associated with it. Homocysteine is degraded by two enzymes; both of these enzymes require vitamins to work efficiently.

Researchers have noticed that people with high levels of homocysteine also tend to have low levels of these vitamins. Low levels of folate especially seem to correlate with elevated homocysteine in the blood. If the body isn't getting enough of these vitamins, the enzymes that control homocysteine cannot function at peak efficiency. The deficit of enzymatic activity leads to accumulation of homocysteine, which in turn causes vascular damage and could lead to serious problems associated with cardiovascular disease.

The majority of major medical studies conducted so far with homocysteine have been retrospective and epidemiologic. A retrospective study simply tests the level of homocysteine in a participant's blood and then follows these participants over a long period of time to see what happens. Epidemiologic studies look at present levels of homocysteine in the blood and compare that data with the current presence or absences of cardiovascular disease.

These types of studies have helped us understand the general relationship between cardiovascular disease and homocysteine, but

---

Green Leafy Vegetables Guard Against CHD

In a 2001 study of over 84,000 women aged 34–59 and over 42,000 men aged 40–75 the researchers concluded, "Consumption of fruits and vegetables, particularly green leafy vegetables, appears to have a protective effect against coronary heart disease."

they are unable to indicate how to prevent homocysteine from causing problems. Preventing homocysteine's adverse effects is the problem the scientific community is working on now. Retrospective and epidemiologic studies have been conducted that link homocysteine with cardiovascular disease and current research is now focusing on intervention trials. One of the things that scientists are investigating is whether dietary supplementation with vitamins B6, B12, and folate can lower homocysteine levels in the blood and prevent cardiovascular disease. Reports from large studies will be coming over the next several years. Preliminary results from smaller studies are positive. It appears that folate supplementation significantly reduces plasma homocysteine levels. Vitamin B12 also decreases the amount of homocysteine in the blood, but not nearly as much as folate. Current tests with vitamin B6 show minimal and frequently insignificant effects. From the results of these studies it is evident that, of the three, folate does the most good in the battle against heart disease.

Researchers propose that people should eat 400 micrograms of folate per day in order to maintain low, stable levels of homocysteine. The current RDA is 200 micrograms a day, a level recently lowered by the Committee on Dietary Allowances. Estimates indicate only about half of American adults get 200 micrograms of folate per day, while 88 percent consume less than 400 micrograms. As one researcher put it, "There is ample scope for intervention."

In a review published in the *Journal of the American Medical Association* dealing with twenty-seven studies on homocysteine, researchers calculated that even a minor increase of folate intake by the American public could potentially prevent over 26,000 deaths a year caused by homocysteine related heart disease. They also suggest that increased folate fortification of flour and cereals by the FDA could possibly prevent as many as 50,000 deaths a year!

There are many foods rich in folate including: green leafy vegetables, asparagus, broccoli, beans, lentils, oranges, nuts, seeds and liver. Many breads and cereal products are now fortified with folate. For the most part, researchers do not suggest dietary folate supplementation with pills and multivitamins. Extremely high levels of folate can cause insomnia, irritability, diarrhea, and may mask B12 deficiency. Women who might get pregnant are advised to take a multivitamin that provides at least 400 micrograms of folate.

Although vitamin B12 didn't lower homocysteine levels as much as folate did, it has still been shown to help. Vitamin B12 is found almost exclusively in animal products such as meat, fish, poultry, eggs, cheese, milk, and yogurt. Thus conscientious consumption of these foods will provide the necessary amount of vitamin B12.

Even though much research has yet to be completed, there is ample evidence showing that a diet high in fruits and vegetables with meats in moderation can help prevent heart disease.

References

Anderson JW, Hanna TJ. Impact of Nondigestible Carbohydrates on Serum Lipoproteins and Risk for Cardiovascular Disease. J Nutr. 1999 Jul; 129(7 Suppl): 1457S–66S.

Aviram M, Fuhrman B. Polyphenolic Flavonoids Inhibit Macrophage-Mediated Oxidation of LDL and Attenuate Atherogenesis. Atherosclerosis. 1998 Apr; 137 Suppl: S45–50.

Boushey CJ, Beresford SAA, Omenn GS, Motulsky AG. A Quantitative Assessment of Plasma Homocysteine as a Risk Factor for Vascular Disease. JAMA. 1995; 274: 1049–1057.

Cao G, Booth SL, Sadaeski JA, Prior RL. Increases in Human Plasma Antioxidant Capacity After Consumption of Controlled Diets High in Fruit and Vegetables. Am J Clin Nutr 1998; 68: 1081–7.

Chen C, Halkos ME, Surowiec SM, Conklin BS, Lin PH, Lumsden AB. Effects of Homocysteine on Smooth Muscle Cell Proliferation in Both Cell Culture and Artery Perfusion Culture Models. J Surg Res. 2000 Jan; 88(1): 26–33.

Chopra M, Thurnham DI. Antioxidants and Lipoprotein Metabolism. Proc Nutr Soc. 1999 Aug; 58(3): 663–71.

Emmert DH, Kirchner JT. The Role of Vitamin E in the Prevention of Heart Disease. Arch Fam Med. 1999 Nov–Dec; 8(6): 537–42.

Ford ES, Giles WH. Serum Vitamins, Carotenoids, and Angina Pectoris: Findings from the National Health and Nutrition Examination Survey III. Ann Epidemiol. 2000 Feb; 10(2): 106–16.

Fraser GE. Associations Between Diet and Cancer, Ischemic Heart Disease, and All-Cause Mortality in Non-Hispanic White California Seventh-day Adventists. Am J Clin Nutr. 1999 Sep; 70(3 Suppl): 532S–538S.

Gaziano JM. Antioxidant Vitamins and Cardiovascular Disease. Proc Assoc Am Physicians. 1999 Jan–Feb; 111(1): 2–9.

Hininger I, Chopra M, Thurnham DI, Laporte F, Richard MJ, Favier A, Roussel AM. Effect of Increased Fruit and Vegetable Intake on the Susceptibility of Lipoprotein to Oxidation in Smokers. Eur J Clin Nutr. 1997 Sep; 51(9): 601–6.

Hu FB, Stampfer MJ, Colditz GA, Ascherio A, Rexrode KM, Willett WC, Manson JE. Physical Activity and Risk of Stroke in Women. JAMA. 2000; 283: 2961–7.

Jacob RA. Evidence that Diet Modification Reduces In Vivo Oxidant Damage. Nutr Rev. 1999 Aug; 57(8): 255–8.

Joshipura KJ, et al. Fruit and Vegetable Intake in Relation to Risk of Ischemic Stroke. JAMA. 1999 Oct 6; 282(13): 1233–9.

Joshipura KJ, et al. The Effect of Fruit and Vegetable Intake on Risk for Coronary Heart Disease. Annals of Internal Medicine. June 2001: 134(12):1106-1114.

Klipstein Grobusch K, Launer LJ, Geleijnse JM, Boeing H, Hofman A, Witteman JC. Serum Carotenoids and Atherosclerosis. The Rotterdam Study. Atherosclerosis. 2000 Jan; 148(1): 49–56.

Kushi LH, Folsom AR, Prineas RJ, Mink PM, Wu Y, Bostick RM. Dietary Antioxidant Vitamins and Death from Coronoary Heart Disease in Postmenopausal Women. N Engl J Med. 1996; 334: 1156–62.

La-Vecchia C, Decarli A, Pagano R. Vegetable Consumption and Risk of Chronic Disease. Epidemiology. 1998 Mar; 9(2): 208–10.

Law MR, Morris JK. By How Much Does Fruit and Vegetable Consumption Reduce the Risk of Ischaemic Heart Disease? Eur J Clin Nutr. 1998 Aug; 52(8): 549–56.

McCully KS. Vascular Pathology of Homocysteinemia: Implications for the Pathogenesis of Arteriosclerosis. Am J Pathol. 1969; 56: 111–28.

McDowell IF, Lang D. Homocysteine and Endothelial Dysfunction: A Link with Cardiovascular Disease. J Nutr. 2000 Feb; 130(2S Suppl): 369S–372S.

Miller ER 3rd, Appel LJ, Risby TH. Effect of Dietary Patterns on Measures of Lipid Peroxidation: Results From a Randomized Clinical Trial. Circulation. 1998 Dec 1; 98(22): 2390–5.

Moat SJ, Bonham JR, Cragg RA, Powers HJ. Elevated Plasma Homocysteine Elicits an Increase in Antioxidant Enxyme Activity. Free Rad Res. 2000 Feb.; 32(2): 171–9.

Pryor WA. Vitamin E and Heart Disease: Basic Science to Clinical Intervention Trials. Free Radic Biol Med. 2000 Jan 1; 28(1): 141–64.

Rimm EB, Ascherio A, Giovannucci E, Spiegelman D, Stampfer MJ, Willett WC. Vegetable, Fruit, and Cereal Fiber Intake and Risk of Coronary Heart Disease Among Men. JAMA. 1996 Feb 14; 275(6): 447–51.

Rimm EB, Stampfer MJ, Acherio A, Giovannucci E, Colditz GA, Willett WC. Vitamin E Consumption and the Risk of Coronary Heart Disease in Men. N Engl J Med. 1993; 328: 1450–6.

Selhub J, Jacques PF, Bostom AG, D'Agostino R, Wilson PWF, Belanger AJ, O'Leary DH, Wolf PA, Schaefer EJ, Rosenberg IH. Association Between Plasma Homocysteine Concentrations and Extracranial Carotid –Artery Stenosis. N Eng J Med. 1995 Feb. 2; 332(5): 286–91.

Stampfer MJ, Hennekens CH, Manson JE, Colditz GA, Rosner B, Willett WC. Vitamin E Consumption and the Risk of Coronary Disease in Women. N Eng J Med. 1993; 328:1444–9.

Stampfer MJ, Hu FB, Manson JE, Rimm EB, Willett WC. Primary Prevention of Coronary Heart Disease in Women Through Diet and Lifestyle. N Engl J Med. 2000; 343:16–22.

Stampfer MJ, Malinow MR, Willett WC, Newcomer LM, Upson B, Ullmann D, Tishler PV, Hennekens CH. A Prospective Study of Plasma Homocysteine and Risk of Myocardial Infarction in U.S. Physicians. JAMA. 1992; 268: 877–881.

Stephens NG, Parsons A, Schofield PM, Kelly F, Cheeseman K, Mitchinson MJ. Randomised Controlled Trial of Vitamin E in Patients with Coronary Disease: Cambridge Heart Antioxidant Study (CHAOS). Lancet. 1996 Mar 23; 347(9004): 781–6.

Suzuki YJ, Lorenzi MV, Shi SS, Da RM, Blumberg JB. Homocysteine Exerts Cell Type-Specific Inhibition of AP-1 Transcription Factor. Free Rad Biol Med. 2000 Jan 1; 28(1): 39–45.

Swain RA, Kaplan-Machlis B. Therapeutic uses of Vitamin E in Prevention of Atherosclerosis. Altern Med Rev. 1999 Dec; 4(6): 414–23.

Todd S, Woodward M, Tunstall-Pedoe H, Bolton-Smith C. Dietary Antioxidant Vitamins and Fiber in the Etiology of Cardiovascular Disease and All-Causes Mortality: Results from the Scottish Heart Health Study. Am J Epidemiol. 1999 Nov 15; 150(10): 1073–80.

Yusuf S, Dagenais G, Pogue J, Bosch J, Sleight P. Vitamin E Supplementation and Cardiovascular Events in High-Risk Patients. The Heart Outcomes Prevention Evaluation Study Investigators. N Engl J Med. 2000 Jan 20; 342(3): 154–60.

CHAPTER 14

Phytonutrition and Cancer Prevention

Uncontrolled cell proliferation, or cancer, kills more Americans per year than any other disease except heart disease. In the U.S. more than 1,500 people are expected to die from cancer every day. That adds up to at least 552,200 deaths this year alone. The real tragedy is that an estimated 60 percent of these deaths might have been prevented. During your lifetime, one in two men and one in three women will develop cancer, and one in four people will eventually die of some kind of cancer. Every year more than a million various cancers are diagnosed. The cost of combating cancer is estimated at approximately 107 billion dollars a year.

When we discuss measures of cancer prevention it should be noted that there is no way to guarantee that a diet rich in fruits and vegetables will prevent cancer. At present, it is impossible to ensure that you will never get cancer, regardless of how carefully you watch your diet. However, we can confidently claim that a diet rich in fruits and vegetables can drastically reduce your risk of cancer based on rigorous scientific tests and principles.

So how do you decrease your odds of dying of cancer? A recent book puts it perfectly:

"Researchers now estimate that 60 to 70 percent of all cancers are directly linked to the foods we eat and related lifestyle factors, including smoking, exercise, and obesity. The federal government's National Cancer Institute reports that as many as 35 percent of cancer deaths are diet related. If you add to that those that are related to smoking and alcohol, as many as three quarters of all cancer deaths are diet or lifestyle related."

Lets take a look at some diet-related studies.

A study involving 42,254 women found that those who ate the largest amounts of healthy foods such as: fruits, vegetables, whole grains, low-fat dairy products, and lean meats had a 30 percent lower risk of death from cancer, heart disease, and stroke. Another huge study involving 47,909 men, researchers found that men who ate more cruciferous vegetables (broccoli and cabbage) had a decreased risk of bladder cancer.

You can do a lot of things to decrease the risk of getting cancer: eat at least five servings of fruits and vegetables every day, a good variety of vegetables of various colors: green, yellow, red etc. You should also eat a variety of grains and cereal products such as beans, corn, and breads. Whole grain products are more nutritious and provide the fiber you need. You should limit fat intake, especially saturated fat, and limit the consumption of red meat. You should exercise and keep your calorie intake in balance. You should avoid alcohol and tobacco products because both individually, and especially combined, lead to greatly increased risks for certain cancers. By doing these things you can drastically improve your odds of not getting cancer.

We will proceed in this chapter focusing on cancer. We will discuss things you should avoid as well as things you should embrace in reducing the risk of cancer. In the end we will simply encourage you to make and maintain basic lifestyle changes that will help you live a long and healthy life.

Tobacco Products, Lung Cancer and Other Cancers

One of the best ways to avoid cancer is to avoid tobacco products. (This information on tobacco products is gleaned from the American Cancer Societies web page) The American Cancer Society reports that one in five deaths in the U.S. is a result of smoking. Male smokers are twenty-three times more likely to die

of lung cancer than male nonsmokers. Female smokers are thirteen times more likely to die of lung cancer then female nonsmokers. Smoking killed approximately 419,000 people in 1990
in the U.S alone. In 1995, smoking killed 2.1 million people in
developed countries around the world. Smoking is responsible for
87 percent of all lung cancers and at least 30 percent of all cancer
deaths. Smoking is expected to kill 171,000 people due to cancer
this year. This estimate is actually lower than previous years due
to a decline in smoking.

Smoking increases the risk for lung, mouth, throat, uterine,
kidney, bladder, and various other cancers. It also increases the
risk of heart disease and a number of other health problems like
pneumonia, bronchitis, and emphysema. Smoking cigars
increases the risk of dying from oral, throat or esophageal cancers by four to ten times. Men who smoke cigars are 34 percent
more likely to die of cancer than men who do not smoke cigars.
There is no available data on cancers in women caused by cigar
smoking, though we can comfortably assure you that the risk is
greatly increased.

Smokeless tobacco also causes cancer. In fact long term use of
snuffs and chews increases the risk of oral cancers nearly fifty times
that of a nonuser! Which means if an ordinary user had a chance
of 1 in 100, a person who uses smokeless tobacco would have a
chance of one in two of developing cancer!

The only nice thing about smokeless tobacco is that you don't
share the increased risk for cancer with others. About 3,000 people die every year as a result of breathing someone else's smoke.
Secondhand smoke is a serious matter. This is particularly true of
smoking around children. In the U.S., secondhand smoke causes
150,000 to 300,000 cases of lower respiratory infections in infants
and very small children under the age of eighteen months every
year. These serious infections include pneumonia and bronchitis
and result in at least 7,500 to 15,000 hospitalizations every year.
Second hand smoke also increases the number and severity of
asthma attacks in older children. Second hand smoke is filled with
a large number of carcinogens, increasing the risk of cancer for
anyone who inhales them.

Alcohol

Alcohol is also connected to an increased risk of cancer. Alcohol is estimated to be responsible for as many as 19,000 cancer deaths in America. Alcohol is especially dangerous when combined with smoking.

Sunlight

Extended exposure to the sun increases the risk for developing skin cancers. This risk is multiplied if your skin burned. This increased risk can be largely avoided by wearing clothing and/or sunscreen. About 1.3 million skin cancers will be diagnosed this year alone. A little caution in the sun could prevent most of them.

Overcooking Meat

If you want to avoid a higher risk for cancer, don't burn the beef, or any other kind of meat for that matter. Protein cooked at high temperatures can warp into by products called heterocyclic amines. Heterocyclic amines are mutagens that increase the risk of breast, colon, lung, prostate, liver and many more cancers. The best way to avoid them is to either avoid meat, or make sure to cook your meat until it is well done (to avoid bacteria etc) at a lower but acceptable temperature.

What Increases Risk for Breast Cancer?

Though not well known, not all breast cancer occurs in women. Men can get breast cancer, though the risk for breast cancer is 100 times greater for women than for men. So how do you prevent it? Not all of the risks of breast cancer are preventable. Some increased risks are due to genetics. People who have family histories of breast cancer are more likely to develop it.

Here are a list of things that increase the probability of getting breast cancer: a prior history of breast cancer, a previous abnormal breast biopsy, previous exposure to irradiation, people whose menstrual periods started at an early age (under twelve) or who went through menopause at a late age, estrogen replacement therapies, race (whites are more likely), taking oral contraceptives, not having children before the age of thirty, experiencing an induced abortion, not breast feeding, alcohol consumption, smoking, high-fat diets, eating few fruits and vegetables, obesity, low physical activity, and environmental risk factors such as pollutants and pesticides.

Your risk of dying from breast cancer increases if you do not undergo regular self-examinations and mammograms. You have a much greater chance of surviving if cancer is found early and can be removed before it begins to invade other tissues.

According to the results of numerous studies, diet can have a drastic impact on the risk of breast cancer. In one study, involving 34,388 postmenopausal women, researchers found that women who ate large amounts of fat had an increased risk for breast cancer. In a later and much larger study involving 322,647 women, higher total fat intake was marginally indicated to a slightly increased risk for breast cancer.

Decreased Risks for Breast Cancer

Milk is a rich source of a fatty acid called conjugated linoleic acid that has been shown in animal experiments to prevent breast cancer.

In a study at the Saitama Cancer Research Center in Japan researchers followed 472 women after they had breast cancer surgery. Those that drank at least 5 cups of green tea every day were less likely to experience a recurrence than other women. Researchers suggest the antioxidants in green tea were responsible for this preventative activity.

A study involving 83,234 women, researchers found that increased intake of the vitamins alpha-carotene, beta-carotene, vitamin C, vitamin A, and lutein/zeaxanthin from food or supplements was associated with a decreased risk for breast cancers. In addition, women who ate five or more serving of fruits and vegetables every day had less risk than those who ate two or less servings.

What Increases Risk for Prostate Cancer?

Prostate cancer is second only to lung cancer in causing death among men who die of cancer. The American Cancer Society estimated that approximately 31,900 men will die of prostate cancer in the U.S. during the year 2000.

Here are a list of things that increase the risk of prostate cancer: being over the age of sixty-five, having a history of prostate cancer in your family, smoking, being African-American, having sex frequently with a large number of sexual partners, living in North America or Europe, being exposed to carcinogenic chemicals at work or at home, eating a lot of fat, red meat and dairy products, lacking exercise, and eating few fruits and vegetables.

Decreased Risk for Prostate Cancer

Consumption of fruits and vegetables rich in lycopene, (such as tomatoes), lowers the risk of prostate cancer. Decreasing the amount of saturated fat, dairy products, and red meat in your diet to quantities within recommended amounts would also decrease risk. Supplementation with Vitamin E and Vitamin A, could be beneficial if you do not get enough in your diet. The proper intake of vitamins and minerals can also decrease your risk.

What Increases Risk for Colon Cancer?

A diet high in fat and low in fiber place you in the highest risk category for colon cancer. You can improve your risks by either decreasing the amount of fat or increasing the amount of fiber in your diet. Of course, you can significantly reduce the risk of colon cancer by reducing the amount of fat and increasing the amount of fiber in your diet.

The main risk-increasing factor for colon cancer is fat intake. Not only is it important to watch how much fat you are eating, it is also important to pay attention to the kind of fat you are eating. Saturated fat and fats derived from animal products are more likely to cause colon cancer than other fats (unsaturated fat and polyunsaturated fat). Saturated fats cause an increase in the production of secondary bile acids, which damage cell membranes and cause the production of other negative by-products that induce cell proliferation and increase the risk of cancer.

A lack of dietary fiber is the second biggest risk-increasing factor for colon cancer. Dietary fiber can even reduce the risk of colon cancer in high-fat diets. This preventative activity varies according to the type of fiber eaten. Cellulose and guar gum are fibers that have not been found to be useful in decreasing colon cancer. The best source of fiber has been cereal bran, (such as wheat bran), and the soluble fibers from fruits and vegetables.

Decreased Risk for Colon Cancer

It is much healthier to eat polyunsaturated and monounsaturated fats, especially those that are rich in omega-3 fatty acids (found in fish, such as tuna). Omega-3 fatty acids are incorporated into the cell membranes at the expense of omega-6 fatty acids and apparently inhibit the pathways that lead to cellular proliferation and increase the cells resistance to developing cancer. Ingestion of omega-3 fatty acids does not stimulate the production of secondary bile acids.

Olive oil and other oils that are rich in monounsaturated fatty acids are better choices than corn or safflower oil, which are rich in omega-6 fatty acids. However, it is important to have a balance of both kinds of fatty acids for good health.

Eating lots of whole grain foods may decrease your risk of cancer by increasing fiber. Eating fruits and vegetables add not only fiber but also powerful anticancer antioxidants.

So what does bran do that makes it useful in preventing cancer of the colon? Fiber is not digestible by you or any of your enzymes, but that does not mean that it is nutritionally or functionally useless to you. Inside of your colon is a huge gathering of millions of

---

Fruits and Vegetables Protect Against Cancer

Researchers reporting on a February 2002 study of stated that "Fruits and vegetables appear to confer protection against several cancers, but most adults eat substantially less than the recommended amounts."

microflora, or native bacteria of your lower GI tract. All animals have them and need them for survival. They live on fiber, and in turn make vitamins and short chain fatty acids: acetic, propionic and butyric acid.

Butyric acid is important in preventing colon cancer; it acts like a regulator of intestinal epithelium. Butyric acid's unique properties appear to encourage the epithelium to proliferate and triggers apoptosis in abnormal cells. This has come to be known as the butyrate "paradox" as no one knows how it could have such differing effects on cells. It is worth noting that the bacteria in your colon naturally produce butyric acid, provided they have enough fiber. However, butyric acid is extremely toxic if taken orally. Butyric acid cannot be supplemented. Simply be sure to eat enough fiber, and leave the production of butyric acid to the bacteria.

Low-fat milk may also be helpful in preventing colon cancer. As mentioned in the section on breast cancer, milk is a rich source of conjugated linoleic acid, which has been shown in animal experiments to prevent breast cancer and may prove helpful in other cancers. However, a great deal of research has yet to be done. Milk also provides Vitamin D and Calcium, both of which have been shown to protect the colon epithelium from damage and inhibit the formation of cancer. Calcium seems to induce apoptosis and has a direct antiproliferative effect on colon cells.

The Final Analysis: Reducing the Risk

The single greatest thing you can do to reduce the risk of cancer is eat a balanced diet, including plenty of fruits and vegetables. You can make a difference by changing your lifestyle to avoid unnecessary risks. Of course this is also the single greatest thing you can do to reduce the risk of the nation's biggest killer: cardiovascular disease. It also happens to be the single greatest thing you can do to reduce the risk of diabetes, arthritis, Alzheimer's and other lifestyle diseases. And finally, it is the single greatest thing you can do to ensure health and fitness.

References

American Institute for Cancer Research. Stopping Cancer Before It Starts.

Baker AH and Wardle J. Increasing Fruit and Vegetable Intake Among Adults Attending Colorectal Cancer Screening: The Efficacy of a Brief Tailored Intervention. Cancer Epidemiology, Biomarkers and Prevention. Feb. 2002: 11(2):203–206.

Clinton SK, Giovannucci E. Diet, Nutrition, and Prostate Cancer. Annu. Rev. Nutr. 1998. 18:413–40.

http://usaweekend.com/98_/980927/980927eat_smart.html

Hunter DJ, et al. Non-Dietary Factors as Risk Factors for Breast Cancer, and as Effect Modifiers of the association of fat intake and risk of breast cancer. Cancer-Causes-Control. Jan 1997. 8(1): 49–56.

Kushi LH, et al. Dietary Fat and Postmenopausal Breast Cancer. J-Natl-Cancer-Inst. Jul 15, 1992. 84(14): 1092–9.

Lipkin M, Reddy B, Newmark H, Lamprecht SA. Dietary Factors in Human Colorectal Cancer. Annu. Rev. Nutr. 1999. 19:545–86.

Michaud DS, et al. Fruit and Vegetable Intake and Incidence of Bladder Cancer in a Male Prospect Cohort. Journal of the National Cancer Institute. 1999. 91(7): 605–13.

Nagao M. A New Approach to Risk Estimation of Food-Borne Carcinogens—Heterocyclic Amines—Based on Molecular Information. Mutat. Res. 1999. 431(1)–3–12.

Schatzkin A, et al. A Prospective Study of Diet Quality and Mortality in Women. JAMA. 2000. 283(16): 2109–15.

Williams JA, et al. Pathways of Heterocyclic Amine Activation in the Breast: DNA Adducts of 2-Amino-3-Methylimidaso[4,5-f] Quinoline (IQ) Formed by Peroxidases and in Human Mammary Epithelial Cells and Fibroblasts. Mutagenesis. 2000. 15(2): 149–54.

www.cancer.org/statistics

www.cancer.org/statistics/cff98/tobacco.html, www.cancer.org/statistics/cff2000/tobacco.html

www.cancer.org/statistics/cff98/tobacco.html, www.cancer.org/statistics/cff2000/tobacco.html

www3.cancer.org/cancerinfo/load_cont.asp?st=pr&ct=36&language=english

www3.cancer.org/cancerinfo/load_cont.asp?st=pr&ct=5&language=English

Zhang S, et al. Dietary Carotenoids and Vitamins A, C, and E and Risk of Breast Cancer. Journal of the National Cancer Institute. 1999. 91(6): 547–56.

CHAPTER 15

Phytonutrition, Aging and Lifestyle Diseases

As we progress through life, our bodies age. Aging is nothing more nor less than the natural process of change, though many have compared it to disease. People have wondered if there is a maximum biological limit to the human life span. A Japanese man named Shirechiyo Izumi reportedly lived to be 120 years 237 days old, finally dying of pneumonia. Is 120 years the maximum limit to human lifespan? Whether or not there is such a limit, what happens as we age? What are the dynamics of this process, and what makes a lifespan short, average, or long? Once we understand these dynamics, could we be able to extend everyone's life span to 120 years or even, as some scientists speculate, much longer? Answers to these and other fundamental questions about aging may now be within reach.

Aging is often described in terms of two major theories; one emphasizing internal biological clocks or "programs," and the other focusing on external or environmental forces that damage cells and organs until they can no longer function adequately. The first theory claims every body has a genetic program that predetermines how long it can live. Aging therefore is the inevitable process of an internal timer ticking away the remaining days, hours, and minutes of life. The second theory proposes that there is no intrinsic limit to life in itself. Instead, it emphasizes the concept that the cumulative effect of a lifetime of environmental assaults to our systems is what gradually causes things to go wrong and ultimately ends life. Intimately coupled to this second way of thinking is the idea that if we can find ways to avoid damage to our bodies, we can extend life. That, in essence, is what much of modern science is about.

The average lifespan has grown dramatically in the United States over the last 100 years. In 1900 the life expectancy was only forty-seven years, compared to seventy-five years in 1990—an increase in twenty-eight years of life! What's more, not only has the actual quantity of life increased, but the quality of life has risen as well. People live longer with less disease and illness. This dramatic increase in the quantity and quality of life is due in large part to improvements in sanitation, antibiotics, and medical care. The chief menaces of the elderly are now chronic diseases like cancer and cardiovascular disease. As scientists in all areas of research turn their attention to these diseases many believe that the average life expectancy will continue to extend.

Much of what we have assumed are the inevitable consequences of aging—wrinkles, memory loss, an escalating risk for heart disease, osteoporosis and cancer—result more from the lifestyle choices we make than from the natural aging process. For many years, medical professionals assumed nutrient need decreased as individuals aged because they get smaller, had less muscle and bone, and were generally less active. In the last ten years however, many studies on older people have been conducted and scientists are realizing that many nutritional requirements increase with age. These studies indicate that our dietary choices are just as important as getting exercise and other preventive programs in forestalling aliments associated with aging. The need for additional dietary nutrients in affording the body protection for aging-related disease is beginning to be fully appreciated at last.

Although gerontologists (scientists who study aging) once looked for a single, all-encompassing reason to explain why we age—a single gene, for instance, or the decline of the immune system—they are now finding multiple processes that combine and interact on many levels. Proteins, cells, tissues, and organ systems are all involved, and gerontologists are now able to discern more and more of the mechanisms by which they cause or react to aging. In fact, today, the biological picture of aging is emerging in much greater detail than ever before. And as more and more of the fundamental mechanisms of aging come to light, they promise to explain and lead to cures for the health problems that often accompany old age.

What is the secret of long life? Gerontologists talk of aging in terms of three variables: heredity, environment, and lifestyle. Is the secret to long life in your genes, the place in which you live, or the lifestyle you choose? It is important to note that many of these ideas about aging are not mutually exclusive. In other words, gerontologists are beginning to recognize that aging is a complex process related to all of these factors.

Heredity

The link between genes and life span is unquestioned. The simple observation that some species live longer than others—humans longer than dogs, tortoises even longer than humans—is one convincing piece of evidence. While humans seem to have a maximum life span of about 120 years, for dogs it's around 20 and tortoises can live about 150 years. In laboratories around the world, scientists are isolating specific genes to learn what they do and how they influence aging and longevity. Some tests are demonstrating that aging is partially the result of the sequential switching on and off of certain genes. Some think that the aging process is controlled through the production of hormones. Your genetic material contains instructions for the production of hormones that cause changes in your body associated with aging. Still others believe that there is a programmed decline in the effectiveness of the immune system, causing your body to be less resistant to infectious disease, eventually causing death and aging.

We think the single greatest hope for increasing your life span is to make appropriate lifestyle choices. The food you eat and the amount of exercise you get can have a tremendous affect on the process of aging. In fact, this is the main thrust of this book. We have tried to indicate how an appropriate shift in your lifestyle, focusing on changes in your diet, can help you live a longer, healthier, happier life.

In the United States, deaths from heart disease have declined 45 percent since 1950, partly due to lower-fat, lower-cholesterol diets, and other behavioral factors (like declines in smoking and an increase in exercise). Diet and exercise, in particular, are known to have a major impact on changes common with advancing age. We are beginning to amass solid scientific understanding of the aging process and the affect of diet on the changes associated with age. We want to look now a little more closely at the aging process and some of the changes and diseases that frequently accompany it. In the course of this discussion we will review the dietary and lifestyle changes that are known to prevent, minimize, and delay these aging processes.

As we age the heart grows slightly larger. Maximum oxygen consumption during exercise declines in men by about 10 percent with each decade of adult life and in women, by about 7.5 percent. Without exercise, muscle mass declines an estimated 22 percent for women and 23 percent for men between the ages of thirty and seventy. In the lungs, maximum breathing capacity may decline by about 40 percent between the ages of twenty and seventy. The brain loses some cells (neurons) and others become damaged as we age. Eyesight is also affected by age. Many have difficulty focusing close up in their forties; while most lose the ability to distinguish fine details in the seventies. From age fifty on, there is greater difficulty in seeing at low levels of illumination. The ability to hear high frequencies also diminishes over time.

Beyond these general changes, there are several diseases that are more frequently seen as we age. These are known as lifestyle diseases because, more often than not, the lifestyle that a person chooses to lead determines in great measure the relative risk of acquiring them.

Diabetes Mellitus

More than sixteen million Americans are currently afflicted with diabetes, a disease characterized by high levels of sugar in the blood. That number accounts for about 6 percent of the total national population and almost 800,000 new patients are diagnosed annually! This disease is so prevalent that it is the sixth leading cause of death in the United States. Diabetes manifests itself through a variety of life-threatening complications causing blindness, kidney disease, cardiovascular disease and stroke, as well as nerve disease frequently leading to lower limb amputation. The direct and indirect costs of diabetes are enormous, estimated at 100 billion dollars annually.

There are two types of diabetes: type I diabetes, also known as juvenile diabetes; and type II diabetes, sometimes called adult-onset diabetes. Only 5 percent of diabetes sufferer's have juvenile diabetes, while the remaining 95 percent have adult-onset diabetes. Diabetes is a disorder in which the body does not regulate sugar well. When sugar is digested, it is most frequently broken down to the simple sugar glucose. Glucose is absorbed in the blood stream and transported throughout the body. Cells use it as their basic source of energy. In order to take glucose from the bloodstream, cells utilize a hormone called insulin. Under normal circumstances insulin is produced by the pancreas in amounts equivalent to the quantity of sugar digested. Among many other functions, insulin helps the cells take glucose from the blood. Without this signal from insulin, most cells would be unable to absorb glucose. Consistently inadequate blood sugar levels leads to diabetes.

Juvenile diabetes begins in childhood or adolescence. In extreme cases, the pancreas does not produce any insulin at all. Adult-onset diabetes, on the other hand, usually begins after forty and is caused by resistance of the insulin receptors on our cells to insulin. This insulin resistance is frequently correlated with obesity, especially when there is considerable fat accumulation around the lower torso. Because the cells do not take up glucose, blood sugar levels rise to excessive levels. The symptoms of the two diseases are practically identical because high blood sugar levels are present in both types.

Urination becomes excessive as the body tries to excrete all the extra glucose in the blood. Diabetics will often feel thirsty because of the increased fluid excretion. Diabetics are prone to rapid weight loss because the body consumes protein and fat in order to satisfy energy requirements. Diabetes often causes fatigue because of the breakdown of the proteins in the muscles and other parts of the body.

If people suffering from diabetes have high blood sugar levels for a long time they can develop other serious complications, including damage to the eyes (retinopathy), nerves (neuropathy) and kidneys (nephropathy). Diabetic retinopathy can eventually cause blindness. Neuropathy can cause tingling, numbness, and even pain in the arms and legs. Diabetic nephropathy can result in kidney failure and can cause many symptoms related to the build-up of waste products that are normally cleared from the blood.

Another very serious consequence of diabetes is that it frequently contributes to the development of atherosclerosis. Because fat is often used for fuel it is released with LDLs into the blood stream. Because the levels of circulating fat and cholesterol thus increase markedly, so does the rate of fat deposition in atherosclerotic plaques. The blockage of blood flow caused by the build-up of atherosclerotic plaques can lead to heart attacks, strokes, and other disorders of the circulatory system. One such disorder, called peripheral vascular disease or PVD, decreases circulation to the extremities, often causing ulcers in the lower legs and feet. Diabetic ulcers may become infected, leading to gangrene. Normally a good supply of blood and an active immune system will combat gangrene to protect the body. However, diabetic plaques slow blood flowing toward infected areas, hampering the immune system. Persistent infections in conjunction with neuropathy often causes the need for limb amputation.

JUVENILE DIABETES
Juvenile diabetes develops quickly. The only treatment for juvenile diabetes is to regularly inject insulin. Patients must keep close track of their blood sugar levels and give themselves injections of insulin at meals or when their blood sugar levels rise. In the past, the insulin used in these injections was obtained from animals. This caused problems because some people developed resistance to animal insulin while others had adverse immune reactions to it. Fortunately, through genetic engineering, scientists have now found a way to produce human insulin.

Compared with juvenile diabetes, adult-onset diabetes develops gradually. Treatment for type II diabetes usually does not begin with insulin shots. In fact, changes in the diet and exercise habits of patients usually ward off many of the symptoms for a time. However, despite dietary and exercise modifications, the disease often progresses until medication becomes necessary. The most common medications used to relieve symptoms of type II diabetes decrease cellular resistance to insulin while increasing pancreatic production of insulin. Ultimately, most people suffering from adult-onset diabetes require insulin injections.

HYPOGLYCEMIA
A frequent danger associated with treatments for both type I and type II diabetes is hypoglycemia. Hypoglycemia occurs when

blood glucose levels are too low. Because the brain and nerve cells rely on glucose for energy, hypoglycemia rapidly affects the ability of the nervous system to function properly. Primary symptoms of hypoglycemia are dizziness, headache, blurred vision, and difficulty concentrating. These symptoms often progress to other more serious neurologic symptoms. Hypoglycemia triggers the release of hormones that work to raise blood sugar levels. These hormones induce symptoms of their own, including: trembling, sweating, rapid heartbeat, anxiety and hunger. These symptoms can be triggered by a number of different things, including: not eating enough sugar, excessive exercise, injecting too much insulin, or taking too many antidiabetic drugs. Treating diabetes requires one to walk a fine line between hypoglycemia and hyperglycemia. This can be a complicated thing to manage.

DIABETES RISK FACTORS

The risk factors for type I and type II diabetes are very different because of their different causes. Type I diabetes is an autoimmune disorder that is essentially genetic in origin, therefore siblings and children of people with type I diabetes are at an increased risk. Type II diabetes results in part from the eating and exercise habits of individuals as they age. Risk factors for type II diabetes include: an age over forty-five, obesity, physical inactivity, a diet high in fat and cholesterol, and a family history of type II diabetes. Some racial groups are disposed to develop type II diabetes. This disease occurs frequently in African Americans, Latinos, Asian & Pacific Islanders, and Native Americans.

Recent research has confirmed the belief that diets high in fruits and vegetables coupled with adequate exercise decrease the risk of type II diabetes. A study conducted in Finland on over 500 adults showed that modest weight losses; appropriate high-fiber, low-fat diets; and regular exercise dropped the risk of developing type II diabetes by 58 percent. Another study with over one thousand participants showed that individuals who consumed vegetables frequently throughout the year did not develop type II diabetes as often as those who consumed vegetables infrequently. One reason for that decrease in risk is likely because of the benefits of fiber in the diet. A branch of the Iowa Women's Study that included nearly 36,000 women studied the effect that fiber has on the development of diabetes. The study showed that women who had a greater dietary fiber intake had a greatly reduced chance of acquiring diabetes. Grains and whole grain products showed the strongest cor-relation between fiber intake and reduced risk of diabetes.

There isn't a great deal that can be done to avoid contracting type I diabetes. Type II diabetes however, is different. When people at risk for developing type II diabetes consume a diet high in fruits and vegetables and get regular exercise they can effectively prevent or delay the onset of this disease. In essence, taking some of the advice and suggestions in the previous sections of this book may be the most productive thing you can do to prevent type II diabetes.

Arthritis

Arthritis and its more serious counterpart, rheumatoid arthritis, are diseases that afflict millions of people across the nation. It is estimated that over thirty-seven million people in America suffer from arthritis. The majority of people suffering from arthritis are women. Arthritis is a disease of the joints caused by any of a variety of problems. Before getting into the details of how joints are affected by arthritis it will be important to discuss the basic make-up of joints.

A joint is composed of bones, ligaments, fluid, and cartilage. The bones making up joints are bound together in specific arrangement by ligaments. Ligaments are tough, nonelastic, connective tissues that support the joint and provide rigidity while allowing flexibility within a specific range of motion. Surrounding the joint is a sac of fluid called the synovium. The fluid within the synovium, appropriately termed synovial fluid, acts as a cushion and a shock absorber in the joints. The synovial fluid also provides nutrients and oxygen to the cartilage that lines the ends of the bone. Cartilage is slippery tissue that decreases friction between the bones when they move. Cartilage also adds a measure of support within the joint. When all of these components function appropriately the bones slide past each other easily and without friction or discomfort.

Arthritis is essentially a chronic, inflammatory disease of the joints. The joint inflammation can be caused by injury, bacterial or viral infection, and, in the case of rheumatoid arthritis, an overactive immune system. Arthritis frequently causes pain, stiffness, warmth, redness, and swelling in and around the joints of the body. In rheumatoid arthritis other organs may become inflamed in addition to the joints. The synovial membrane is the site of inflammation. This constant inflammation does several things.

It destroys the cartilage coating the bones, thus destroying a layer of lubrication in the joints. The destruction of the cartilage narrows the space between the bones of the joint. In time the bones begin to wear on each other. Constant inflammation also attracts the attention of the immune system, which sends white blood cells to the joints. These cells promote the inflammatory process and speed up the break down of both the cartilage and the bone of the afflicted joint. The chemicals released by these cells can also cause fever, shock, and damage to other organs of the body. Another result of the inflammation is the growth of the synovial membrane. It grows to fill the joint, increasing the stiffness. An enlarged synovial sac also deforms the joint, causing the frequent misshapen appearance of arthritic joints.

Arthritis and its more serious counterpart, rheumatoid arthritis, are diseases for which there is no cure. Most people suffering from arthritis do not suffer constantly, and the severity of discomfort fluctuates. There are many treatments alleviating symptoms of arthritis. The majority of these treatments include some form of anti-inflammatory medication or immuno-suppressant drugs. In some cases where the arthritis has progressed extensively, surgery may be required to reconstruct or even replace joints.

What causes arthritis? Nobody really knows the answer, but here are some of the leads that scientists and doctors are currently studying. As mentioned earlier, arthritis can be caused by joint damage such as fractures, sprains, and infectious diseases. These causes of arthritis are temporary and the joint disease will often disappear when the body heals. It appears that inflammations characteristic of rheumatoid arthritis, on the other hand, begin with the body's own immune system.

RHEUMATOID ARTHRITIS

Rheumatoid arthritis is characterized as an auto-immune disease because the body's defense system attacks the body. How the process starts and why it doesn't control itself as in other immune responses is where science is having trouble finding an answer.

Some think rheumatoid arthritis is caused by the same bacterial or viral infection causing temporary arthritis. They say the immune system gets turned on to fight either a bacterial or viral invader and then doesn't shut itself off properly. Proponents of this theory have yet to identify an organism that acts as a primary trigger for the auto-immune response. Others say people have a genetic predisposition toward arthritis. Many people suffering from arthritis produce a molecule called HLA-DR4. This molecule may stimulate the immune system to attack the collagen of the joints. A problem with this idea is that there are many people who have the same molecule, but do not have arthritis. Still other researchers think that a deficiency of corticotropin-releasing hormone, a hormone that suppresses the inflammatory response, is the root of arthritis. Other research has shown that a mutated tumor suppressor gene, which controls cellular division, might play a factor in the growth of the synovial membrane. The answer to the question about the cause of arthritis could be one of these, none of these, or all of these and something more.

ARTHRITIS RISK FACTORS

Whatever be the cause, there are several things that we can do to decrease our chances of developing arthritis. One of the things that we can do is to eat a healthy diet and maintain an appropriate weight. Research has shown that people that are obese have a greater chance of getting arthritis. Maintaining a healthy weight though isn't the only benefit of a nutritious diet. When we eat a diet high in fruits and vegetables we consume many phytochemicals that can decrease our arthritis risk.

As we discussed in the chapter on phytochemicals, several kinds of flavonoids have the capability to reduce the inflammatory response. Flavonoid compounds inhibit the enzymes that produce the chemicals that contribute to inflammation. The flavonoid nobiletin, found in citrus fruit, performs the same function of inhibiting the production of inflammatory chemical messengers, and also decreases the amount of an enzyme that is known to degrade cartilage. Because this enzyme is not present in large quantities, it is proposed that the loss of cartilage will progress much more slowly. Thus, by consuming foods that are high in flavonoids, it is likely that we can decrease our risk for developing arthritis.

Other recent studies have shown a correlation between the types of fats consumed and the incidence of rheumatoid arthritis. It is a well-known fact that we need to avoid saturated fatty acids, but there are different kinds of unsaturated fatty acids that can do us much good. Current research has shown that a diet high in omega-3 and omega-6 fatty acids as well as vitamin E supplementation can reduce the risk of arthritis significantly. These types of fatty acids are found mostly in fatty fish such as salmon and tuna. Another study on rheumatoid arthritis with over 300 participants showed that those who had a high intake of olive oil had lower chances of getting arthritis.

Vitamins B6, B12, and folate may also help prevent arthritis. Several studies over the last few years have shown a correlation between high levels of homocysteine in the blood and the incidence of arthritis.

Alzheimer's Disease

Early in this century, Dr. Alois Alzheimer, a psychiatrist, discovered two unusual properties in the brain of a woman who had died with what he thought was a mental disorder. The first was deposits of an unknown substance he called "senile plaques". The second was an uncharacteristic twisting and tangling of some brain cell fibers. These two properties are now known as neurotic plaques and neurofibrillary tangles. They remain the hallmark of the disease that was named after Dr. Alzheimer. Today, Alzheimer's is the focus of intense study. Almost two million Americans (and nearly half of all Americans over age eigthy-five) currently suffer from Alzheimer's. These numbers are projected to increase dramatically in the coming decades, as the Baby Boomer population gets older.

Despite the fact that we know much more now about Alzheimer's disease than we did years ago, there is still a great deal left to learn. Alzheimer's disease is a chronic condition for which there is no cure. It is the most common cause of dementia among older people. It involves the slow deterioration of the parts of the brain related to memory, orientation, calculation, and other intellectual functions. Early symptoms include mild forgetfulness and confusion. However, eventually patients have difficulty carrying out routine, everyday tasks. In the later stages of the disease there may be much more progressive memory loss, impaired judgment, disorientation, confusion, and other behavioral changes. The disease usually begins later in life, most often after age sixty, but in rare cases it may begin as early as thirty years of age.

WHAT CAUSES ALZHEIMER'S DISEASE?

Doctors and scientists do not know exactly what causes Alzheimer's disease. There are two main causes currently under investigation. Both have to do with the initial observations made by Dr. Alzheimer. The first of these is called neurofibrillary tangles. Pieces of the cellular skeleton in charge of giving structure to nerve cells and transporting nutrients around nerve cells get jumbled up. The cause of neurofibrillary tangles is still unknown, but researchers do know that it causes these cells to become sick and less capable of transmitting information around the brain. Eventually these cells die and the functions they performed and the memory they stored are lost.

BRAIN PLAQUE—BETA AMYLOID

The second cause of brain deterioration involves a protein called beta amyloid. Beta amyloid is a sticky protein that builds up in the diseased parts of the brain, the parts that Dr. Alzheimer called "senile plaques." The build-up of beta amyloid is associated with a decrease in a chemical messenger molecule called acetylcholine that is used by the nerve cells to transmit signals. As levels of this neurotransmitter decrease, it becomes increasingly difficult for nerve cells to communicate with one another. This symptom is treated with drugs that increase the concentration of acetylcholine in the brain. This medication slows the progress of Alzheimer's, but the disease still progresses. Beta amyloid may do two other things directly damaging nerve cells, leading to cell death. First, as beta amyloid breaks down it releases free radicals that can damage sensitive nerve cells.

The second way beta amyloid damages cells is by turning on the body's inflammatory response. White blood cells accumulate around diseased parts of the brain, releasing chemicals that damage surrounding tissues, and further damage diseased tissue, leading to nerve cell death. Scientists don't yet know why this happens, but many think anti-inflammatory medications may help in slowing disease progress. In the end, it seems that science is beginning to find ways to slow the progress of symptoms of Alzheimer's, but they are a long way from understanding the root causes of Alzheimer's or finding a cure.

VASCULAR DAMAGE

One of the current hypotheses is that vascular damage contributes to the development of Alzheimer's disease. Thus, things

that contribute to the injury of our blood vessels, like high cholesterol, smoking, and a lack of fruits and vegetables are also likely to
promote the development of Alzheimer's disease.

Another factor that we discussed extensively in the chapter on
cardiovascular disease was that of homocysteine. A great deal of
current research is also pointing at this amino acid as a major contributor to Alzheimer's disease. It appears that homocysteine is
toxic to nerve cells and thus contributes directly to the degeneration of brain tissue. This nerve cell toxicity is a likely reason why
children of women with high levels of homocysteine have a greater
incidence of neural tube defects. Researchers do not know the
exact mechanisms through which homocysteine does its damage,
but several studies have indicated that people with high levels of
homocysteine are at a much greater risk of Alzheimer's disease. As
well, elderly people who have deficiencies in the vitamins B12 and
folate are much more likely to have Alzheimer's than elderly people who don't. Vitamins B12 and folate together with vitamin B6
are involved in enzymes that convert homocysteine to other amino
acids that are not so dangerous.

Yet another link between homocysteine and Alzheimer's disease
is that an enzyme whose function is to remove homocysteine from
the blood works as a much slower pace in people with Alzheimer's
and other similar mental disorders than in those who don't.
Because that enzyme functions more slowly, levels of homocysteine
are likely to build up and contribute to the progress of the disease.

These studies reconfirm our need to eat a balanced diet and
consume sufficient quantities of fruits and vegetables to ward off
this illness. If we make sure that our fat intake is low and that we
get enough of the vitamins B6, B12, and folate, our risks for developing Alzheimer's disease may be reduced.

Mild Cognitive Impairment (MCI)

MCI is characterized by memory impairment. Unlike
Alzheimer's disease, MCI does not adversely affect all cognitive
functioning, though it is often confused with Alzheimer's. Normal
memory changes associated with aging are characterized by
momentary lapses, such as misplacing an item, forgetting someone's name, or forgetting to pick up something at the store. In
contrast, memory loss associated with MCI is a more persistent

and troublesome problem. In cognitive testing, people with MCI remember significantly less of a paragraph they have read or details of simple drawings they have seen compared to people with normal memory changes associated with aging. A person with MCI is likely to forget important events repeatedly.

Is there a relationship between MCI and Alzheimer's disease? As its name indicates, MCI is a condition of mild impairment, specifically in the area of memory. Dementia, on the other hand, is characterized by additional, severe problems in other areas of cognition, such as orientation, language, and attention. MCI differs from Alzheimer's in some significant ways. Alzheimer's is a degenerative disease, meaning it gets progressively worse over time. MCI on the other hand does not always get worse. Scientists have been interested in MCI in part because a significant number of people over the age of sixty-five with MCI eventually develop Alzheimer's disease. In some studies approximately 12 to 15 percent of people with MCI develop Alzheimer's per year (or about 40 percent after three years). This is much higher than the 1 percent or so per year in a normal population of people sixty-five and older. As such, MCI is a risk factor for developing Alzheimer's. Researchers are examining the possible relationship between the two conditions.

NUTRITION AND MCI RISK FACTORS

For years, scientists have searched for answers for the observed decline in mental capacity so often accompanying aging. Until recently, medical authorities dismissed the idea that nutrition played a pivotal role in the physical and mental health of the elderly. However, several recent studies published in major medical and nutritional journals have shown that symptoms such as dementia, mental disorientation, and memory loss, may actually be due to nutritional deficiencies. One such study showed that the amino acid, homocysteine, found at high levels in the blood of people who eat a lot of meat, is linked with a type of mental disorientation frequently seen in the early stages of Alzheimer's disease. The study demonstrated that eating foods rich in folic acid such as beans, greens, and brewer's yeast, or taking folic acid supplements lowers blood levels of homocysteine and improves mental functioning.

Other studies implicate vitamin B12 deficiency as a cause of senile dementia in elderly people, due both to poor diets and poor protein digestion. Older people tend to be less efficient in digesting because they produce too little stomach acid to break down protein. Many have difficulty with the absorption of vitamin B12 from food. Vitamin B12 supplements can be more easily absorbed than vitamin B12 in food. Nonetheless, experts recommend eating foods rich in vitamin B12 for added insurance.

Other exciting studies indicate that vitamin E has properties capable of countering destructive damage that occurs during normal body activities. The progressive loss of brain cells that occurs in dementia and Alzheimer's disease may be related to this damage. In a 1997 study, vitamin E was shown to slow down functional decline of patients with moderate Alzheimer's disease by about seven months. Vitamin E also seems important in the body for stabilizing membranes. In one study, vitamin E was demonstrated to slow some aspects of functional deterioration in patients with Alzheimer's disease. However, this study has not yet been replicated.

Osteoporosis

Osteoporosis is a debilitating disease caused by the progressive degeneration of an individual's bones. The name literally means "porous bone" and was given to the disease because of the characteristic low bone mass of its sufferers. Osteoporosis is a disease that affects twenty-eight million people in the United States, 80 percent of whom are women. One in two women over the age of fifty can expect to have an osteoporosis-related fracture in her lifetime. The direct cost alone for treating such fractures totals over fourteen billion dollars nationally per year.

WHAT CAUSES OSTEOPOROSIS?

To understand osteoporosis we first need to know just how our bones are made up. Besides supporting the weight of our bodies, bones function to produce both our red and white blood cells. They also serve to store calcium and phosphorous for long and short terms. Calcium and phosphorous perform multiple functions in your body, and move in and out of your bones as necessary. Calcium, for example, is needed for the heart, nerves, and blood clotting mechanisms to work appropriately.

Our bones are consisted of a tough, fibrous matrix formed with collagen. Within this matrix calcium phosphate crystals assemble themselves to build the solid part of the bone. The concept is not unlike that of concrete reinforced with steel bars, only that bone material has much greater strength. Cells called osteoclasts within our bones constantly degrade bone material while other cells known as osteoblasts continually build it up. As a person grows, the activity of the osteoblasts and other bone forming cells far exceeds that of the osteoclasts resulting in the generation of new bone material. That is how we grow as children and young adults. Once we have matured and our bodies are no longer growing, the activity of the osteoblasts balances with the work of the osteoclasts resulting in the perpetual recycling of bone material.

As we age, osteoblasts become increasingly less active, while osteoclasts continue working. The bone is thus degraded faster than it is built up, resulting in osteoporosis. This action usually begins at about age thirty. Up until that point the body is more or less continually depositing new bone. The discrepancy of activity between the osteoblasts and the osteoclasts is especially pronounced in postmenopausal women. In women, the hormone estrogen stimulates osteoblastic activity. In men, the hormone testosterone does the same thing. When a woman undergoes menopause she stops producing estrogen and her osteoblasts lose a major stimulant. Men, under normal circumstances, never stop producing testosterone. As a result, women's bones degrade faster than those of men.

Osteoporosis is characterized by low bone density, causing the bones to become weak and brittle. Sufferers of osteoporosis can fracture bones doing common activities. Sometimes mild falls will break bones. Bones that normally don't break, such as the hip-bones, become especially susceptible to fractures that cause great pain. Often such injuries can immobilize the victim. People who suffer from osteoporosis can experience a loss of height and develop a curvature of the spine known as Dowager's Hump. This is brought about by compression fractures in the weakened vertebrae that cause them to collapse vertically. Osteoporosis is known as the "Silent Killer" because one usually does not know that they have it until a minor bump or fall causes a fracture.

OSTEOPOROSIS RISK FACTORS

There are several risk factors for osteoporosis. Primary among them is being a woman. As we have mentioned, once women go through menopause, the cells that build up the bone do not function as actively as those in men. Women can lose up to 20 percent of their bone mass in the first five to seven years following menopause. Thus small, thin-boned women are at a largely increased risk of developing osteoporosis in old age. Age is another risk factor. The older you get, the more likely you are to have lost considerable bone mass. Other risk factors include a family history of osteoporosis, a diet low in calcium, the use of certain medications, an inactive lifestyle, cigarette smoking, the excessive use of alcohol and coffee, and high-protein diets.

Many things can be done to prevent the onset of osteoporosis. First and foremost among them is to assure that you are getting an adequate dietary intake of calcium and vitamin D. As we have mentioned, calcium helps to form the solid, crystalline portion of the bone. Vitamin D is needed to absorb the calcium from the intestines. Regardless of how much calcium you consume, if you do not have adequate levels of vitamin D, the body cannot use it. Calcium is found in dark green leafy vegetables and dairy products. Vitamin D has two principal sources. One source is the skin where it is formed following direct exposure to sunlight. Another way that we can get vitamin D is by consuming dairy products fortified with vitamin D. When we assure ourselves of a high intake of calcium and vitamin D through appropriate dietary sources we decrease substantially our risk of developing osteoporosis.

One can further prevent the onset of osteoporosis with regular and frequent weight-bearing exercise. These activities include such things as walking, dancing, jogging, racquet sports, and weight lifting. These kinds of activities place stress on the bones, stimulating them to continually build themselves up. The bone becomes thicker and its density is increased as new bone material is deposited.

Smoking has also been implicated in the development of osteoporosis. Tobacco seems to antagonize the function of estrogen and can cause premature menopause. Women who smoke have a higher chance of developing osteoporosis. However, as soon as they stop smoking, the risk decreases. Anti-inflammatory drugs such as corticosteroids contribute to the development of osteoporosis because they interfere with calcium absorption. It is therefore wise, when possible, to avoid them when possible.

Another way to prevent osteoporosis is to limit consumption of caffeine and alcohol. Caffeine and alcohol act as diuretics. As more urine is excreted from the body, more calcium and phosphorus are lost, too. As we have mentioned before, calcium is important in many physiologic processes. When calcium levels in the blood drop, the body seeks to correct that decrease by replacing the lost calcium with calcium taken from the bones. In essence the bones are dissolved to make up for what is lost. Now, this process is a very slow one, but over the years it can be a contributing factor to the development of osteoporosis. The National Osteoporosis Foundation has said that even as little as two or three ounces of alcohol per day can damage bones. High-protein diets also increase the excretion of calcium from the body having a similar effect as caffeine and alcohol.

An interesting study recently reported in the *American Journal of Clinical Nutrition* shows that older women who drink tea have higher bone mineral density than others that don't. The results are surprising in light of the fact that caffeine is known to reduce bone mineral density. Researchers propose that flavonoids found in the tea are likely responsible for the observed effect on bone strength. Thus flavonoids obtained from other dietary sources are likely to strengthen bones as well. One that we mentioned in the section on flavonoids was genistein, which directly influences bone deposition.

Other recent studies show that vitamin K can also have a positive effect on bone health. Research has revealed the vitamin K is necessary for the addition of carbon and oxygen molecules to bone proteins. The addition of those molecules is thought to strengthen the bone. Indeed, low levels of vitamin K in the blood are related to an increase in hip fractures in women.

In general, a diet high in fruits and vegetables and low in fat and cholesterol improves bone strength. Without isolating any one component of fruits or vegetables one study showed that people who eat many fruits and vegetables experience fewer symptoms of osteoporosis than those who don't. Another study has shown that diets high in saturated fat decreases bone strength.

Hormone replacement therapy for postmenopausal women can be very effective against the onset of osteoporosis. Even though women do not produce the estrogen needed to stimulate the osteoblasts in the bones, the estrogen therapy can make up for it. Phytoestrogens act in a similar fashion as estrogen and may be instrumental in maintaining healthy bones.

Although osteoporosis is a serious disease common in our society, you can reduce your risk significantly by eating fruits, vegetables, and dairy products rich in calcium and vitamin D. In addition to a healthy diet, regular exercise is essential in preventing osteoporosis.

All of the diseases we have discussed are not caused by foreign pathogens. Some are connected to cellular deterioration that simply accompanies aging. Others are the result of the kind of food we eat, or the types of chemicals we take into the body. In the end it seems there are no quick fixes for these diseases. We believe that eating smart and living right are the only ways to help curb the destructiveness of these diseases at present. In essence, this is the primary goal of this book: to promote healthy living to prevent premature death and the pain and discomfort associated with these debilitating diseases. It is possible to live longer and happier with a little effort directed at diet, exercise and lifestyle.

Immune System Decline

As we age our immune system does not function as well as it used to. We have lower numbers of white blood cells in our blood. Our body does not produce as many new white blood cells as it used to. As well, the amount of protective antibodies that are circulating in our system also declines leaving us susceptible to diseases to which we were previously immune. Many people believe that the decline in our immune systems contributes significantly to aging and ultimately causes a great deal of chronic disease. For example, misdirected inflammatory responses contribute to arthritis and Alzheimer's disease while a decrease in immunosurveillance leads to cancer when our own cells get out of control. What can be done to slow, stop, or even reverse this process? The answer lies again in fruits and vegetables. Several exciting studies show the potential in healthy eating to improve our immune function—whether in young, middle, or advanced age.

A study conducted with carotenoid-rich vegetables showed that a diet low in carotenoids adversely affects the function of white blood cells. These cells did not divide as fast or excrete as great a quantity of signaling molecules necessary for an adequate response as did cells of people who consumed a diet rich in carotenoids. This loss of immune function was restored when individuals who were consuming a low-carotenoid diet ate carotenoid rich foods. Other epidemiological research supports the concept that carotenoids improve immune function.

Another group of researchers studying the immune system sought to test the effects of dietary supplementation with the antioxidant vitamins C and E on aged women. They found that after sixteen weeks of supplementations with both vitamins, the immune systems of the women who received the supplements was significantly improved over those who didn't. Specifically, their white blood cells proliferated faster, the activity of their macrophages increased, and all cells of the immune system demonstrated greater ability to home in to sites of infection. Another study that measured just the effects of vitamin E on the immune system reported that vitamin E can increase white blood cell proliferation as well as stimulate the secretion of chemical messengers needed for an immune response. This effect of vitamin E has been seen in other studies as well. A great deal of research supports the concept that antioxidant vitamins play a strong role in improving immune function. These studies are powerful indications of our need to incorporate into our diets foods that are rich in these antioxidant compounds.

Vitamin A has recently been shown to have an effect on the progression of viral, bacterial, and parasitic diseases. Clinical trials have suggested that vitamin A supplementation reduces the morbidity and mortality of several infections diseases such as measles, some forms of diarrhea, HIV infection, and malaria. A specific study on the effects of vitamin A on malaria showed that children infected with the malaria parasite had a 36 percent reduction in parasite density in their blood if they were given vitamin A. As well, they experienced 30 percent fewer episodes of acute illness.

An interesting fact about vitamin D is that it may be able to help prevent auto-immune disorders. Auto-immune disorders are when the immune system turns on its own body and attacks it instead of invading pathogens. As we have discussed, an immune system misguided in such a way probably contributes to a variety of chronic diseases such as rheumatoid arthritis, diabetes, and Alzheimer's disease. Researchers first noted the correlation between vitamin D and auto-immune disorders because they observed that parts of the world that consistently experience vitamin D deficiencies also have increased rates of these diseases of the immune system. In later research vitamin D was shown to suppress the development of autoimmunity.

A nutritious diet full of fruits and vegetables has repeatedly been demonstrated to improve overall immune system function and enhance the quality of life. Studies have shown that elderly people who eat a healthy, well-balanced diet do not demonstrate the decline in immune function that others do. Because of this, we need to be sure to eat a balanced diet of fruits and vegetables now and plan to continue to eat right for the rest of our lives.

References

Breteler MM, Bots ML, Ott A, Hofman A. Risk Factors for Vascular Disease and Dementia. Haemostasis. 1998 May–Aug; 28(3–4): 167–73.

Camplani A, Saino N, Moller AP. Carotenoids, Sexual Signals and Immune Function in Barn Swallows from Chernobyl. Proc R Soc Lond B Biol Sci. 1999 Jun 7; 266(1424): 1111–6.

Cantorna MT. Vitamin D and Autoimmunity: Is Vitamin D Status an Environmental Factor Affecting Auto-immune Disease Prevalence? Proc Soc Exp Biol Med. 2000 Mar; 223(3): 230–3.

Cornuz J, Feskanich D, Willett WC, Colditz GA. Smoking, Smoking Cessation, and Risk of Hip Fracture in Women. Am J Med. 1999 Mar; 106(3): 311–4.

De-la-Fuente M, Ferrandez MD, Burgos MS, Soler A, Prieto A, Miquel J. Immune Function in Aged Women is Improved by Ingestion of Vitamins C and E. Can J Physiol Pharmacol. 1998 Apr; 76(4): 373–80.

De-la-Fuente M, Victor VM. Anti-Oxidants as Modulators of Immune Function. Immunol Cell Biol. 2000 Feb; 78(1): 49–54.

Eriksson J, Lindstrom J, Valle T, Aunola S, Hamalainen H, Ilanne Parikka P, Keinanen Kiukaanniemi S, Laakso M, Lauhkonen M, Lehto P, Lehtonen A, Louheranta A, Mannelin M, Martikkala V, Rastas M, Sundvall J, Turpeinen A, Viljanen T, Uusitupa M, Tuomilehto J. Prevention of Type II Diabetes in Subjects with Impaired Glucose Tolerance: The Diabetes Prevention Study (DPS) in Finland. Study Design and 1-Year Interim Report on the Feasibility of the Lifestyle Intervention Programme. Diabetologia. 1999 Jul; 42(7): 793–801.

Feskanich D, Weber P, Willett WC, Rockett H, Booth SL, Colditz GA. Vitamin K Intake and Hip Fractures in Women: A Prospective Study. Am J Clin Nutr. 1999 Jan; 69(1): 74–9.

Gallagher JC. The Role of Vitamin D in the Pathogenesis and Treatment of Osteoporosis. J Rheumatol Suppl. 1996 Aug; 45: 15–8.

Gao YH, Yamaguchi M. Inhibitory Effect of Genistein on Osteoclast-Like Cell Formation in Mouse Marrow Cultures. Biochem Pharm. 1999; 58: 767–772.

Gomes-Trolin C, Regland B, Oreland L. Decreased Methionine Adenosyltransferase Activity in Erythrocytes of Patients with Dementia Disorders. Eur Neuropsychopharmacol. 1995 Jun; 5(2): 107–14.

Grimble RF. Effect of Antioxidative Vitamins on Immune Function with Clinical Applications. Int J Vitam Nutr Res. 1997; 67(5): 312–20.

Han SN, Meydani SN. Vitamin E and Infectious Diseases in the Aged. Proc Nutr Soc. 1999 Aug; 58(3): 697–705.

Hegarty VM, May HM, Khaw KT. Tea Drinking and Bone Mineral Density in Older Women. Am J Clin Nutr. 2000 Apr; 71(4): 1003–7.

Hernanz A, Plaza A, Martin Mola E, De-Miguel E. Increased Plasma Levels of Homocysteine and Other Thiol Compounds in Rheumatoid Arthritis Women. Clin Biochem. 1999 Feb; 32(1): 65–70.

Hughes DA. Effects of Carotenoids on Human Immune Function. Proc Nutr Soc. 1999 Aug; 58(3): 713–8.

Hughes DA. Effects of Dietary Antioxidants on the Immune Function of Middle-Aged Adults. Proc Nutr Soc. 1999 Feb; 58(1): 79–84.

Ishiwa J, Sato T, Mimaki Y, Sashida Y, Yano M, Ito A. A Citrus Flavonoid, Nobiletin, Suppresses Production and Gene Expression of Matrix Metalloproteinase 9/Gelatinase B in Rabbit Synovial Fibroblasts. J Rheumatol. 2000 Jan; 27(1): 20–5.

Joosten E, Lesaffre E, Riezler R, Ghekiere V, Dereymaeker L, Pelemans W, Dejaeger E. Is Metabolic Evidence for Vitamin B-12 and Folate Deficiency More Frequent in Elderly Patients with Alzheimer's Disease? J Gerontol A Biol Sci Med Sci. 1997 Mar; 52(2): M76–9.

Kaufman JM. Role of Calcium and Vitamin D in the Prevention and the Treatment of Postmenopausal Osteoporosis: An Overview. Clin Rheumatol. 1995 Sep; 14 Suppl 3: 9–13.

Kerstetter JE, O'Brien KO, Insogna KL. Dietary Protein Affects Intestinal Calcium Absorption. Am J Clin Nutr. 1998 Oct; 68(4): 859–65.

Kim HK, Cheon BS, Kim YH, Kim SY, Kim HP. Effects of Naturally Occurring Flavonoids on Nitric Oxide Production in the Macrophage Cell Line RAW 264.7 and Their Structure-Activity Relationships. Biochem Pharmacol. 1999 Sep 1; 58(5): 759–65.

Krause D, Mastro AM, Handte G, Smiciklas Wright H, Miles MP, Ahluwalia N. Immune Function Did Not Decline with Aging in Apparently Healthy, Well-Nourished Women. Mech Ageing Dev. 1999 Dec 7; 112(1): 43–57.

La-Vecchia C, Decarli A, Pagano R. Vegetable Consumption and Risk of Chronic Disease. Epidemiology. 1998 Mar; 9(2): 208–10.

Liang YC, Huang YT, Tsai SH, Lin-Shiau SY, Chen CF, Lin JK. Suppression of Inducible Cyclooxygenase and Inducible Nitric Oxide Synthase by Apigenin and Related Flavonoids in Mouse Macrophages. Carcinogenesis. 1999 Oct; 20(10): 1945–52.

Linos A, Kaklamani VG, Kaklamani E, Koumantaki Y, Giziaki E, Papazoglou S, Mantzoros CS. Dietary Factors in Relation to Rheumatoid Arthritis: A Role for Olive Oil and Cooked Vegetables? Am J Clin Nutr. 1999 Dec; 70(6): 1077–82.

Meydani M. Dietary Antioxidants Modulation of Aging and Immune-Endothelial Cell Interaction. Mech Ageing Dev. 1999 Nov; 111(2–3): 123–32.

Meyer KA, Kushi LH, Jacobs DR Jr, Slavin J, Sellers TA, Folsom AR. Carbohydrates, Dietary Fiber, and Incident type II Diabetes in Older Women. Am J Clin Nutr. 2000 Apr; 71(4): 921–30.

Miller JW. Homocysteine and Alzheimer's Disease. Nutr Rev. 1999 Apr; 57(4): 126–9.

Moriguchi S, Muraga M. Vitamin E and Immunity. Vitam Horm. 2000; 59: 305–36.

Parsons RB, Waring RH, Ramsden DB, Williams AC. In Vitro Effect of the Cysteine Metabolites Homocysteic Acid, Homocysteine and Cysteic Acid Upon Human Neuronal Cell Lines. Neurotoxicology. 1998 Aug–Oct; 19(4–5): 599–603.

Pedersen BK, Bruunsgaard H, Jensen M, Krzywkowski K, Ostrowski K. Exercise and Immune Function: Effect of Ageing and Nutrition. Proc Nutr Soc. 1999 Aug; 58(3): 733–42.

Pettersson T, Friman C, Abrahamsson L, Nilsson B, Norberg B. Serum Homocysteine and Methylmalonic Acid in Patients with Rheumatoid Arthritis and Cobalaminopenia. J Rheumatol. 1998 May; 25(5): 859–63.

Ravaglia G, Forti P, Maioli F, Bastagli L, Facchini A, Mariani E, Savarino L, Sassi S, Cucinotta D, Lenaz G. Effect of Micronutrient Status on Natural Killer Cell Immune Function in Healthy Free-Living Subjects Aged >/=90 y. Am J Clin Nutr. 2000 Feb; 71(2): 590–8.

Roubenoff R, Dellaripa P, Nadeau MR, Abad LW, Muldoon BA, Selhub J, Rosenberg IH. Abnormal Homocysteine Metabolism in Rheumatoid Arthritis. Arthritis Rheum. 1997 Apr; 40(4): 718–22.

Sahyoun NR, Hochberg MC, Helmick CG, Harris T, Pamuk ER. Body Mass Index, Weight Change, and Incidence of Self-Reported Physician-Diagnosed Arthritis

Among Women. Am J Public Health. 1999 Mar; 89(3): 391–4.

Semba RD. The Role of Vitamin A and Related Retinoids in Immune Function. Nutr Rev. 1998 Jan; 56(1 Pt 2): S38–48.

Semba RD. Vitamin A and Immunity to Viral, Bacterial and Protozoan Infections. Proc Nutr Soc. 1999 Aug; 58(3): 719–27.

Shankar AH, Genton B, Semba RD, Baisor M, Paino J, Tamja S, Adiguma T, Wu L, Rare L, Tielsch JM, Alpers MP, West KP Jr. Effect of Vitamin A Supplementation on Morbidity Due to Plasmodium Falciparum in Young Children in Papua New Guinea: A Randomized Trial. Lancet. 1999 Jul 17; 354(9174): 203–9.

Swaminathan R. Nutritional Factors in Osteoporosis. Int J Clin Pract. 1999 Oct–Nov; 53(7): 540–8.

Tucker KL, Hannan MT, Chen H, Cupples LA, Wilson PW, Keil DP. Potassium, Magnesium, and Fruit and Vegetable Intakes are Associated with Greater Bone Mineral Density in Elderly Men and Women. Am J Clin Nutr. 1999 Apr; 69(4): 727–36.

Venkatraman JT, Chu WC. Effects of Dietary Omega-3 and Omega-6 Lipids and Vitamin E on Serum Cytokines, Lipid Mediators and Anti-DNA Antibodies in a Mouse Model for Rheumatoid Arthritis. J Am Coll Nutr. 1999 Dec; 18(6): 602–13.

Wang XB, Zhao XH. The Effect of Dietary Sulfur-Containing Amino Acids on Calcium Excretion. Adv Exp Med Biol. 1998; 442: 495–9.

Watzl B, Bub A, Brandstetter BR, Rechkemmer G. Modulation of Human T Lymphocyte Functions by the Consumption of Carotenoid-Rich Vegetables. Br J Nutr. 1999 Nov; 82(5): 383–9.

Weber P. The Role of Vitamins in the Prevention of Osteoporosis—A Brief Status Report. Int J Vitam Nutr Res. 1999 May; 69(3): 194–7.

Williams DE, Wareham NJ, Cox BD, Byrne CD, Hales CN, Day NE. Frequent Salad Vegetable Consumption is Associated with a Reduction in the Risk of Diabetes Mellitus. J Clin Epidemiol. 1999 Apr; 52(4): 329–35.

Wohl GR, Loehrke L, Watkins BA, Zernicke RF. Effects of High-Fat Diet on Mature Bone Mineral Content, Structure, and Mechanical Properties. Calcif Tissue Int. 1998 Jul; 63(1): 74–9.

Wu D, Meydani M, Beharka AA, Serafini M, Martin KR, Meydani SN. In Vitro Supplementation with Different Tocopherol Homologues can Affect the Function of Immune Cells in Old Mice. Free Radic Biol Med. 2000 Feb 15; 28(4): 643–51.

CHAPTER 16

Exercise, Diet
and Well-Being

Exercise is an essential element in a healthy lifestyle. Of course this is not ground-breaking news. In fact, dieticians and nutritionists have been encouraging people to exercise regularly for years. Exercise has been praised for its positive influence on physical, mental and spiritual health. A regular exercise regimen has tremendous benefits in all areas of life. Eating healthy foods works well with a regular exercise program to ensure health. It is important to incorporate both a balanced diet and regular exercise in your lifestyle to ensure optimum fitness and well-being. We hope to convince you that a regular exercise program positively impacts your ability to eat a balanced diet, and that eating a balanced diet will also help motivate you to exercise regularly. In other words, we hope to show how diet and exercise influence one another.

Physical Activity—Thirty Minutes Daily

The Surgeon General warns that "a lack of physical activity is detrimental to health," and recommends a minimum of thirty minutes of exercise daily. Many experts recommend thirty minutes of exercise daily, but just what constitutes "exercise"? Technically speaking, exercise is the voluntary movement of muscles. In this sense, you probably do more exercise than you think. One could consider activities like typing on a keyboard, switching channels on the television, or eating a candy bar exercise. However, it seems that the Surgeon General had a little more in mind than things like this when recommending thirty minutes of exercise. As a general rule of thumb, you should plan to spend at least thirty uninterrupted minutes a day doing something that requires big movements from your major muscle groups.

The following guidelines were issued by the Centers for Disease Control and Prevention and the American College of Sports Medicine, in cooperation with the President's Council on Physical Fitness and Sports in 1997:

"It is recommended that every American adult accumulate thirty minutes or more moderate exercise at least on most days of the week to maintain health. There are multiple activities that can be done to achieve this moderate exercise, for example, walking up and down the stairs instead of taking the elevator, gardening, dancing."

What Kind of Physical Activity?

One specific way to get thirty minutes of exercise is to walk two miles briskly. These recommendations are targeted to the 24 percent of American adults that are entirely sedentary and the 54 percent of Americans who are almost inactive.

Activities like walking, jogging, aerobics, weightlifting, or playing any of a wide variety of sports that require you to move your arms and legs will suffice. You should elevate your heart rate when exercising. Exercise prepares the heart and blood vessels for other incidents of stress. When the heart performs regularly at an increased level, as it does during exercise, it can react more efficiently in an emergency.

There are two kinds of movement: active and passive. Active movement is the conscious movement of the muscle, like walking up the stairs or hitting a ball, while passive movement is the jiggling of an arm or leg. Active movement builds lean muscle tissue. The more lean muscle tissue you have, the more calories your body burns both when exercising and when at rest.

Because lean muscle tissue increases your body's energy expenditure, a strong weight-loss program should include some form of exercise that will build muscle (weight training, for instance). Increased muscle tissue leads to decreased fat because your body will continue to seek sources of energy in increased quantities even when resting. Physical exercise thus helps maintain an appropriate body weight and will enable you to perform routine tasks without fatigue.

Exercise and Disease Prevention

Many studies indicate that exercise is a major factor in the prevention of certain cancers, heart disease, diabetes, and other chronic diseases. We can significantly decrease the rate of progression, and even prevent, coronary heart disease by including the following in our lifestyles: smoking cessation, blood lipid reduction, weight reduction, reduced caloric intake, and regular physical activity.

A consistent effort is required to be physically fit. Fitness is important in all aspects of life, from cleaning the house or typing up a report or memo, to running a marathon. In the end, physical fitness can help you live a longer life, and help you enjoy the years you are alive. It is not enough to simply live to be 120. We all want to get the most out of the years we live, and being physically fit is absolutely necessary for total wellness. Physical fitness incorporates cardiorespiratory fitness, muscle strength and endurance, flexibility, and an appropriate body composition. We will discuss these elements of physical fitness and how diet and exercise combine to maintain a healthy body.

A healthy lifestyle will ensure that your body takes in and utilizes enough energy to maintain your body's oxygen needs. Cardiorespiratory fitness or endurance determines how long a person can continue to do something that is physically demanding, from walking across the street, to participating in the iron man triathlon. Aerobic exercise is exercise that increases heart rate and requires oxygen in metabolism. This type of exercise improves cardiovascular fitness. Physical activity can have lasting cardiovascular health benefits. While everyone knows that exercise is good for the body, fewer people are aware of the many proven cardiovascular benefits that come with exercise.

Through exercise we can increase the maximum ventilatory oxygen intake by increasing the volume of blood pumped by the heart per minute. When the volume of the blood pumped out of the heart increases, our muscles receive more oxygen. When our heart is used to increased pressure, its response to other stresses will not lead to heart attacks.

Changing the Body's Composition

Regular exercise also changes our body's composition, making us leaner. Exercise increases the rate of metabolism, making you loose fat weight when you exercise: the less excess fat on your body, the better it is for your heart. Remember, exercise benefits your bodies most if it is maintained for at least thirty minutes. The best exercise for you is the one you enjoy the most.

Oxygen is needed for the breakdown of carbohydrates, fats, and proteins into energy, carbon dioxide, and water. When we exercise, we require more oxygen in our bodies, because our muscles are working hard. Without adequate oxygen intake, our performance level decreases significantly. This can be seen in the difficulty of peak performance with higher altitudes. Muscles require oxygen to perform all the difficult functions needed in daily living. In fact, muscles have their own oxygen transporter to speed the supply of oxygen from the blood to the muscles. As more oxygen is released into the blood stream, maximal energy release increases and physical performance reaches its optimum.

Physical exercise will tone and develop your muscles. The more muscle you have, the more calories you burn. Muscle mass also increases your metabolic rate. If your resting metabolic rate increases you will burn more calories while resting than previously. Thus, developing muscle strength is also a great way to lose weight. Those that exercise regularly (building lean muscle tissue) thus burn fat more efficiently, more rapidly and for longer periods of time than sedentary people.

Flexibility and Overall Health

Flexibility is another term for range of motion. Flexibility is very important for your health, because it determines how far you can bend and stretch muscles and ligaments. A healthy diet does little to improve flexibility. The only way to increase your range of motion is to stretch on a regular basis. Flexibility enhances strength and performance by reducing muscle tension. When you increase your flexibility, you decrease your risk of joint injury by absorbing and dissipating force and trauma that occurs at the joints.

Not only will physical activity (moderate to intense) make everyday tasks seem easier, it also actually changes the composition of your body and increases its ability to perform vital functions. Exercise strengthens muscle tissue, increases the efficiency of the circulatory system, and promotes bone density.

First, increased physical activity changes your body composition. Fat percentages decrease as muscle percentages increase. As we have already discussed, this enables you to burn more calories both when exercising and resting. The more calories you burn, the less likely you will be to develop serious chronic conditions like obesity and atherosclerosis. Excess body weight places tremendous stress on your body, particularly on your heart. Regular aerobic exercise can increase the "good" cholesterol (HDL), and lower blood pressure.

Second, physical activity increases the efficiency of your circulatory system. Exercise causes dilation of the blood vessel lining, or endothelium. Routine physical activity leads to more efficient dilation of the blood vessels, which then improves overall blood flow. Blood vessels that do not dilate regularly respond more slowly when called to action.

Blood flow is also affected by exercise through the production of nitrous oxide in the blood stream. When muscle tissue requires additional nutrients, it produces nitrous oxide to signal the blood vessels to dilate, which then allows more blood (and nutrients) to flow to the muscles. This reaction takes place during exercise, but has a lasting effect on the body. Even when resting after exercise, blood vessels may remain dilated, increasing blood flow throughout the day. This in turn reduces blood pressure, and decreases stress on the heart. The circulatory system is further aided by exercise in more mediated ways. A lean body generally has less fat circulating in the blood stream. Exercise tends to lower cholesterol levels, reducing the risk of atherosclerosis significantly. The lower your cholesterol levels the less likely you are to accumulate blockage in your blood vessels.

Exercise and Bone Density

Third, exercise promotes bone density. With healthy bones, you decrease your risk of osteoporosis. We have already discussed this in chapter 15.

Other Benefits that You Don't Always See

A benefit that should not be discounted is the emotional "boost" and satisfaction you will feel as a result of an ongoing exercise routine. During exercise, endorphins are produced which increase one's sense of well-being. This, in turn, should provide encouragement to continue exercise patterns.

Exercise significantly decreases the risk of diabetes, obesity, and cardiovascular disease. According to the American Heart Association, "physical inactivity is recognized as a risk factor for coronary artery disease." Because regular physical activity increases cardiovascular functional capacity, exercise plays a crucial role in both primary and secondary prevention in cardiovascular disease. There are many known benefits that come with regular physical exercise, but none are more valuable than the benefits exercise brings for the heart.

Regular physical exercise can help control blood lipid abnormalities, diabetes, and obesity. The AHA states, "there is a direct relationship between physical inactivity and cardiovascular mortality, and physical inactivity is an independent risk factor for the development of coronary artery disease." Through inactivity, we are jeopardizing our lives. Here are just a few examples of how a good diet and a regular exercise regime can prevent chronic degenerative diseases.

Preventing Cardiovascular Disease

Cardiovascular disease (CHD) is a general term for all the diseases related to the heart and blood vessels, and is the leading cause of death in the United States. CHD is responsible for hundreds of thousands of deaths due to heart disease, stroke, and heart attack. Excess fat, high blood pressure, abnormally high cholesterol levels, diabetes, smoking, estrogen deficiency in women, and a family history of the disease are factors that can lead to CHD. If you have more than one of these factors, your risk of CHD becomes even greater.

Modifying your lifestyle, with diet, exercise and cholesterol lowering drugs, is the only way to prevent the signs of CHD. The only factor over which you have no control is whether your family has a history of CHD. You can take some action on every other factor.

Reducing your body fat percentage is probably the best way to take some initiative in reducing the risk of CHD. The closer you are to your ideal body weight, the lower your risk of heart disease. A combined regimen of exercise and proper nutrition are probably the best ways to prevent and treat CHD. As we have already indicated, blood pressure and blood cholesterol can be lowered through exercise.

The Medizinische Universitatsklinik, in Heidelberg, Germany, demonstrated that those who engage in regular physical activity and consume a low-fat diet, significantly decrease the progression of coronary artery disease.

Smoking is another cause of CHD. Multiple studies indicate that on the first day someone quits smoking, the likelihood of CHD decreases, and continues to decline every day someone refrains from smoking.

We will continue to highlight foods that will make your exercise program more effective in this respect. It is never too late to change your lifestyle to reduce your risk of CHD.

Cancer and Diabetes Prevention

High-fat diets are associated with increased risks of cancers in the breast, colon, and prostate. With exercise, you are able to lose excess fat and reduce the risk of certain cancers. Blood levels of the body's natural killer cells increase and can fight off cancer more efficiently with regular exercise in your lifestyle. People who are physically active have lower rates of deaths from cancer. High estrogen levels are also associated with increased risks of cancer. Exercise can lower estrogen levels in the blood, which reduces the risk of certain cancers (breast and other cancers found in the reproductive tract of women).

Those with diabetes can also benefit from a regular exercise routine. Exercise can lower the amount of insulin a person with diabetes needs. People who are not overweight are much less likely to develop noninsulin dependent diabetes.

An important part of arthritis treatment is physical therapy and exercise. Range-of-motion exercise (yoga) can increase and maintain mobility and decrease pain.

A study in *Circulation: Journal of the American Heart Association* indicates that exercise can keep blood vessels young. Exercise can help counter the damaging affects of free radicals.

Starting Your Exercise Regimen

Exercise regimens should begin slowly and build up gradually, particularly if you have gone for a long time without exercising. Research has shown that heavy physical activity (e.g. shoveling snow) can trigger a heart attack in previously sedentary individuals, so please be cautious. Doctors agree that careful attention to a warm-up period (to avoid muscle strain) and a gradual increase in the level of activity are important aspects of any exercise program. Consult a qualified physician when beginning an exercise program. Again, the most important thing is to make changes in your

---

Heart Health and the FIT Formula

To improve your health, the American Heart Association recommends following the F.I.T. formula.

F = frequency (days per week)
I = intensity (how hard; easy, moderate, vigorous) or percent heart rate
T = time (amount for each session or day)

This formula will allow you to reach optimal performance. For most healthy people the AHA recommends at least thirty minutes of vigorous activity three to four times a week. It doesn't matter the intensity of the work out. What matters is that you are making it part of a new healthy lifestyle. Start off doing low intensity workouts, and build your way up. It is important to remember not to exercise too heavily because too much exercise can lead to injury.

lifestyle that will be life long. When it comes right down to it, the most important thing you can do as far as exercise goes, is to make sure you are increasing your heart rate for thirty minutes a day by moving your major muscle groups.

Nutrition and Exercise

The relationship between exercise and diet has been important throughout history. The Chinese, Indians, Persians, Sumerians, and the Egyptians were deeply concerned with issues of nutrition and physical strength and endurance. Greek athletes were often restricted to diets of fresh fruits, figs, cheeses, grains, and meats when training. Cladius Galenus (Galen) (129–201 AD), taught his patients to "breathe fresh air, eat proper foods, drink the right beverage, exercise, get adequate sleep, have a daily bowel movement, and control one's emotion."

It has been suggested that physical exercise utilizes all the natural antioxidants produced in your defense system in the body. Some studies indicate that exercise can make an individual more susceptible to free-radical-induced muscle damage, muscle soreness, infection, and other such things without additional protection.

Studies indicate that regular physical exercise can increase the activity of a number of antioxidant enzymes in multiple tissues, which then provides greater protection. But other studies indicate that regular physical activity can increase the production of reactive oxygen molecules. This can outstrip the body's natural defense system. Regular exercise thus increases the body's need for antioxidants.

When you increase your physical activity, you have to make sure you are consuming adequate amounts of nutrients. The amount of nutrients you need when exercising depends on the duration and the type of exercise, as well as your body weight and fitness level. Your diet should reflect the level of your energy expenditure. If you are very active, your diet ought to supply you with plenty of calories. On the other hand, if you are not very active your diet should not supply too many calories. Regardless of whether you are active or sedentary, however, your diet ought to provide plenty of phytochemicals.

Make sure that you are drinking plenty of fluids when you exercise. Dehydration leads to poor performance. Consuming more carbohydrates and less fat before and during training will also help improve performance. When you exercise regularly, you deplete the amount of sugar available for your body to convert into energy. A diet rich in carbohydrates (complex carbohydrates) can help maintain sugar supplies to ensure you have enough energy to make it through the day.

It is important to incorporate exercise into a healthy lifestyle. Coupled with a diet based in fruits and vegetables, exercise can help prevent disease, combat aging, and improve the quality of your life. In the end, it is not only a matter of living longer, but of enjoying the years in which you live.

References

Alternative and Complementary Therapies: Tai Chi. 6/21/00 http://www.cancer.org/alt_therapy/taichi.htm

Alternative and Complementary Therapies: Yoga. 6.21.00 http://www.cancer.org/alt_therapy/yoga.htm

American Medical Association 1997. The Centers for Disease Control and Prevention and the American College of Sports Medicine, in cooperation with the President's Council on Physical Fitness and Sports.

Chandan K, Sen, Lester Packer, Osmo Hänninen. Elsevier Science BV, Exercise and Oxygen Toxicity. Amsterdam 1994.

Committee on Exercise and Cardiac Rehabilitation of the Council on Clinical Cardiology, American Heart Association. Gerald F. Fletcher, MD, Chair; Gary Balady, MD; Steven N. Blair, PED; James Blumenthal PhD; Carl Caspersen, PhD; Bernard Chaitman, MD; Stephen Epstein, MD; Erika S. Sivarajan Froelicher, PhD, MPH, RN; Victor F. Froelicher, MD; Ileana L. Pina, MD; Michael L. Pollock, PhD. Statement on Exercise: Benefits and Recommendations for Physical Activity programs for all Americans. http://wwww.americanheart.org/Scientific/statements/1996/0815_exp.html

Department of Food Science and Human Nutrition in the College of Agriculture, Forestry, and Life Sciences at Clemson University and the South Carolina Council, South Carolina State University and Tri-County Technical College. Cardiovascular Disease: FAQ.

Edmund R Burke, Ph.D., and Jacqueline R Berning, Ph.D., R.D. Training Nutrition: The Diet and Nutrition Guide for Peak Performance. Cooper Publishing Group LLC. IN 1996.

Exercise Nutrition: From Antiquity to the Twentieth Century and Beyond-Frank I Katch, William d McArdle, Victor L Katch, James A Freeman.

Frances Sienkiewicz Sizer and Eleanor Nose Whitney. Nutrition Concepts and Controversies. West/Wadsworth. Boston 1997.

G. Shuler, R Hambrecht, G Schlieerf, J Niebauer, K Hauer, J Neumann, E Hoberg, A Drinkmann, F Bracher, and M Grunze. Regular Physical Exercise and Low-Fat Diet. Effects on Progression of Coronary Artery Disease. Department of Cardiology, Medizinische Universitatsklinik, Heidelberg, Germany. Circulation, Vol 86, 1–11 Copyright 1992 by American Heart Association.

Gordoon M. Wardlaw, Ph.D., R.D., L.D. Contemporary Nutrition. Brown and Benchmark. Chicago 1997.

Grattan Woodson, M.D., FACP. Prevention of Cardiovascular Disease.

Harvard Heart Letter, March, 1997. Why is Exercise So Good for the Heart?

Health & Wellness Information

Health Pages–Diet and Exercise in Disease Prevention.htm. Diet and Exercise in Disease Prevention.

I-Min Lee, MBBS, ScD; Chrales H Hennekens, MD, DrPH; Klaus Berger, MD; Julie E Buring, ScD; JoAnn E. Manson, MD, DrPH. Exercise and Risk of Stroke in Male Physicians. Division of Preventive Medicine, Department of Medicine, Brigham and Women's Hospital and Harvard Medical School, Boston, Mass; The Department of Epidemiology, Harvard Medical School of Public Health, Boston, Mass; Institute of Epidemiology and Social Medicine, University of Muenster, Muenster, Germany; and the Department of Ambulatory Care and Prevention Harvard Medical School, Boston, Mass. Stroke 1999; 30:1–6. 1999 American Heart Association, Inc.

Ira Wolinsky; Professor of Nutrition, University of Houston. Nutrition in Exercise in Sport. Houston, Texas. CRC Press 1998 New York.

Jaqueline R Berning and Suzanne Nelson Steen. Nutrition for Sports and Exercise. An Aspen Publication. Maryland 1998.

Judy A Driskel. Sports Nutrition. CRC Press, Boca Raton 1999.

Katrina Woznicki. Stay Young With Exercise. Lifestyle News, Tuesday June 27th, 2000. http://about.onhealth.com

Lori A Smolin, Ph.D. and Mary B. Grosvenor, M.S., R.D. Nutrition Science and Applications. Saunders College Publishing. San Diego 2000.

Nutritional antioxidants and Physical Activity-Mitchell M Kanter.

P.M. Kris-Etherton, PhD, RD, Professor of Nutrition, Pennsylvania State University and Debra Krummel, PhD, RD. Role f Nutrition In The Prevention and Treatment of Coronary Heart Disease In Women. Hershey Food Corporation. Journal of the American Dietetic Association, September, 1993.

Relaxation and Meditation. http://www.members.xoom.com/_XMCM/duranman/2.relaxation-and-med.html

Therapies: Tai Chi. Wholehealthmd.com6/20/00 http://www.wholehealthmd.com/refshelf/substances_view/0,1525,737,00.html

Therapies: Yoga. Wholehealthmd.com 6/20/00 http://www.wholehealthmd.com/refshelf/substances_view/0,1525,746,00.html

Vincent Hegarty, Ph.D. Nutrition, Food, and the Environment. Eagan Press, St. Paul 1995

CHAPTER 17

The Scientific Approach to Phytonutrition

Those hoping to stay current on the issues raised and discussed in this book will face a unique situation: there is simply more information available than any individual can read. This overload of information promises to increase, as science becomes more and more interested and capable of discovering the function of vitamins, minerals, and phytochemicals. How can you distinguish between fact and fiction, between folklore and remedy, and between myth and reality when it comes to the myriad of "fads" and "diets" springing up daily? We will present you with some basic ways to discern between valid and false claims.

Valid Claims vs. False Claims

We will class claims according to three basic criteria: substantiated claims, experimental claims, and invalid claims. Substantiated claims have been scientifically proven according to strict criteria, often employing replicable tests. Experimental claims have not been proven according to strict scientific criteria, but these claims are often logically plausible and carry some evidence according to preliminary research and testing. Finally, invalid claims lack scientific proof or may have been proven false when tested. It is important to note that some invalid claims may nonetheless be effective—however, they lack rigorous testing and scientific research. In the end we simply hope you will exercise healthy skepticism with regard to experimental and invalid claims in the health industry. Your health is too important to trust to unsubstantiated claims and anecdotal evidence.

In the scientific community, those making claims bear the burden of proof. They must conduct careful studies and report them in sufficient detail to allow scientific evaluations and confirmation by other scientists. Generally, clinical tests involve trials involving a sample of human subjects. These trials ought to be designed in order to demonstrate the appropriateness of a given treatment, while at the same time ensuring the safety of those involved. Clinical trials are widely employed for evaluating the safety and ethical value of many pharmaceutical products, medical devices, surgical procedures, food additives, medical foods, and dietary supplements.

Guidelines for Good Clinical Research

The Food and Drug Administration (FDA) has issued specific guidelines for good clinical practice as well as recommendations for clinical trial designs. According to the FDA, a good clinical trial will have a focused, explicit research question; a well-defined hypothesis; and specific, appropriate controls. Substantiated claims generally require clinical trials with a few other important criteria, including: a large sample size, random selection, as well as double-blind and cross-over methodologies.

A large sample size is necessary to draw conclusions from a clinical trial for many reasons. In order for a test to be valid, researchers must try to control any factor that may interfere with the results of a test. Unfortunately, it is impossible to completely control all of the possible factors contributing to a result. In order to balance out all of the possible extraneous variables, researchers use a large number of participants. The hope is that all of the individual differences between participants will be balanced out over a large sample size. For example, if testing a dietary supplement, researchers should use at least several hundred patients. We will discuss some of the other reasons large sample sizes are necessary for substantiated claims in discussing random selection, blind and double-blind research and cross-over studies.

In good clinical trials, patients are totally randomized. At least two groups are established: one group receives a treatment while another receives a placebo. The age, sex, ethnic background, and physical health of each patient ought to be matched as closely as possible between groups and within groups. The patients should be placed into the groups in a totally random manner, thus ensuring that a group does not demonstrate a biased result. Studies should be large enough to detect important differences between treatments and treatment sequences.

Blind and Double-Blind Studies

Clinical trials where the person administering the trial is unaware of which group receives the placebo and which receives the treatment until after the results have been evaluated are called "blind" studies. Blind studies help prevent invalid testing due to researcher bias. Blind studies are necessary because researchers often begin a study hoping to discover a treatment for a particular problem. Sometimes this desire may influence how a researcher administers the test or evaluates the results. Even the most honest researcher may unwittingly skew the results of a study by knowing which group receives the placebo and which receives the treatment.

Another type of blind study is called a "double blind" study. In a double-blind trial neither researchers nor subjects are aware of whether they are administering or receiving the treatment or placebo. This controls the bias of both researchers and subjects, further adding credibility to results of the study. Often, however, it is difficult to maintain a double-blind study because it is difficult to make a placebo that is identical to a treatment. Small differences in color, taste, smell, or feel may allow either a patient or a researcher to distinguish between placebos and treatments. This is another important reason for a large sample size. A large number of subjects tend to balance out the few times that subjects and researchers distinguish between a placebo and a treatment.

Cross-Over Studies

A technique often employed in good clinical trials to help control researcher or subject bias is called "cross over." Cross-over studies are carried out when one patient is started on a particular treatment and after several months of the treatment is switched to a placebo or vice versa. This adds credibility to the clinical trial, particularly when used in conjunction with a double-blind methodology.

One of the biggest problems with crossover studies is that a treatment may continue to have an effect on the subject for a period of time after switching to a placebo. This is called the "carry-over" effect. Many cross-over trials attempt to control the carry-over effect by incorporating an appropriate time period without treatment before switching.

Researchers deciding not to employ a cross-over methodology will often conduct parallel studies. In parallel studies one group is given a placebo while the other group is given a treatment. This is not as effective as a cross-over study because it is unable to distinguish between the possible bias of one group for or against the treatment. In order to control this, parallel studies use a larger number of subjects than cross-over studies to draw meaningful conclusions.

Other Factors in Clinical Research

There are many other factors that need to be taken into consideration. The medical condition of the subjects involved in the study, any therapies and supplementation they may already be on, and changes in the subject's personal situation (i.e. severe stressful situations such as divorce, recently stopping smoking, or pregnancy). Things such as alcohol and drug abuse should exclude subjects from most studies.

When conducting trials with phytochemicals or dietary supplements, several issues must be considered. If a food is added to a diet, its energy content must be correctly matched in the placebo. Care should also be taken to insure that addition of the product does not imbalance the natural diet of the subject. In an ideal study, control foods should be indistinguishable from the treatment.

Clinical trials do not end with the last administration of the treatment to subjects. Trial findings must be reported and scrutinized by scientists, clinicians, and the general public before it is appropriate to make claims that a treatment improves health or fights disease. It is imperative that the results of clinical trials are submitted to recognized scientific journals with a rigorous peer review process. This will allow the data to be exposed to other well-trained scientists in the field, who will make critical judgments on the claims of the research trial.

There are many journals available today that are not peer reviewed, despite the fact that they have titles similar to well-respected journals. It is therefore important to have a good understanding of the scientific literature that is available and the peer-review process in order to make sure that a study or report you encounter is substantial.

When reading literature on clinical trials involving phytochemicals, it is important to note the source of the information (the journal in which it is published) and the manner in which the research was carried out. Careful consideration must be given to the research questions. Some questions you may want to ask include: did the researchers conclusively prove their hypothesis true or false? Did they use appropriate controls and did they use randomization in their choice of subjects? Were the studies carried out blind? Did they have inclusion/exclusion criteria, such as age, sex, and weight? Did they exclude those that were on medication, alcohol, or drugs? Were the statistics analyzed appropriately? Can the test be repeated with similar results? And finally, do the results have sufficient scientific foundation to be considered valid?

Many of the phytochemicals and dietary supplements that are on the market have claims made for them based on very little scientific evidence or few appropriate clinical trials. These claims are supported by anecdotal evidence, or testimonials. Often, manufacturers use this evidence for marketing purposes rather than to add to the growing body of knowledge about health and nutrition. There are a few characteristics of these types of products.

Many have no scientific validation and make unbelievable claims such as, "will cure many cancers!" These claims are often backed by testimonies of apparently believable people, many standing to benefit financially from the sale of the product. In fact the term 'quack' medicine has often been applied to those preying on the public's desire to eat healthily and live well, by convincing them that a particular product is necessary. Many people believe that if something appears in newspapers or on television it must be true. Others are seeking for an easy solution to complex problems and believe that claims of a particular product, as unbelievable as they may seem, are nonetheless true.

Some people with serious health conditions are desperate to try anything, regardless of how believable the claims made by a manufacturer may be. These people are often the most vulnerable to false and misleading claims. We fear patients suffering from cancer, arthritis, multiple sclerosis, AIDS, heart disease, and diabetes all too often fall into this category. They hear of a miracle cure and feel they could be hurting themselves by not at least trying the treatment for themselves. Some companies standing to gain from the sale of their products take advantage of this way of thinking.

One of the most common tricks of unscrupulous companies is to market "organically grown" foods as "safer" or more "nutritious" than foods grown with the aid of fertilizers and pesticides. Though these "natural" foods are usually indistinguishable from foods grown with pesticides and fertilizers, they cost significantly more. Studies comparing organic and conventional fruits have found that their pesticide content is similar. The Food and Drug Administration indicates that pesticide residues are insignificant to our overall diet. It is important to understand that nutrients are absorbed by the plant in an inorganic chemical state, regardless of whether the soil has been prepared with manure or synthesized-artificial fertilizer. Plants are concerned with the supply of nutrients not the source. However, consideration must be given to the source of the soil in which plants are cultivated because many fields are polluted by heavy metals and other contaminants. These factors could adversely affect the health and nutritional quality of a plant product.

Many studies have compared the taste of different fruits and vegetables between organic and conventional foods. No significant differences have been noted in the taste quality between any of the fruits and vegetables studied. This may be due to the fact that plants do not distinguish between atoms of manure and atoms of synthetic fertilizers. As far as the plant is concerned, nutrients are nutrients.

The Market's Influence on You

Every year Americans are bombarded with new supplements. Often the most revolutionary aspect of these products is the manner in which they are marketed. Techniques gaining in popularity in the marketing of food supplements are scare tactics and false promises. Many have begun claiming it is difficult to eat a balanced diet. This is not true. It may be difficult to eat a balanced diet if you tend to eat candy bars all day every day, but reasonably interested and motivated people should have no difficulty obtaining and eating foods that ensure a balance of necessary nutrients. It is not as hard to obtain a balanced diet as it is to have the discipline to eat a balanced diet. Many of the amazing claims made by some manufacturers are made to get you to buy a product. We simply urge you to take a moment and skeptically analyze the validity of claims made by these companies.

"Experts" and "Practitioners"

In an effort to appear legitimate, many of the companies making claims for their products employ "experts" who have credentials that appear impressive. It is important to note that the field of nutritional science is still relatively young and lacks some of the traditional controls of the medical profession as a whole. There are a lot of institutions that offer seemingly rigorous degrees accrediting individuals with sufficient qualification to make appropriate judgments on food and nutrition. Perhaps the most prevalent are the initials C.N. (Certified Nutritionist). This is issued by the nonaccredited National Institution for Nutritional Education. Such degrees and diplomas have no scientific merit, but can be advertised in states that do not regulate nutritionists, giving credibility to the recipient and alluring patients into a false sense of security.

Some nutrition experts will try to appear to be highly qualified by using apparently "scientific" methods of diagnosis and analysis. One of the most common is a hair analysis test. These tests almost always return from the "lab" indicating a deficiency in several critical vitamins and minerals. Of course the required supplements are available through the practitioner (and often only through the practitioner). However, many of these kinds of practices have been the subject of increased scrutiny. The hair sample test was has been generally disqualified as a reliable measure. The results of tests are too inconsistent to be capable of supporting an accurate diagnosis of nutrient deficiency.

Chinese Traditions: Myth or Medicine?

Many companies have now turned to traditional Chinese medicine, which is based on the belief that the body has vital energy, or chi, which flows through all areas of the body. Illnesses and diseases can be attributed to changes in the chi or energy of the body and can be restored by correct supplementation or acupuncture. Recently, a national council against health fraud task force concluded that acupuncture has not been proven to be effective for the treatment of any disease. You may have read or heard material indicating that acupuncture is an effective treatment for arthritis, and other chronic conditions. Generally, the greater the benefit claimed in such reports, the worse the experimental design. In other words, the national council against fraud found that studies supporting acupuncture were poorly planned and performed. The council did find, on the other hand, that well-controlled experiments employing large samples, found no significant difference between the effects of acupuncture on those of the control or placebo group.

Iridology

Another dubious technique often employed to diagnose nutritional deficiencies is called "iridology." Iridiology is based on the notion that each spirit of the body is represented by a corresponding area of the iris (the colored area surrounding the pupil of the eye). Iridologists claim that states of health and disease can be diagnosed from the colored texture and location of various pigment flecks in the eye. They claim they can find imbalances and vitamin deficiencies by looking into a patient's eyes. They claim these eye markings are very accurate at diagnosing, not only present but past illnesses. However, recent probes have demonstrated they could not predict patients with recognizable disease from healthy patients. In fact, different iridologists differed in their diagnoses.

The Imbalance Theory

Many natural healers claim disease is a poison caused by imbalances. Some claim a cleansing process is necessary in removing the imbalance to restore the patient's normal metabolism. They also claim many diseases are caused by the build-up of toxins and anti-bodies. Removing the toxins therefore remove or prevent diseases. Generally, these toxins are never defined, thus it is difficult if not impossible to objectively measure them.

It is quite possible that many diseases are the product of toxic build-up. In such a case, a cleansing process would be an appropriate treatment. The problem lies not within the logic of these practices, but in the impossibility of objective measurement.

Questionable Cancer Treatments

There are many claims of questionable cancer therapies. The proponents of these questionable cancer therapies typically explain their approach in a very common sense manner. Most indicate that the use of their product will help enhance the body system to fight these cancer symptoms and therefore cure the patient. When someone is suffering from cancer, they have a tendency to reach out and clutch at any particular reported treatment.

The American Cancer Society advises that although dietary measures, such as eating more vegetables and fruits can help prevent certain cancers, there is no scientific evidence that any dietary regime is substantially appropriate as a primary treatment of cancer. Fruits and vegetables and other dietary factors are thus effective in preventing cancer from starting, but they do not appear to stop cancer from growing once it has already begun. Therefore, qualified medical intervention is recommended.

In recent years some have claimed that powdered shark cartilage was able to contain and inhibit the growth of certain cancers. This was based on the mistaken belief that sharks do not get cancer. Since then, it has been demonstrated that sharks do get cancer, including cancer of the cartilage. Although clinical trials are supposedly ongoing, none have been published to date in any respectable scientific journal.

Vitamin C was also reported to fight cancer. This claim is attributed to Linus Pauling, who claimed that large doses of vitamin C could be useful in fighting cancer. It was thought that those people in advanced stages of cancer could be treated by large doses of vitamin C. However, in a double blind study carried out by the Mayo clinic using a total of 300 patients, it was found that patients receiving vitamin C did no better than patients receiving a placebo.

Money and the Cure of Disease

Wherever people are sick, there is money to be made in finding a cure. Sometimes, however, people are more concerned about making money than they are in affecting a cure. As a result, many terminally ill patients spend vast fortunes that do very little to extend or even improve their quality of life. Our advice is to look at the scientific evidence (research and studies). Pay attention to where they are produced and who is producing them, looking closely at the qualifications of those producing them. Was the study conducted correctly? Did they use sufficient numbers? Was it a double-blind randomized study? Was there an appropriate age and sex match, and was it published in an appropriate peer review journal? Finally, is it generally accepted by the scientific community or based solely on testimonies of people using the product. There are certain products that have made many claims in regard to curing cancer. However, until scientific evidence is there to substantiate these claims, we consider them interesting, but not recommended.

Conclusion

We would encourage our readers to consider the evidences presented and adjust their lifestyle eating habits in such a way that their diet will contain a large variety and substantial amounts of fruit and vegetables everyday. This will help prevent many of the biggest killers in the world from continuing to kill, as well as improve the quality and vitality of life. It is best to make important changes in your diet before facing disease, rather than searching for a wholistic answer to a life-threatening condition. Diets rich in fruits and vegetables have stood the test of time. They have withstood scientific scrutiny, and are highly recommendable.

References

Barrett. S. and Jarvis, W.T. The Health Robbers: A Close Look at Quackery in America. 1993. Amherst, NY: Promtheus Books.

Barrett, S. et al. Cosumer Health: A Guide to Intelligent Decisions 6th Ed. 1997. Madison, WI. Brown and Benchmark.

Pocock, S.J. Clinical Trials: A Practical Approach. NYC, NY. J. Wiley and Sons.

Yetiv, J. Popular Nutritional Practices. 1987. San Carlos, CA.Popular Nutr. Press.

Appendices

The appendices that follow contain information relevant to the discussion of the health benefits of phytonutrition. Some of it is a bit more technical in nature than the rest of the book, which is why we've placed it in an appendix. However, some readers will find the material informative and supportive of the overall idea of making one's diet largely a plant-based one.

Appendix A

Cellular Function

Fats

In all biological systems there are two general kinds of fats or lipids: those containing fatty acids, and those that belong to the steroid family. The steroid family includes precursors to, and final products of, bile acids, cholesterol, steroid hormones, and vitamins A, D, E, and K. Fatty acids are long carbon chains with hydrogen atoms attached to each carbon and an acid group at one end of the molecule. A great deal of potential energy is contained within the bonds of such hydrocarbons when electrons are removed from the carbon atoms in a process called oxidation which will be discussed later in this section.

Fatty acids and lipids are used as energy storage molecules. They are produced when the body has an excess of energy and used when there is an energy deficit. There are two principle kinds of fatty acids: saturated and unsaturated. Saturated fatty acids have all the hydrogen atoms possible bound to their carbon atoms. Saturated fats are efficient energy storage molecules because they use as many bonds as they can. However in some fatty acids a few of the carbon atoms have two bonds between them. This is referred to as an "unsaturated fatty acid" since fewer hydrogen atoms can bond to the carbon atoms with a double bond between them. Double bonded carbon atoms and the number of double bonds in dietary fatty acids can have an important impact on human health since they play key roles in the onset of cardiovascular diseases, including atherosclerosis, coronary heart disease, and stroke.

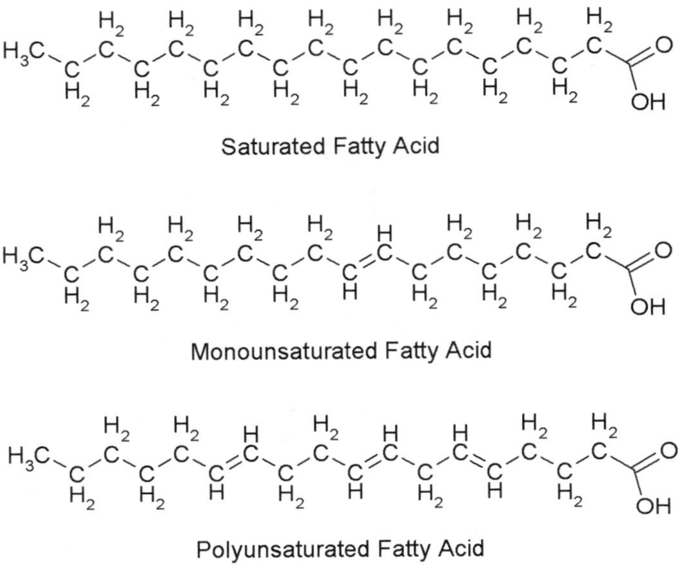

Saturated Fatty Acid

Monounsaturated Fatty Acid

Polyunsaturated Fatty Acid

Figure A.1 Fatty Acids

There are two main kinds of unsaturated fatty acids: monounsaturated fatty acids and polyunsaturated fatty acids. Monounsaturated fatty acids, as the name implies, have only one double bond and are missing only two hydrogens. Polyunsaturated fatty acids contain multiple double bonds and lack several hydrogen molecules. Lipids rich in saturated fatty acids are usually solid at room temperature while lipids rich in unsaturated fatty acids are liquid. Because of the fluid nature of unsaturated fatty acids, we often call them oils. An important property of fatty acids, whether they are saturated or not, is that they are non-polar molecules. That means that the electrons are distributed evenly over the whole molecule, and they do not have both a positive and negative charge.

Dietary fatty acids rarely occur as individual fatty acids, rather they are found in complexes with a molecule called glycerol. Monoglycerides contain one fatty acid, diglycerides are composed of two fatty acids, and triglycerides are made of three fatty acids. In fact, a commonly used indicator of serum lipid levels is obtained by measuring serum triglyceride concentrations.

We also either ingest or produce another class of lipids and lipid-related compounds, which include such diverse molecules as cholesterol, cholesterol derivatives, steroid hormones, vitamins A, E, D, K, and other antioxidant molecules including carotenoids and terpenes. Of these compounds, we are probably most familiar with cholesterol, steroid hormones, and the vitamins. Cholesterol is an essential component of cell membranes. Our bodies produce about 80 percent of the cholesterol we require. A high level of serum cholesterol, often resulting from the consumption of dietary cholesterol, is associated with the onset of cardiovascular diseases. Vitamins A, E, D, and K are known as fat- or lipid-soluble vitamins because they share the molecular structure of lipids.

Proteins

Proteins are essential molecules involved with the structure and function of our bodies. They are sometimes referred to as peptides or polypeptides. Proteins are made up of long strings of smaller molecules called amino acids. This string of amino acids folds into a specific shape that determines the function of the protein. Our bodies use the twenty basic amino acids in unlimited combinations to form proteins. Each amino acid has a unique structure allowing it to contribute to the overall configuration and function of whole proteins. For example, small proteins may contain only five, ten, or twenty amino acids, while large proteins may contain upwards of two hundred amino acids. These chains of amino acids fold and twist into special shapes that allow them to perform important structural and mechanical duties. Keratin, for example, is a fibrous protein that contributes to the structure of our hair, nails, and skin. Hemoglobin is a protein in the blood whose special shape allows it to carry oxygen from the lungs to the outer parts of the body. Some proteins have functions to help perform the chemical reactions needed to maintain life. In essence, they do all the hard molecular labor that keeps us alive.

Enzymes do their work by catalyzing reactions within our bodies. To catalyze a reaction means to speed up the rate at which one or more molecules, known as reactants, interact to produce different products. Enzymes have a pocket called an active site. Enzymes bind reactants and hold them in a specific orientation to facilitate reactions, or the sharing of electrons, in the active site. Sometimes the enzymes twist, pull, and stretch the bonds within the reacting molecules to speed up the process. At other times, the enzyme helps the reaction by passing electrons from one molecule to another. Whatever the reaction may be, enzymes do the "grunt" work to make reactions possible and fast. Once reactants become products they are released from the active site of the enzyme. The enzyme then quickly moves on to bind other reactants in order to perform other reactions. There are literally thousands of different kinds of enzymes in our bodies catalyzing numerous reactions.

Some enzymes cannot function alone. They require the help of other molecules called cofactors or coenzymes. Cofactors bind to enzymes and allow them to function correctly. Some will attach themselves directly to an enzyme's active site and participate in the reaction that the enzyme catalyzes. Other cofactors bind to other parts of an enzyme and change its shape to allow reactions to occur. Many vitamins, including all of the B vitamin group, and phytochemicals are cofactors. For example, vitamin C acts as a cofactor for an enzyme that modifies amino acids found in collagen, an important part of the connective tissues of our body. When there is no vitamin C in the diet, that enzyme cannot form functional collagen to support the tissues of the body, resulting in scurvy. Merely ingesting vitamin C reverses the effects of scurvy because the enzyme-producing collagen begins to function properly.

Two important kinds of reactions that are often catalyzed by enzymes are termed oxidation and reduction reactions. In oxidation reactions an atom or molecule loses electrons, while in a reduction reaction an atom or molecule gains an electron. Something that has lost electrons is oxidized while a compound that has gained electrons is reduced. Rusting iron is a process that we are all familiar with. As iron is exposed to oxygen and moisture, the oxygen molecules take electrons from the iron. This oxidizes the iron because it loses electrons and reduces the oxygen because it gains electrons. As this exchange of electrons occurs, iron and oxygen are bound together to form ferric oxide, or rust.

Nucleic Acids

Living organisms contain two kinds of nucleic acids, DNA and RNA. RNA is a copy of DNA and has a number of biological roles in our cells. The one we are most familiar with is the "messenger" RNA made from DNA as our genetic code is "read." We mention RNA to note that there are different types of nucleic acid. For our purposes in this book we will confine our discussion of nucleic acids to DNA.

DNA, short for deoxyribonucleic acid, is the molecule that carries all of our genetic information and which we refer to as our genome. It ultimately determines how our bodies are put together and how they function. DNA is a double helical molecule made up of two strands that wind around each other in a configuration similar to that of a twisted ladder. Ringed molecules known as bases are attached to each sugar and phosphate group and directed inward toward the axis, or center, of the helix. A base bound to a sugar molecule and phosphate group is called a nucleotide. These bases bind with the bases of the opposing strand and make up the rungs of the ladder. In DNA there are four bases: adenine, guanine, cytosine, and thymine, represented respectively as A, G, C, and T. The sequence of these bases on each strand make up what is called the genetic code. This code governs the processes that keep us alive and maintain our health. Recently, the entire nucleotide sequence of the human genome, billions of nucleotides, has been mapped. Specific lengths of DNA with unique sequences make up what are known as genes. Our genes encode the instructions needed to produce our body's proteins. For instance we have a gene that codes for keratin, a protein found in hair and in fingernails. Scientists estimate we have around one hundred thousand genes in our DNA.

When the genetic code is altered the body may have trouble functioning properly. Many diseases result from mutations, or alterations of the genetic code. In fact, cancer is the most well-known disease resulting from changes to the structure of DNA. We will discuss later how free radicals are a part of the process of altering DNA. For now we only wish to lay the groundwork.

Carbohydrates

Carbohydrates, also known as sugars, are relatively small compounds of carbon, hydrogen, and oxygen that form the basic source of fuel for our bodies. Sugar molecules are also frequently referred to as saccharides. A single sugar molecule is known as a monosaccharide, while many sugar molecules linked together into polymers are called polysaccharides or complex carbohydrates (starch). Sucrose, or common table sugar, is really a disaccharide, or molecule of two sugars, consisting of a molecule of glucose and a molecule of fructose. Carbohydrates are important because they provide energy. In times of need the body can use other molecules for fuel, but it prefers carbohydrates. As a general rule, animals consume sugars while plants specialize in making them. This is because plants have the ability to harness the sun's energy to create carbohydrates.

Cell Biology

Two of the primary components of cells are the plasma membrane, which forms the outer structure of a cell and is the cellular equivalent to skin, and the cytoplasm, which is the liquid portion inside of the cell containing a collection of various components called organelles. It is important to understand these two elements of cells in order to appreciate the need for proper nutrition. A basic understanding of the composition and function of the cell membrane and organelles will also better inform our discussion of disease, aging, and free radicals. It will also help us to more completely explain why a diet relying heavily on fruits and vegetables is essential for good health.

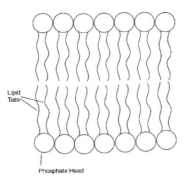

Lipid
Tails

Phosphate Head

Figure A.2 The Cellular Membrane

Cell Membranes

A membrane called the "cellular membrane" or plasma membrane holds cells together. It functions much like skin on your body. The core of the cell membrane is composed of fatty acids, in the form of various lipid molecules. The lipids that make up the cell membrane consist of three parts: a head and two tails. The head is comprised of a molecule of glycerol, a phosphate group, and a variety of other molecules. Because of the large electron charge on the phosphate group, this group of atoms is hydrophilic and thus will dissolve in water. The tails of the lipid molecule, on the other hand, are long fatty acid chains that are hydrophobic and will not dissolve in water. Because the tails will not mix with water while the heads will, the cellular membrane actually forms a sandwich of two rows of lipid molecules. This structure is referred to as a lipid bilayer. In addition to the lipid bilayer, a complete cell membrane also contains cholesterol and a variety of proteins and carbohydrates.

The cell membrane serves a vital role in the maintenance of the body. It regulates the flow of molecules coming into the cell as well as those leaving. Only small, non-polar molecules like oxygen and carbon dioxide can easily pass through the cell membrane. Larger molecules like sugars, fats, and proteins, must get into the cell through pores or via special structures called membrane receptors. If the cell membrane is damaged it becomes brittle and leaky and loses its ability to decide what to let in and what to keep out. Because of that loss of control, a chemical imbalance can occur in the cell causing it to die. Cells try to quickly repair any damage done to their membranes by clipping out any damaged lipid molecules and replacing them with new ones. If the damage is too extensive to be repaired, the cell dies. We discuss how the cellular membrane is damaged by free radicals in Chapter 4.

Organelles

The cytoplasm contains many different components called organelles. Organelles function much like organs in the body. Each organelle has a specific function and special job to keep the cell alive. Some specialize in nutrient digestion and storage, while others work to build and transport new molecules. There are about ten principle kinds of organelles, but we will focus primarily on two: the nucleus and the mitochondria. These organelles have a direct relation to the food we eat.

The Nucleus

Perhaps the most important organelle in the cell is the nucleus. The nucleus is like the brain of the cell and houses all the genetic information necessary for life. In the nucleus the DNA molecules, which contain all of our genetic information, are wound into twenty-three separate pairs of bundles called chromosomes. Each chromosome carries a specific set of genes. From the nucleus our DNA directs everything that the cell is and does. If the DNA of a cell is damaged, vital functions can be lost or changed, or the cell can die or become cancerous. We will return to this in a moment. For now we will only emphasize that damage to the DNA of a cell can have disastrous effects.

Mitochondria

The mitochondria specialize in the production of high-energy molecules that serve as the fuel for all of the cell's activities. These molecules are called "ATP." The mitochondria ultimately use compounds from the food we eat to create ATP. Each cell has numerous of these mini-power plants to provide for its energy needs. Without them, the cell would die in a matter of seconds. A mitochondrion, in some respects, is a little cell within a cell. Its function is so important that it has its own DNA. The DNA in a mitochondrion contains instructions to produce the specialized proteins and enzymes that only mitochondria use. Mitochondria have two membranes, an outer and an inner. The outer membrane has a similar function to the cellular membrane. The inner membrane, though, has a vital role in energy production.

A p p e n d i x   B

Free Radicals

Superoxide Ion

The superoxide ion is essentially an oxygen molecule with an extra electron. The superoxide ion can be produced in a variety of ways. First, in reactions between iron and oxygen, electrons are transferred from iron to oxygen, forming a superoxide ion. Second, superoxide ions are intentionally generated by white blood cells to combat invading bacteria. This is an interesting and very important beneficial use of free radicals by the body. White blood cells use a noxious mixture of various ROS and toxic chemicals to attack and kill invading bacteria and other pathogens that might be present in our bodies. In these cases, white blood cells are pretty sloppy. This mixture also damages some of the body's healthy cells. In fact, the redness and soreness that accompany infections come, in part, from damage done to our tissues by our very own white blood cells. It is evident that the immune system gets the job done from the fact that we survive in a world full of bacteria. However, the whole defense mechanism could use a bit more finesse. Thus an overactive or misdirected immune reaction can be a source of oxidative damage.

Another one of the principle sources of superoxide is the electron transport chain (ETC). Oxygen sits at the end of the ETC and receives the electrons from the last protein electron carrier. The process of converting oxygen into water in the mitochondria actually creates a series of free radicals. The reaction proceeds roughly in the following fashion with the addition of one electron at each step.

For oxygen to become water it must pass through three steps as a ROS, two of which are radical molecules. The radical molecules carry a dot in the superscript. (see Appendix E) If this chain aborts in any of these two steps a free radical is produced rather than water. These ROS can then cause damage to both the mitochondria and other important cellular components. Seeing this process in light of the billions of ETC reactions taking place at any given moment in your body, there are literally millions of opportunities for free radicals to damage the cells and tissues of the body.

Hydroxyl Radical

The hydroxyl radical ($OH\bullet$) is the most reactive and dangerous of all the ROS. This species reacts aggressively with almost every molecule in our cells and is so reactive that it can only travel an average of 5 to 10 molecular diameters from its site of generation before attacking some other compound. $OH\bullet$ can be generated in the human body by four main mechanisms. First, hydroxyl radicals are formed through the reduction of O_2 in the ETC. Some estimate that as much as 5 percent of all the terminal oxygen in the ETC is converted to free radicals, amounting to millions and millions of free radicals generated each day. Second, hydroxyl radicals are produced from hydrogen peroxide (H_2O_2) reacting with UV light. The single bond between the two oxygen atoms is broken and each oxygen molecule takes one electron from the bonding orbital. Such a reaction forms two hydroxyl radicals.

This event is likely to occur in skin exposed to intense sunlight. Third, $OH\bullet$ is produced through the action of transition metals on hydrogen peroxide. Oxidation of the metal and reduction of the oxygen-oxygen bond in H_2O_2 produces hydroxyl radicals. The extra electron taken from the metal is paired in the bonding orbital of one of the oxygen atoms, thus displacing the electron of the other oxygen. The O-H group that received the extra electron becomes a hydroxyl ion, while the other group is left as a hydroxyl radical.

The last principle mechanism of $OH\bullet$ generation involves the reaction of superoxide with hypochlorous acid.

Singlet Oxygen

Singlet O_2 is produced in two principle ways. First, it can be generated by the protective cells of our immune system through the reaction of hydrogen peroxide and hypochlorite. Singlet oxygen is also produced by light. Other chemicals in our bodies absorb light energy and then transfer it to oxygen to produce the singlet oxygen state. The reason that our bodies are not overrun by singlet oxygen species is because the majority of our tissues are protected by skin.

Singlet oxygen undergoes two general types of reactions. The first type of reaction does not cause any damage to the body, but the second type of reaction is responsible for many problems. First, singlet oxygen can collide with other molecules surrounding it, transferring energy to them. Receptor molecules first become excited and then give off the extra energy as heat. These collisions, known as singlet oxygen quenching reactions, convert singlet oxygen molecules into normal oxygen molecules without damaging surrounding molecules. Water is an effective singlet oxygen quencher.

The second and more serious type of reaction involves interaction with molecules that have carbon-carbon double bonds. The oxygen molecule disrupts the double bond and inserts itself randomly. For example double bonds between carbon atoms in saturated fatty acids are damaged in this way in a process called lipid peroxidation.

Hydrogen Peroxide

Though not specifically a free radical itself, hydrogen peroxide is an important ROS because of its involvement with the generation of so many of the other ROS. As we have seen, hydrogen peroxide can be split by UV light or reduced by metals to form hydroxyl radicals.

Reactive Nitrogen Species (RNS)

Two major RNS exist in the body. The first is nitric oxide (NO?), which is used principally by our nervous system as a signal molecule. Nerve endings in the arteries release nitric oxide into the muscular layer of the arteries to help it relax. This relaxation causes a widening, or dilation, of the arteries. Nitric oxide is fairly stable and relatively unreactive. It does, however, react with the superoxide ion to form peroxynitrite, which is the second major RNS in the body and the one that does serious damage. Peroxynitrite is a very dangerous chemical. It is a powerful oxidant and nitrating agent because it can attach nitrate compounds (-N=O) to other molecules.

Herb Glossary

Aloe Vera *(Aloe vera/Aloe barbadensis)*

Common names: aloe, barbados aloe, burn plant, Curacao aloe, medicine plant, Mediterranean aloe, saqal, true aloe

PRESENT DAY KNOWLEDGE

There is a considerable amount of research data on the usefulness of aloe vera in treating minor burns. Placing aloe gel on normal skin you can feel the cooling sensation that is so relieving in a burn situation. The effect may be caused by extended evaporative cooling from the gel or other properties of the herb in addition to this. Aloe vera may also promote healing via mechanisms that promote new tissue growth, restore tissue that was damaged and enhance immune response to damaged tissues. Aloe vera has also been found to be effective in reducing discomfort related to psoriasis, a very uncomfortable skin disorder.

NEGATIVE ASPECTS/SIDE EFFECTS

Aloe vera, like any other herb, may cause allergic reactions. Aloe vera is recommended only for minor burns, meaning first and possibly lesser second degree.

REFERENCES

http://www.aloeveraproducts.com/about_aloe_vera.htm
http://www.blakees.com/house/plants/aloe_b.htm
http://www.res.agr.ca/cgi-bin/brd/poisonpl/ddplant5?plant=Aloe+barbadensis

&info=all&name=sci

Lee KC, et al. Prevention of ultraviolet radiation-induced suppression of contact hypersenstitiviy by Aloe vera gel components. International Journal of Immunopharmacology. 1999. 21:303-10.

Syed TA, et al. Management of psoriasis with Aloe vera extract in a hydrophilic cream: a placebo-controlled, double-blind study. Trop Med Int Health. 1996. 1(4):505-9.

Williams MS, et al. Phase III double-blind evaluation of an aloe vera gel as a prophylactic agent for radiation-induced skin toxicity. Int J Radiat Oncol Biol Phys. 1996. 36(2):345-9.

Zhang L, Tizard IR. Activation of a mouse macrophage cell line by acemannan: The major carbohydrate fraction from Aloe Vera gel. Immunopharmacology. 1996. 35:119-28.

Black Cohosh (Cimicafuga racemosa, Actaea racemosa)

Common names: actaea, baneberry, bugbane, black snakeroot, bugwort, cimicifuga, cohosh, rattle root, rattle weed, and squaw root.

PRESENT DAY KNOWLEDGE

Black cohosh has gained notoriety for relieving discomfort related to menopause. The plant contains phytoestrogens which are structurally or functionally related to animal estrogens. They have been shown to have the ability to bind to estrogen receptors in the body. Phytoestrogens are able to relieve hot flashes brought on by menopause for some people. It is possible that they may produce the other estrogen therapy benefits, including reduced risk of heart disease and osteoporosis.

Phytoestrogens from soybeans have been shown in animal models to reduce bone loss, though not as effective as estrogen therapy. The other benefits of estrogen therapy, including reduced risk of heart disease, are also thought to apply. Some phytoestrogens are also thought to have antioxidant effects. Phytoestrogens may constitute a new class of medications for treating menopause.

NEGATIVE ASPECTS/SIDE EFFECTS

Do not confuse black cohosh with blue cohosh as they are unrelated to each other and have very different effects. Since blue cohosh has a long list of side effects and has been connected to birth defects, most good herbal companies will not supply it. Both plants are listed as potentially unsafe.

There have been reports of miscarriages and premature labor in connection with this herb.

REFERENCES

Dixon-Shanies D, Shaikh N. Growth inhibition of human breast cancer cells by herbs and phytoestrogens. Oncology Reports. 1999. 6:1383-87

Draper CR, et al. Phytoestrogens Reduce Bone Loss and Bone Resorption in

Oophorectomized Rats. The Journal of Nutrition. 1997. 127(9):1795-9.

Duker EM, Kopanski L, Jarry H, Wuttke W. Effects of Estracts from Cimicifuga racemosa on Gonadotropin Release in Menopausal Women and Ovariectomized Rats. Planta Med. 1991. 57: 420-24.

Fremont-L. Biological effects of resveratrol. Life-Sci. 2000 Jan 14; 66(8): 663-73.

Hutchens, Alma R. 1983. Indian Herbalogy of North America. 9th ed. Ann Arbor, Michigan. pg 45.

Moerman, Daniel E. 1986. Medicinal plants of native America. University of Michigan Museum of Anthropology, Technical Reports 19. pg 121-2.

Turner and Szczawinski. 1991. Common Poisonous Plants and Mushrooms of North America. Timber Press Inc. pg 276-7.

Chamomile

(Matricaria chamomilla, Chamomilla recutita, Anthemis nobelis, Chamaemelum nobile)

Common names: anthemis, garden chamomile, German chamomile, ground apple, matricary, pinheads, roman camomile, and sweet false chamomile.

PRESENT DAY KNOWLEDGE

Chamomile has a reputation of being able to settle the stomach and relieve gastrointestinal discomfort. It has a scent that some may find pleasant and that has been shown to promote relaxation in aromatherapy experiments.

Chamomile has been indicated to reduce the duration of severe diarrhea in young children. The benefits of chamomile have been associated with its electrolyte composition when in solution. Chamomile has shown some promise as an anti-inflammatory agent when applied topically. Chamomile may also help stimulate healing of wounds.

NEGATIVE ASPECTS/SIDE EFFECTS

Besides allergies no side effects are known. Chamomile is considered a very safe herb. Individuals who are allergic to any plants of the Compositae or Asteraceae family, which includes plants such as the chrysathumum, asters, mayweed, dog fennel, pineapple weed and ragweed may wish to avoid using chamomile.

REFERENCES

de-la-Motte S, Bose-O'Reilly S, Heinisch M, Harrison F. [Double-blind comparison of an apple pectin-chamomile extract preparation with placebo in children with diarrhea]. Arzneimittelforschung. 1997. 47: 1247-9.

Grimme H, Augustin M. [Phytotherapy in chronic dermatoses and wounds: what is the evidence?]. Forsch-Komplementarmed. 1999. 6 Suppl 2: 5-8.

Korting HC, Schafer-Korting M, Hart H, Laux P, Schmid M. Anti-inflammatory activity of hamamelis distillate applied topically to the skin. Influence of vehicle and dose. Eur-J-Clin-Pharmacol. 1993. 44: 315-8.

Wilkinson S, Aldridge J, Salmon I, Cain E, Wilson B. An evaluation of aromatherapy massage in palliative care. 1999. Palliat-Med. 13: 409-17.

Chaste Tree Berry *(Vitex agnus castus)*

Common names: Abraham's balm, agnus castus, chaste tree, hemp tree, monk's pepper tree, monk's tree, and safe tree.

PRESENT DAY KNOWLEDGE
The most common use for chaste tree berry has been for the relief from premenstrual syndromes and various discomforts related to menstruation. Premenstrual syndromes (PMS) are extremely complex and involve many hormone fluxuations and various psychological and physiological symptoms. Symptoms of PMS include the following: mood swings, irritability, depression, weight gain, food cravings, water retention, cramps, diarrhea, headaches, breast tenderness, back pain, low blood sugar, acne, bloating, and fatigue. Many of these symptoms occur at the same time. Needless to say this can be the cause of a great deal of discomfort for many women.

NEGATIVE ASPECTS/SIDE EFFECTS
A preliminary observation report has indicated that chaste tree berry may cause abnormal ovulations.

REFERENCES
Cahill CJ, Fox R, Wardle PG, Harlow CR. Multiple follicular development associated with herbal medicine. Human Reproduction. 1994. 9(8):1469-70.

Lauritzen CH, Reuter HD, Repges R, Bohnert KJ, Schmidt U. Treatment of premenstrual tension syndrome with Vitex agnus castus. Controlled, double-blind study verses pyridoxine. Phytomedicine. 1997. 4(3):183-9.

Milewicz A, et al. Vitex agnes castus extract in the treatment of luteal phase defects due to latent hyperlactinemia. Results of a randomized placebo-controlled double blind study. Arzneimittelforschung. 1993. 43(7):752-6.

Sliutz G, Speiser P, Schultz AM, Spona J, Zeillinger R. Agnus Castus Extracts Inhibit Prolactin Secretion of Rat Pituitary Cells. Horm. Metab. Res. 1993. 25(5):253-55.

Cranberry *(Vaccinium macrocarpon)*

Common names: bear berry, bounce berry, cranberry, crane berry

PRESENT DAY KNOWLEDGE
Cranberries are naturally high in vitamin C, containing 130 percent of the recommended daily allowance in an 8-ounce glass of juice. Cranberries have been shown to reduce the likelihood of urinary infec-

tions and the formation of kidney stones. Research data has shown that cranberries contain compounds which have the ability to prevent bacteria from adhering to the epithelium of the bladder.

One substance that could be aiding in the function of cranberry juice is vitamin C, which has been shown to have a facilitative effect in inhibiting bacteria adhesion to the bladder epithelium, though it is not as effective alone as when included in cranberry juice. Another compound being investigated in cranberry juice is proanthocyanidin.

NEGATIVE ASPECTS/SIDE EFFECTS

Reasonable consumption of cranberries would normally have no side effects, unless a person is allergic to the berries.

REFERENCES

Avorn J, Monane M, Gurwitz JH, Glynn RJ, Choodnovskiy I, Lipsitz LA. 1994. Reduction of Bacteriuria and Pyuria After Ingestion of Cranberry Juice, JAMA 271:751-4.

Duke, James A. and Steven Foster, Peterson Field Guides: Eastern/Central Medicinal Plants and Herbs. Houghton Mifflin Company, 2000. in addition to multiple Internet sites and photographs.

Fleet JC. New Support for a Folk Remedy: Cranberry Juice Reduces Bacteriuria and Pyuria in Elderly Women. Nutrition Reviews. 1994. 52:168-78.

Habash MB, Van der Mei HC, Busscher HJ, Reid G. The effect of water, ascorbic acid, and cranberry derived supplementation on human urine and uropathogen adhesion to silicone rubber. Can. J. Micorbiol. 1999. 45:691-4.

http://agri.gov.ns.ca/pt/hort/berrycrops/cranberry/cranfact.htm

http://www.oceanspray.com/cran_health.htm

Jackson B, Hicks LE. Effect of Cranberry Juice on Urinary pH in Older Adults. Home Healthcare Nurse. 1997. 15:199-202.

Schlager TA, Anderson S, Trudell J, Hendley J. Effect of cranberry juice on bacteriauria in children with neurogenic bladder receiving intermittent catheterization. The Journal of Pediatrics. 1999. 135:698-702.

Echinacea *(Echinacea angustifolia/purpurea/pallida)*

Common names: black sampson, indian head, narleaf purple, purple cone flower, red sunflower, and snake root.

PRESENT DAY KOWLEDGE

The most common use of echinacea is in the treatment of colds and flu. Some research does indicate that echinacea reduces the amount of time a person is sick after they catch a cold or flu. Echinacea contains cichoric acid, which may have antiviral effects, alkamides and various polysaccharides that are indicated to have immune stimulating effects. Echinacea also contains a compound known as echinacoside, which is an antioxidant and has been shown to protect the skin from damage from the sun.

NEGATIVE ASPECTS/SIDE EFFECTS
Side effects including fever, nausea and vomiting occur in a few rare individuals.

REFERENCES

Bauer R, Remiger P, Wagner H. Alkamides from the roots of Echinacea Angustifolia. Phytochemistry. 1989. 28(2):505-8.

Cheminat A, et al. 1988. Caffeoyl Conjugates From Echinacea Species: Structures and Biological Activity. Phytochemistry. 27(9):2787-94.

Duke, James A. and Steven Foster. Peterson Field Guides: Eastern/Central Medicinal Plants and Herbs. Houghton Mifflin Company. 2000. in addition to many Internet pages and pictures.

http://www.herbalgram.org/

Miller LG. Herbal medicinals: selected clinical considerations focusing on known or potential drug-herb interactions. Arch Intern Med. 1998. 158(20): 2200-11.

Wagner H, et al. 1988. Immunologically Active Polysaccharides of Echinacea Purpurea Cell Cultures. Phytochemistry. 27(1):119-26.

Feverfew
(Tanacetum parthnium, Chrysanthemum parthenium)

Common names: manzanilla, featherfew, featherfoil, and febrifuge plant.

PRESENT DAY KNOWLEDGE
Feverfew has gained notoriety for being effective in preventing migraine headaches. Feverfew contains the flavonol methyl ethers of 6-hydroxykaempferol and quercetagetin. These hydroxyflavonols have been shown to function as cyclooxygenase and 5-lipoxygenase inhibitors. Aspirin is also a cyclooxygenase inhibitor. Feverfew contains a flavonoid called tanetin or santin, which has been indicated to have anti-inflammatory effects. Feverfew has been used to treat arthritis in connection to its anti-inflammatory effects.

NEGATIVE ASPECTS/SIDE EFFECTS
Feverfew is known to cause mouth sores, ulcers and irritations for those that consume unencapsulated herb. Feverfew can cause rashes and other allergy symptoms to those who are allergic to this herb. Allergies are not uncommon.

REFERENCES

Williams CA, Harborne JB, Geiger H, Hoult JRS. The flavonoids of Tanacetum parthenium and T. vulgar and their anti-inflammatory properties. Phytochemistry. 1999. 51(3):417-23.

Garlic *(Allium sativum)*

Common name: garlic, allium

PRESENT KNOWLEDGE

Garlic is well known in recent years for its possible reduction in arteriosclerosis and heart disease. In early research, garlic and one of its constituents, allicin, were shown to reduce cholesterol and blood pressure *in vitro*, and in animal models. Other studies generated a great deal of interest in the possible blood lipid and cholesterol lowering effects of garlic products. Other research shows that the organosulfur compounds in garlic (in order of decreasing effectiveness: allicin, diallyl disulfide, allyl mercaptan, and vinyl dithiin) inhibit the biosynthesis of cholesterol in the liver. Other possible beneficial effects that deserve further research are antibacterial and antifungal properties as well as a blood thinning effect that may be beneficial for lowering blood pressure. There have been reports that indicate allicin also acts as an antioxidant. Antiviral effects against both RNA and DNA viruses have been shown. The evidence for an anticarcinogenic effect of garlic has support. There are an absolutely huge number of reports, both *in vitro* and *in vivo*, that indicate diallyl sulfate (DADS), a component of garlic, may inhibit the growth of several different kinds of cancer cells of both animals and humans. There are a few other garlic compounds that are also postulated to have anticarcinogenic effects, Ajoene, S-allylmercaptocysteine and S-allylcysteine

Allicin and the thiosulfinates of garlic have also been indicated to have antimicrobial abilities against several strains of gram-positive and gram-negative bacteria.

NEGATIVE ASPECTS/SIDE EFFECTS

Garlic oil is very concentrated and can be very irritating to mucus membranes, causing a burning sensation, Garlic is also well known for having a very strong and often considered offensive odor.

Allicin and the other sulfur-containing chemicals thought to be responsible for the beneficial effects of garlic are also the source of garlic's characteristic smell. Scentless garlic supplements are of questionable value.

REFERENCES

Abramovitz D, et al. Allicin-induced decrease in formation of fatty streaks (atherosclerosis) in mice fed a cholesterol-rich diet. Coron Artery Dis. 1999. 10(7):515-9.

Al-Qattan KK, Alnaqeeb MA, Ali M. The antihypertensive effect of garlic (Allium sativum) in the rat two-kidney—one-clip Goldblatt model. J Ethnopharmacol 1999. 66(2):217-22.

Ankri S. Antimicrobial properties of allicin from garlic. Microbes Infect. 1999. 1(2):125-9.

Balasenthil S. et al. Effects of Garlic on 7,12-dimethylbenz[a]anthracine-Induced

Hamster Buccal Pouch Carcinogenesis. Cancer Detect Prev. 1999. 23(6):534-8.

Berthold HK, Sudhop T, von-Bergmann K. Effect of a garlic oil preparation on serum lipoproteins and cholesterol metabolism: a randomized controlled trial. JAMA. 1998. 279(23):1900-2.

Byrne DJ, Neil HA, Vallance DT, Winder AF. A pilot study of garlic consumption shows no significant effect on markers of oxidation or sub-fraction composition of low-density lipoprotein including lipoprotein (a) after allowance for non-compliance and the placebo effect. Clin Chim Acta. 1999. 285(1-2):21-33.

Chung JG. Effects of garlic components diallyl sulfide and diallyl disulfide on arylamine N-acetyltransferase activity in human bladder tumor cells. Drug Chem Toxicol. 1999. 22(2):343-58.

Dirsch VM, Gerbes AL, Vollmar AM. Ajoene, a compound of garlic, induces apoptosis in human promyeloleukemia cells, accompanied by generation of reactive oxygen species and activation of nuclear factor kappaB. Mol Pharmacol. 1998. 53(3):402-7.

Gebhardt R, Beck H. Differential Inhibitory Effects of Garlic-Derived Organosulfur Compounds on Cholesterol Biosynthesis in Primary Rat Hepatocyte Cultures. Lipids. 1996. 31(12):1269-76.

Issacsohn JL, et al. Garlic powder and plasma lipids an lipoproteins: a multicenter, randomized, placebo-controlled trial. Arch Intern Med. 1998. 158(11):1189-94.

Knowles LM, Milner JA. Depressed p34 Kinase activity and G2/M Phase Arrest Induced by Diallyl Disulfide in HCT-15 Cells. Nutrition and Cancer. 1999. 30(3):169-74.

Li G, Qiao CH, Lin RI, Pinto J, Osborne MP, Tiwari RK. Anti-proliferative effects of garlic constituents in cultured human breast cancer cells. Oncology Reports. 1995. 2:787-91.

McCrindle BW, Helden E, Conner WT. Garlic extract therapy in children with hypercholesterolemia. Arch Pediatr Adolesc Med. 1998. 152(11):1089-94.

Munday R, Munday CM. Low doses of diallyl disulfide, a compound derived from garlic, increase tissue activities of quinone reductase and glutathione transferase in the gastrointestinal tract of the rat. Nutr Cancer 1999. 34(1):42-8.

Neil HA, et al. Garlic powder in the treatment of moderate hyperlipidaemia: a controlled trial and meta-analysis. J R Coll Physicians Lond. 1996. 30(4):329-34.

Ohta R, et al. In vitro inhibition of the growth of Helicobacter pylori by oil-macerated garlic constituents [letter] Antimicrob Agents Chemother. 1999. 43(7):1811-2.

Orekhov AN, Tertov VV. In Vitro Effect of Garlic Powder Extract on Lipid Content in Normal and Atherosclerotic Human Aortic Cells. Lipids. 1997. 32(10):1055-60.

Prasad K, Laxdal VA, Yu M, Raney BL. Antioxidant activity of allicin, an active principle in garlic. Mol Cell Biochem. 1995. 148(2):183-9.

Sakamoto K, Lawson LD, Milner JA. Allyl Sulfides from garlic suppress the in vitro proliferation of human A549 lung tumor cells. Nutr Cancer. 1997. 29(2):152-6.

Siegers CP, Steffen B, Robke A, Pentz R. The effects of garlic preparations against human tumor cell proliferation. Phytomedicine. 1999. 6(1):7-11.

Sigounas G, Hooker JL, Li W, Anagnostou A, Steiner M. S-allylmercaptocysteine, a stable thioallyl compound, induces apoptosis in erythroleukemia cell lines. Nutr Cancer. 1997. 28(2):153-9/

Simons LA, et al. On the effect of garlic on plasma lipids and lipoproteins in mild hypercholesterolaemia. Atherosclerosis. 1995. 113(2):219-25.

Singh SV, et al. Novel anti-carcinogenic activity of an organosulfide from garlic: inhibition of H-RAS oncogene transformed tumor growth in vivo by diallyl disulfide is associated with inhibition of p21H-ras processing. Biochem Biophys Res Commun. 1996. 225(2):660-5.

Steiner M, Khan AH, Holbert D, I-San Lin R. A double-blind crossover study in moderately hypercholesterolemic men that compared the effect of aged garlic extract and placebo administration on blood lipids. Am J Clin Nutr. 1996.

64:866-70.

Superko HR, Krause RM. Garlic powder, effect on plasma lipids, postprandial lipemia, low-density lipoprotein particle size, high-density lipoprotein subclass ditribution and lipoprotein(a). Journal for the American College of Cardiology. 2000. 35(2):321-6.

Weber ND, Andersen DO, North JA, Murray BK, Lawson LD, Hughes BG. In vitro virucidal effects of Allium sativum (garlic) extract and compounds. Planta Medica. 1992. 58(5):417-23.

Yoshida H et al. Antimicrobial activity of the thiosulfinates isolated form oil-mar ated garlic extract. Biosci Biotechnol Biochem. 1999. 63(3):591-4.

Ginger *(Zingiber officinalis)*

Common names: Asian ginger, Canton ginger, common ginger, culinary ginger

PRESENT DAY KNOWLEDGE

Ginger, garlic and cholesterol. Ginger has been used in addition to garlic to experimentally reduce cholesterol and blood lipids. Both garlic and ginger have statistically measurable effects on cholesterol and lipid reduction and they seem to act in an additive effect, producing increased results when used together. The two herbs may work through different pathways so they can each have their effects at the same time. Even the combination of these two beneficial spices does not appear to have a great effect on lowering cholesterol. The effect appears to be there but is quite minimal.

Two traditional uses of ginger are now backed up by scientific studies. The first is ginger's long traditional use for nausea, in this particular case, nausea related to seasickness. The second is the claim is that ginger can increase gastrointestinal motility and thus aid in digestion.

Ginger and cancer. Other observations have brought forth new and surprising properties of ginger compound. In a 1998 report the ginger components 6-gingerol and 6-paradol were shown to induce apoptosis, or programmed cell death, in cancer cells *in vitro*. 6-gingerol has been shown have antioxidative activity which may be related to this function.

6-gingerol and 6-paradol are components of ginger and seem to help end the continuous cycles of cancer cells, inducing their death. Another study done in 1998 tested these chemicals on living mice. A carcinogenic substance was applied to the skin of mice to induce inflammation and cancer. The ginger components were later applied to the skin of the mice to see if they could reduce the effects of the carcinogen. Mice that had the ginger components applied to their skin had statistically significant reduction in inflammation and cancer compared to mice in the control group.

Anti-platelet and anti-inflammatory effects of ginger. There have been studies done *in vitro* that show ginger to have cyclooxygenase and thromboxane inhibiting activity. These characteristics would cause blood thinning as a result.

NEGATIVE ASPECTS/SIDE EFFECTS

Used in normal quantities this is a very safe herb that is often considered a flavorful seasoning.

REFERENCES

Ahmed RS, Sharma SB. Biochemical studies on combined effects of garlic (Allium sativum) and ginger (Zingiber officinale) in albino rats. Indian J Exp Biol. 1997. 35(8):841-3.

Grontved A, Brask T, Kambskard J, Hentzer E. Ginger root against seasickness. A controlled trial on the open sea. Acta Otolaryngol (Stockh) 1988. 105:45-9.

Janssen PL, et al. Consumption of ginger (Zingiber Offininale Roscoe) does not affect ex vivo platelet thromboxane production in humans. European Journal of Clinical Nutrition. 1996. 50:772-4.

Lee E, Surh YJ. Induction of apoptosis in HL-60 cells by pungent vanilloids [6]-gingerol and [6]-paradol. Cancer Letters 1998. 134:163-168.

Park KK, et al. Inhibitory effects of [6]-gingerol, a major pungent principle of ginger, on phorbol ester-induced inflammation, epidermal ornithine decarboxylase activity and skin tumor promotion in ICR mice. Cancer Letters. 1998. 129:139-44.

Sharma SS, Gupta YK. Reversal of cisplatin-induced delay in gastric emptying in rats by ginger (Zingiber officinale) Journal of Ethnopharmacology. 1998. 62:49-55.

Turner and Szczawinski. 1991. Common Poisonous Plants and Mushrooms of North America. Timber Press Inc. pg. 269.

Ginkgo Biloba

Common names: ginkgo, maidenhair tree

PRESENT DAY

The main use listed for ginkgo is improved memory and alertness.

Ginkgo and blood thinning. Research has shown that ginkgo has a blood thinning property much like that of aspirin. This blood thinning property makes ginkgo a possible treatment for lowering blood pressure and improving circulation for those whom have circulation deficiencies. The substances that give *Ginkgo biloba* its blood thinning ability are called ginkgolides. Ginkgolides inactivate a substance in the blood called PAF or platelet activating factor. PAF is the molecule responsible for activating platelets. Platelets are the components in blood that cause stickiness and are key in forming clots.

Ginkgo and disorder and disease of the brain. Ginkgo has been shown to help lessen the damage and improve the outlook for patients suffering from cerebral blood flow insufficiencies, Alzheimer's, and stroke. The effect is not a curative one.

Some forms of depression are also caused by cerebral blood flow insufficiencies and ginkgo has the potential to help people who are afflicted with this condition when used in connection with other drugs as directed by a physician.

Ginkgo the antioxidant. Ginkgo also contains flavonoid components that are very good antioxidants. Through elimination of free radicals these components are able to preserve the body from oxidative forces that may otherwise damage the brain and other tissues. One of these flavonoids, a specific ginkgolide, called ginkgolide B, has been shown in experiments to work as a neuroprotector against different forms of oxidative stress. Damage done by free radicals has been linked in some studies to age-related dementias and other cognitive diseases such as Alzheimer's.

Ginkgo and impotence. Because of ginkgo improving blood flow and being an antidepressant *Ginkgo biloba* has the possibility to be ideal for use by men who suffer from impotence and from depression-induced sexual dysfunction.

Other possible benefits currently being researched that may benefit from ginkgo supplementation are: fatigue, anxiety, moodiness, protection of the inner ear, and anti-inflammatory properties.

NEGATIVE ASPECTS/SIDE EFFECTS

The outside of the seeds, or the fruit flesh, contains a toxin appropriately called ginkgotoxin (4-O-methylpyridoxine). This toxin is a vitamin B6 derivative and causes symptoms of vitamin B6 deficiency. The main symptom of ginkgotoxin ingestion is convulsions, though death may result.

Reported adverse effects of *Ginkgo biloba* supplement use are rare. In the less serious cases, patients complained of mild gastrointestinal problems (such as diarrhea), headache, dizziness, and allergic skin reactions. It has been reported to cause nausea and vomiting with higher doses. A serious problem or side effect of *Ginkgo biloba* involves spontaneous bleeding or hemorrhage related to drug contraindications. In most cases these people were taking ginkgo in addition another drug that was used to thin the blood. Apparently ginkgo works in an additive fashion with other drugs and bleeding troubles can result. Ginkgo should not be taken with aspirin, warfarin or any other blood-thinning agent.

REFERENCES

Brown, Edwin W. 1998. A world view of dementia- and a study of ginkgo biloba. Medical Update 21(12):5.

Cupp MJ. Herbal Remedies: Adverse Effects and Drug Interactions. American Family Physician. 1999. 59(5):1239-1244.

Curtis-Prior P, Vere D, Fray P. Theraputic value of Ginkgo biloba in Reducing Symptoms of Decline in Mental Function. J. Pharm. Parmacol. 1999. 51:535-41.

Glisson J, Crawford R, Street S. The clinical applications of Ginkgo Biloba, St. John's Wort, Saw Palmetto, and Soy. Nurse Practitioner. 1999. 24(6): 28, 31, 35-6 passim; quiz 47-9.

Kleijnen J, Knipschild P. 1992. Ginkgo biloba. Lancet, 340:1136-1139.

le Bars PL, Catz MM, Berman N, Itil TM, Freedman AM, Schatzberg AF. A placebo-Controlled, Double-Blind, Randomized trial of an Extract of Ginkgo biloba for Dementia. Journal of American Medical Association. 1997. 278(16):1327-39.

Oken BS, Storzbach DM, Kaye JA. The efficacy of Ginkgo biloba on Cognitive Function in Alzheimer Disease. Arch Neurology. 1998. 55:1409-15.

University of California, Berkeley: The museum of Paleontology website: http://www.ucmp.berkeley.edu/seedplants/ginkgoales.html

Ginseng, American *(Panax quinquefolius)*

PRESENT DAY KNOWLEDGE

American Ginseng; fungus and yeasts. American ginseng contains a molecule called quinqueginsin, a protein. This protein appears to have antifungal properties against several different fungal strains.

NEGATIVE ASPECTS/SIDE EFFECTS

No side effects of American ginseng were found to be reported.

REFERENCES

http://www.rxlist.com/cgi/alt/ginseng.htm or
http://www.kingsu.ab.ca/~hank/HDBMfiles/Ginseng%20lecture/Lecture%20on%20gi
nseng.htm

Ginseng, Asian *(Panax ginseng)*

PRESENT DAY KNOWLEDGE

Antioxidant effects of Asian ginseng. An experiment was done that utilized exercise to induce oxidative stress and test the antioxidative effects of ginseng on the liver and its enzymes. Exercise is a physical process that requires oxygen in order to work. The oxygen required by our muscles and other cells during exercise results in the formation of free radicals. Antioxidants protect cells from receiving damage from free radicals, which is why antioxidants are so important in our diet and part of the reason why some of them are required for good health (Vitamines C and E).

Asian ginseng and cancer. Compounds in ginseng have been shown to inhibit the growth of human cancer cells *in vitro*. The compounds that appear to have this ability are polyacetylenic compounds. These compounds effect the expression of certain proteins and the activity of an enzyme called cyclin-dependent kinase.

Asian ginseng and sugar balance. The researchers reported that ginseng supplementation statistically lowered fasting blood glucose, elevated mood and improved physical performance. There is little information on this function and much research remains before it would be feasible to recommend ginseng for regulation of sugar balance.

Studies have indicated that ginseng causes vascular dilation or relaxation. Ginseng appears to have this vasodilator effect by upregulating or increasing the release of nitric oxide (NO) from the lining of blood vessels. Nitric oxide is a vasodilator that is involved in mechanisms related to regulation of blood pressure. Nitric oxide is also a free radical or oxidant possessing an extra electron. It can be both helpful and harmful depending on the pathways that are studied.

Chinese ginseng and exercise. Although exercise is one of the most commonly touted uses of ginseng it is also the most disputed. Current research indicates that ginseng is ineffective in increasing the ability of muscle to perform work.

NEGATIVE ASPECTS/SIDE EFFECTS
Side effects included headache and high blood pressure if taken in large doses. Since ginseng has been indicated to have blood thinning properties it should not be taken with other blood thinning agents, such as the herb ginkgo biloba, asprin or warfarin.

Ginseng, Siberian
(Eleutherococcus senticosus, Acanthopanax senticosus)

Common names: ciwujia, devil's bush (named because of spiky, thorny branches), Siberian ginseng, touch-me-not (do not confuse with impatiens), and Ussurian thorny pepper-bush.

PRESENT DAY KNOWLEDGE
Very little research has been done on this herb.

NEGATIVE ASPECTS/SIDE EFFECTS
Siberian ginseng may cause stomach irritation and diarrhea. Siberian ginseng should not be taken with the drug digoxin as it seems to interfere with appropriate elimination of the drug. Always consult a physician before taking this herb with any current medications.

REFERENCES

Baskin, and Salem. 1997. Oxidants, Antioxidants, and Free Radicals. Taylor and Francis. Pg 35-9.

Bhattacharya SK, Mitra SK. Anxiolytic activity of Panax ginseng roots: an experimental study. J Ethnopharmacol. 1991. 34(1):87-92.

Bittles AH, Fulder SJ, Grant EC, Nicholls MR. The effect of Ginseng on Lifespan and Stress Responses in Mice. Gerontology. 1979. 25:125-131.

Chen X, Salwinski S, Lee TJ. Extracts of Ginkgo biloba and ginsenosides exert cerebral vasorelaxation via a nitric oxide pathway. Clin Exp Pharmacol Physiol. 1997. 24(12):958-9.

Chen X. Cardiovascular protection by ginsenosides ad their nitric oxide releasing action. Clin Exp Pharmacol Physiol. 1996. 23(8):728-32.

Chin RK. Ginseng and common pregnancy disorders [letter]. Asia Oceania J

Obstet Gynaecol 1991. 17(4):379-80.

Choi HK, Seong DH, Rha KH. Clinical efficacy of Korean red ginseng for erectile dysfunction. Int J Impot Res. 1995. 7(3):181-6.

Choi, YD Xin ZC, Choi HK. Effect of Korean red ginseng on the rabbit corpus cavernosal smooth muscle. Int J Impot Res. 1998. 10(1):37-43.

Dowling EA, et al. Effect of Eleutherococcus senticosus on submaximal and maximal eercise performance. Med Sci Sports Exerc. 1996. 28(4):482-9.

Engels HJ, Wirth JC. No ergogenic effects of ginseng (Panax ginseng C.A. Meyer) during graded maximal aerobic exercise. J Am Diet Assoc. 1997. 97(10):1110-5.

http://herbsforhealth.about.com/health/herbsforhealth/gi/dynamic/offsite.htm?site=
http://www.scruz.net/%7Eroque/adapt/bleleur1.htm

http://www.virtualdrugstore.com/endurance/ciwujia.html

Ismail MF, Gad MZ, Hamdy MA. Study of the hypolipidemic properties of pectin, garlic and ginseng in hypercholesterolemic rabbits. Pharmacol Res. 1999. 39(2):157-66.

Kim HJ, Woo DS, Lee G, Kim JJ. The relaxation effects of ginseng saponin in rabbit corporal smooth muscle: is it a nitric oxide donor? Br J Urol. 1998. 82(5):744-8.

Kitts DD, Wijewickreme AN, Hu C. Antioxidant properties of a North American ginseng extract. Mol Cell Biochem. 2000. 203(1-2):1-10.

McRae S. Elevated serum digoxin levels in a patient taking digoxin and Siberian ginseng. CMAJ. 1996. 155(3): 293-5.

Moerman. 1986. Medicinal Plants of Native America. Research Reports in Ethnobotany, Contribution University of Michigan Museum of Anthropology. Technical Reports, Number 19. Ann Arbor. Pg 322-3

Moon J, Yu SJ, Kim HS, Sohn J. Induction of G (1) cell cycle arrest and p27 (KIP1) increase by panaxydol isolated from Panax ginseng. Biochem Pharmacol. 2000. 59(9):1109-16.

Oh M, et al. Anti-proliferating effects of ginsenoside Rh2 on MCF-7 human breast cancer cells. Int J Oncol. 1999. 14(5):869-75.

Park HJ, Lee JH, Song YB, Park KH. Effects of dietary supplementation of lipophilic fraction from Panax ginseng on cGMP and cAMP in rat platelets and on blood coagulation. Biol Pharm Bull. 1996. 19(11):1434-9.

Sotaniemi EA, Haapakoski E, Rautio A. Ginseng therapy in non-insulin dependent diabetic patients. Diabetics Care. 1995. 18(10):1373-5.

Voces J, et al. Effects of administration of the standardized Panax ginseng extract G115 on hepatic antioxidnat function after exhaustive exercise. Comparative Biochemistry and Physiology, Part C 1999. 123:175-84.

Wang BX, et al. Studies on the hypoglycemic effect of ginseng polypeptide. Yao Hsueh Hsueh Pao. 1990. 25(6):401-5.

Wang HX, Ng TB. Quinqueginsin, a novel protein with anti-human inmmunodeficiency virus, antifungal, ribonuclease and cell-free translation-inhibitory activities from American ginseng roots. Biochem Biophys Res Commun. 2000. 269(1)203-8.

Wang LC, Lee TF. 1997. Effect of Ginseng Saponins on Exercise Performance in Non-trained Rats. Planta Medica. 64:130-3.

Yoshimura H, Watanabe K, Ogawa N. Acute and chronic effects of ginseng saponins on maternal aggression in mice. Eur J Pharmacol. 1988. 150(3):319-24.

Yoshimura H, Watanabe K, Ogawa N. Psychotropic effects of ginseng saponins on agonistic behavior between resident and intruder mice. Eur J Pharmacol. 1988. 146(2-3):291-7.

Goldenseal *(Hydrastis canadensis)*

Common names: eye balm, eye root, ground raspberry, hydrastis, indian plant, jaundice root, orange root, turmeric root, yellow eye, yellow Indian paint, yellow paint, yellow puccon, yellow root and wild turmeric.

PRESENT DAY KNOWLEDGE

Goldenseal is able to act as an antibiotic or bacteriostatic substance, and may be useful in preventing or treating infections. It has been shown to have these effects on a broad range of microorganisms. It also appears to have anti-inflammatory capabilities when applied to external chemically induced inflammations. All these characteristics could prove helpful in external wound healing.

Goldenseal's antimicrobial abilities: berberine and berberine sulfate. A chemical constituent of goldenseal, berberine sulfate, is a dye that is commonly used in experiments to identify other molecules and substances, especially a molecule called heparin.

Several studies claim goldenseal has antibiotic or bacteriostatic (non-stick) capabilities against various pathogens. Most of these studies are *in vitro* studies that use the chemical berberine or berberine sulfate.

Berberine may be effective against *Mycobacterium tuberculosis*. A study of the effectiveness of berberine, extracted from a different plant, indicated anti-protozoal activity against *Giardia lamblia, Trichomonas vaginalis*, and *Entamoeba histolytica*.

Berberine sulfate indicated to be bacteriostatic against streptococcus bacteria, making it harder for the bacteria to stick to host cells and become pathogenic. Berberine sulfate also made it harder for *E. coli* bacteria to stick to the host cells apparently by inhibiting the production of fibrial units. Fibria are what allow the bacteria to stick to the host cells where they can cause damage and disease.

NEGATIVE ASPECTS/SIDE EFFECTS

Ingestion of large doses has been connected to hypertension, convulsions and central nervous system damage and should not be risked. It appears to work as a depressant and may slow or stop the functioning of the cardiovascular system, which may result in death.

REFERENCES

&definition+file=chems-in-taxon&arg1=Hydrastis%20canadensis

Eaker EY, Sninsky CA. Effect of berberine on myoelectric activity and transit of the small intestine in rats. Gastroenterology. 1989. 96(6):1506-13.

Gentry EJ, et al. Anti-tubercular natural products: berberine from the roots of commercial Hydrastis Canadensis powder. Isonlation of inactive 8-oxotetrahydorthalifendine, canadine, beta-hydrastine, and two new quinic acid esters, hycandinic acid esters-1 and –2. J Nat Prod. 1998. 61(10):1187-93.

Guandalini S, et al. 1987. Effects of berberine on basal and secretagogue-modified ion

transport in the rabbit ileum in vitro. J Pediatr Gastroenterol Nutr. 6(6):953-60.
http://ars-genome.cornell.edu:80/cgi-bin/WebAce/table-maker?db=phytochemdb
http://my.webmd.com/content/dmk/dmk_article_58932
http://www.vitaminusa.com/pharmacy/00-33984-03868.html
Kaneda Y, Tanaka T, Saw T. Effects of berberine, a plant alkaloid , on the growth of anaerobic protozoa in axenic culture. Tokai J Exp Clin Med. 1990. 15(6):417-23.
McCaleb RS, Leigh E, Morien K. 2000. The Encyclopedia of popular herbs. Your complete guide to the leading medicinal plants. Prima Publishing. Pg. 227.
Nishino H, Kitagawa K, Fujiki H, Iwashima A. Berberine sulfate inhibits tumor-promoting acitivity of teleocidin in two-stage carcinogenesis on mouse skin. Oncology. 1986. 43(2):131-4.
Rabbani GH, Butler T, Knight J, Sanyal SC, Alam K. Randomized controlled trial of berberine sulfate therapy for diarrhea due to enterotoxigenic Escherichia coli and Vibrio cholerae. J Infect Dis. 1987. 155(5):979-84.
Rehman J, et al. Increased production of antigen-specific immunoglobins G and M following in vivo treatment with the medicinal plants Echinacea angustifolia and Hydrastis Canadensis. Immunol Lett. 1999. 68(1-2):391-5.
Schewe, Muller W. 1976. Inhibition of the respiratory chain by the alkaloids berberine sulfate, alpinigenine and tetrahydropalmatine. Acta Biol Med Ger. 35(7):1019-21.
Sun D, Abraham SN, Beachley EH. Influence of berberine sulfate on synthesis and expression of Pap fimbrial adhesin in uropathogenic Esherichia coli. Antimicrob Agents Chemother. 1988. 32(8):1274-7.
Sun D, Courtney HS, Beachey EH. 1988. Berberine sulfate blocks adherence of Streptococcus pyogenes to epithelial cells, fibronectin, and hexadecane. Antimicrob Agents Chemother. 32(9):1370-4.
Swanston-Flatt SK, Day C, Bailey CJ, Flatt PR. Evaluation of traditional plant treatments for diabetes: studies in streptozotocin diabetic mice. Acta Diabetol Lat. 1989. 26(1):51-5.
Zhang MF, Shen YQ. 1989. Antidiarrheal and anti-inflammatory effects of berberine. Chung Kuo Yao Li Hsueh Pao. 10(2):174-6.

Hawthorn *(Crataegus species)*

Common names: bread and cheese tree, gazels, hagthorn, halves, haw, hazels, hedgethorn, holy thorn, ladies meat, may tree, mayblossom, quickset, thorn, and whitethorn.

PRESENT DAY KNOWLEDGE

The hawthorn fruit, though not particularly tasty, contains a number of vitamins, including vitamins C, B1, B2, and E. It also contains carotene and various pigments. Anthocyanin and procyanidin are pigments or flavonoids that are present in appreciable amounts in the brightly colored ripe fruits of some species of hawthorn. There are many other different kinds of these pigments. Some of these pigments have been found to have active biological functions. Herbal merchants recommend hawthorn as a support for heart functions. For this reason hawthorn has come into use as a therapy for hypertension and congestive heart disease.

NEGATIVE ASPECTS/SIDE EFFECTS

In a recent study, a small percentage of subjects experienced side effects from ingesting hawthorn. These side effects included: abdominal discomfort, facial pain and tachycardia, or fast heart beats.

REFERENCES

Chen HB, Jiang JL, Yu L, Gao GY. Comparisons of pharmacological effect and LD50 among four kinds of Hawthorn fruit. Chung Kuo Chung Yao Tsa Chih. 1994. 19(8):454-5, 510.

He G. Effect of the prevention and treatment of atherosclerosis of a mixture of Hawthorn and Motherworm. Chung His I Chieh Ho Tsa Chih. 1990. 10(6):361,326.

Mazza G, Miniati E. 1993. Anthocyanins in Fruits and vegetables and grains. CRC Press. Pg 43.

Popping S, Rose H, Ionescu I, Fischer Y, Kammermeier H. Effect of a hawthorn extract on contraction and energy turnover of isolated rat cardiomyocytes. Arzneimittelforschung. 1995. 45(11):1157-61.

Schussler M, Holzl J, Rump AF, Fricke U. Functional and antiischaemic effects of Monoacetyl-viteninrhamnoside in different in vitro models. Gen Pharmacol. 1995. 26(7):1565-70.

Schussler M, Holzl J, Fricke U. Myocardial effects of flavonoids from Crataegus species. Arzneimitelforschung. 1995. 45(8):842-5.

Tauchert M, Gildor A, Lipinski J. High dose Crataegus extract WS1442 in the treatment of NYHA stage II heart failure. Herz. 1999. 24(6):465-74.

Milk Thistle *(Silybum marianum)*

Common names: marian thistle, Our Lady's thistle, St. Mary's thistle.

PRESENT DAY KNOWLEDGE

The use which milk thistle is most famous for is for detoxification of the kidneys and liver. Milk thistle contains a collection of substances that are collectively called silymarin. Two of these substances, silibinin and silicristin, have been shown to stimulate the proliferation and activities of kidney cells *in vitro*. These effects have been indicated to provide a protective effect from substances that are toxic to the kidneys. Silibinin, a powerful flavonoid antioxidant, has been shown to be anticarcinogenic in a number of cancer cell lines. It has been effective against prostate, breast, and cervical cancers.

Silibinin has been shown to inhibit the growth of prostate cancer cell lines through a reduction in serum prostate-specific antigen (PSA), which causes the growth cell cycle to stop. However, the substance did not cause apoptosis or programmed cell death among the cancer cells. It succeeded in preventing the cells from further growth and proliferation. Silymarin has been shown to be effective in stopping the growth of human breast cancer cells. It appears to have this effect through its antioxidant properties and the inhibition of the enzyme cyclin-dependent kinase (CDK).

Silymarin has also been indicated to be very effective against the development and growth of skin cancers when applied topically. It was shown to reduce edema, hyperplasia, oxidation and cellular proliferation.

NEGATIVE ASPECTS/SIDE EFFECTS

Milk thistle causes allergic reactions in some people. If you experience rashes, nausea, tight throat or any other negative symptoms in association with this herb, stop taking it immediately. Milk thistle may cause diarrhea, gas and upset stomach in some people. It should only be taken in recommended amounts. The part of the plant that is used medicinally is the seeds.

REFERENCES

Bhatia N, Zhao J, Wolf DM, Agarwal R. Inhibition of human carcinoma cell growth and DNA synthesis by silibinin, an active constituent of milk thistle: comparison with silymarin. Cancer Lett. 1999. 147(1-2):77-84.

Feher J, Lengyel G, Blazovics A. Oxidative stress in the liver and biliary tract diseases. Scand-J-Gastroenterol-Suppl. 1998. 228: 38-46.

Ferenci P, et al. Randomized controlled trial of silymarin treatment in patients with cirrhosis of the liver. J-Hepatol. 1989. 9(1): 105-13.

Katiyar SK, et al. Protective effects of silymarin against photocarcinogenesis in a mouse skin model. J Natl Cancer Inst. 1997. 89(8):556-66.

Lahiri CM, et al. A flavonoid antioxidant, silymarin, affords exceptionally high protection against tumor promotion in the SENCAR mouse skin tumorigenesis model. Cancer Res. 1999. 59(3):622-32.

Manna SK, Mukhopadhyay A , Van NT, Aggarwal BB. Silymarin suppresses TNF-induced activation of NF-kappa B, c-Jun N-terminal kinase, and apoptosis. J Immunol. 1999. 163(12):6800-9.

Pares A,et al. Effects of silymarin in alcoholic patients with cirrhosis of the liver: results of a controlled, double-blind, randomized and multicenter trial. J-Hepatol. 1998. 28(4): 615-21.

Sonnenbichler J, et al. Stimulatory effects of silibinin and silicristin from the milk thistle Silybum marianum on kidney cells. J Pharmacol Exp Ther. 1999. 290(3):1375-83.

Trinchet JC, et al. Treatment of alcoholic hepatitis with silymarin. A double-blind comparative study in 116 patients. Gastroenterol-Clin-Biol. 1989. 13(2): 120-4.

Von Schonfeld J, Weisbrod B, Muller MK. Silibinin, a plant extract with antioxidant and membrane stabilizing properties, protects exocrine pancreas from cyclosporin A toxicity. Cell Mol Life Sci. 1997. 53(11-12):917-20.

Zhao J, Agarwal R. Tissue distribution of silibinin, the major active constituent of silymarin, in mice and its association with enhancement of phase II enzymes: implications in cancer chemoprevention. Carcinogenesis. 1999. 20(11):2101-8.

Zi X, Agarwal R. Silibinin decreases prostate-specific antigen with cell growth inhibition via G1 arrest, leading to differentiation of prostate carcinoma cells: implications fro prostate cancer intervention. Proc Natl Acad Sci USA. 1999. 96(13):7490-5.

Zi X, Feyes DK, Agarwal R. Anticarcinogenic effect of a flavonoid antioxidant, silymarin, in human breast cancer cells MDA-MB 468: induction of G1 arrest through an increase in Cip/p21 concomitant with a decrease in kinase activity of cyclin-dependent kinases and associated cyclins. Clin Cancer Res. 1998. 4(4):1055-64.

Zi X, Mukhtar H, Agarwal R. Novel cancerpreventive effects of a flavonoid antioxidant silymarin: inhibition of mRNA expression of an endogenous tumor promoter TNF alpha. Biochem Biophys Res Commun. 1997. 239(1):334-9.

Saw Palmetto
(Serenoa serrulata, Serenoa repens, Sabal serulta)

Common names: dwarf palmetto, fan palm, palmetto scrub, sabal.

PRESENT DAY KNOWLEDGE
Saw Palmetto has most recently gained favor in the herbal and scientific world for it's potential in regard to benign prostatic hyperplasia (BPH), a disorder many men across the world experience. BPH is enlargement of the prostate gland, which surrounds the urethra like a donut around a straw. When the prostate enlarges it causes constriction of the urethra leading to problems such as difficulty urinating, increased urgency for urination, and frequent urination.

NEGATIVE ASPECTS/SIDE EFFECTS
For a few people ingestion of saw palmetto can cause gastrointestinal discomfort. It is generally recognized as a relatively safe herb with very few side effects. Research has indicated that saw palmetto might interfere with the absorption of iron in the diet, so you may wish to avoid ingesting it with iron rich foods or supplements.

REFERENCES
Gholz HL, Guerin DN, Cropper WP. Phenology and productivity of saw palmetto (Serenoa repens) in a north Florida slash pine plantation. Canadian Journal of Forest Research. 1999. 29(8):1248-53.

Marks LS, et al. Effects of a Saw palmetto herbal blend in men with symptomatic benign prostatic hyperplasia. The Journal of Urology. 2000. 163:1451-6.

Miller LG. Herbal medicinals: selected clinical considerations focusing on known or potential drug-herb interactions. Arch Intern Med. 1998. 158(20):2200-11.

Moerman. 1986. Medicinal Plants of Native America vol. 1, Research reports in Ethnobotany, contribution 2, University of Michigan Museum of Anthropology Technical Reports, number 19. Ann Arbor. Pg 426.

Wilt TJ, Ishani A, Stark G, MacDonald R, Lau J, Mulrow C. Saw palmetto extracts for treatment of benign prostatic hyperplasia: a systematic review. JAMA. 1998. 280(18): 1604-9.

St. John's Wort *(Hypericum perforatum)*

Common names: hard hay, hypericum, klamath weed, St. Johnny's wort

PRESENT DAY KNOWLEDGE

St. John's wort is probably the most heavily researched and used herb in Germany. It is most commonly used to treat the symptoms of mild depression. It is prescribed in Germany more often than prescription drugs for the same purpose. Mild depression is the same use it has been marketed for in the United States. St. John's wort is most famous for an ability to reduce depression. Although not conclusive, there are some good studies that indicate that St. John's wort may eventually become a proven therapy for mild depression.

St. John's wort contains hyperforin that is thought to be at least partially responsible for neurotransmitter inhibitions. A study reported in 1999 indicates that this inhibition may be partially caused by hyperforin causing a slight elevation of sodium, which effects serotonin uptake. The study also showed that the inhibition by hyperforin was reversible, indicating that no permanent damage was done in this pathway. They think that there are other constituents in St. John's wort that work together with the hyperforin to have its overall effects. St. John's wort contains a molecule called hypericin which is a photodynamic pigment, which means that it reacts to light.

In recent years studies have been conducted to determine the value of St. John's wort as an antiretroviral agent. Hypericin was found to inactivate retrovirus *in vitro*. Hypericin requires light in order to function but could inactivate a large percentage of the viruses *in vitro*. There are some studies concerning St. John's wort and cancer. Current research is ongoing about whether hypericin may be used to make cancer cells more susceptible to radiation therapy and/or help induce apoptosis.

NEGATIVE ASPECTS/SIDE EFFECTS

St. John's wort generally has a very low occurrence of side effects when used in recommendable amounts, especially when compared to prescription drugs used for the same purpose. Rare side effects that may occur include: allergic reactions, dry mouth, confusion, dizziness, fatigue, gastrointestinal discomfort, nervousness, and sensitivity to light.

St. John's wort is known to cause serious problems when used with some medications. In fact it is the only herb we have come across which the FDA has felt compelled enough to release a Public Health Advisory about the problem.

Note that when St. John's wort has been recommended, it has been for *mild* depression. For those out there who are suffering from more severe depression, St. John's wort may not be effective enough.

REFERENCES

Couldwell WT, et al. Hypericin: A potential Antiglioma Therapy. Neurosurgery. 1994. 35(4):705-10.

Duke, James A. and Steven Foster. Peterson Field Guides: Eastern/Central

Medicinal Plants and Herbs. Houghton Mifflin Company. 2000.

Gulick RM, et al. Phase I Studies of Hypericin, the active compound in St. John's wort, as an Antiretroviral Agent in HIV-Infected Adults. AIDS Clinical Trials Group Protocols 150 and 258. Annals of Internal Medicine. 1999. 130:510-14.

http://students.washington.edu/sarabh/stjohnswort.html

http://www.ednet.ns.ca/educ/museum/poison/stjohn.htm

http://www.ednet.ns.ca/educ/museum/poison/stjohn.htm

http://www.fda.gov/cder/drug/advisory/stjwort.htm

http://www.nimh.nih.gov/publicat/stjohnqa.cfm

http://www.nwgardening.com/stjohnswort.html

Hubner WD, Lande S, Podzuweit H. Hypericum treatment of mild depressions with somatic symptoms. J.Geriatr-Psychiatry-Neurol. 1994. 7 Suppl:S12-4.

Neary, JT. Hypericum 160 inhibits uptake of serotoin and norepinephrine in astrocytes. Brain Research. 1999. 816:358-63.

Prince AM, et al. Strategies for Evaluation of Enveloped Virus Inactivation in Red Cell concentrates Using Hypericin. Photochm and Photobio. 2000. 71:188-195.

Schempp CM, Pelz K, Wittmer A, Schopf E, Simon JC. Antibacterial activity of hyperforin from St. John's wort, against multiresistant Staphylococcus aureus and gram-positive bacteria. The Lancet. 1999. 353:2129.

Singer, A. Hyperforin, a major antidepressant constituent of St. John's wort, inhibits serotonin uptake. J-Pharmacol-Exp-Ther. 1999. 290:1363-8.

Sommer, H. Placebo-controlled double-blind study examining the effectiveness of an hypericum preparation. J-Geriatr-Psychiatry-Neurol. 1994. 7 Suppl:S9-11.

Zhang W, et al. Enhancement of Radiosensitivity in Human Malignant Glioma Cells by Hypericin in Vitro. Clinical Cancer Research. 1996. 2:843-6.

Tea *(Camellia Sinensis, Thea sinensis, Camellia thea)*

Common names: tea plant, tea tree

PRESENT DAY KNOWLEDGE

Powerful antioxidants for inflammation. Green tea contains a group of chemicals called polyphenols, which include flavonoids. The most abundant of the polyphenols in green tea is called (-)epigallocatechin gallate (EGCG). EGCG has been shown to inhibit the production of several inflammation-inducing molecules. EGCG and other polyphenols are potent and durable antioxidants that are also anti-inflammatory. The antioxidants in green tea are particularly powerful. In fact, studies have shown polyphenols have twice the antioxidizing potential of vitamins E or C. Polyphenols inhibit the production of nitric oxide (NO), tumor necrosis factor (TNFa), and other inflammatory intermediates. Because oxidative pathways cause inflammation, strong antioxidants can interfere with and improve inflammatory conditions. Green tea polyphenols have been tested on mice that were induced to have arthritis through chemical means. The same powerful antioxidants that reduce inflammation can also help prevent atherosclerosis and heart disease. For atherosclerosis, oxidation can cause damage in two ways. Oxidative processes cause damage to the tissue of the vessel walls, causing the proliferation of the smooth muscle cells of the arteries out into the middle, which causes them to become narrow and constricted. Also, oxidative damage to LDL lipoproteins in the blood causes their deposition on the artery walls leading to constriction and eventually blockage. Decreased cancer rates among tea drinkers are also attributed to the powerful antioxidants it contains. Caffeine is present in tea in appreciable amounts, though not as much as is present in coffee. There are many studies and reports on the effect of caffeine on blood pressure. Caffeine acts as a stimulant, causing the heart to beat harder. Both caffeine itself and the tannins contained in tea have vasoconstricting effects, narrowing vessel walls. Tea tannins are polyphenol compounds with antioxidant capabilities. Tannins have been shown to interfere with nutrient absorption when ingested with other kinds of foods, which may counteract the positive effects of the polyphenols. For this reason it is highly recommended that tea not be consumed with meals, but rather at a separate time when it will not accompany other foods during digestion.

NEGATIVE ASPECTS/SIDE EFFECTS

A higher incidence of esophageal cancer amongst tea consumers has been reported. Current reports indicate that the carcinogenic effect appears to be caused by the high temperatures at which the tea is often served rather than any other property of the tea itself. The high temperatures of hot tea tend to scald the surface of the mucus membrane of the esophagus causing irritation and cellular proliferation in order to repair the dead and damaged tissues.

REFERENCES

Chung KT, Wong TY, Wei CI, Huang YW, Lin Y. Tannins and human health: a review. Critical reviews in food science and nutrition. 1998. 38(6):421-64.

Daly and Fredholm. 1998. Caffeine—an atypical drug of dependence. Drug Alcohol Depend. 51(1-2):199-906.

Engle et al. 1999. Effects of discontinuing coffee intake on iron deficient Guatemalan toddlers' cognitive development and sleep. Early Human Development. 53(3):251-69.

Ghadirian P. Thermal irritation and esophageal cancer in northern Iran. Cancer. 1987. 60(8):1909-14.

Haqqi TM, et al. Prevention of collagen-induced arthritis in mice by a polyphenolic fraction from green tea. Proc. Natl. Acad. Sci. USA. 1999. 96:4524-9

http://www.ada.org/consumer/fluoride/facts/saf13-22.html#16 (American Dental Association)

Leenen R, Roodenburg AJ, Tijburg LB, Wiseman SA. A single dose of tea with or without milk increases plasma antioxidant activity in humans. European Journal of Clinical Nutrition. 2000. 54:87-92.

Lin JK, Liang YC, Lin-Shiau SY. Cancer Chemoprevention by Tea Polyphenols through Mitotic Signal Transduction Blockade. Biochemical Pharmacology. 1999. 58:911-5.

Nakagawa K, et al. Tea Catechin Supplementation Increases Antioxidant Capacity and Prevents Phospholipid Hydroperoxidation in Plasma of Humans. J. Agric.

Food Chem. 1999. 47:3967-73.

Ohta M, et al. Effects of caffeine on the bones of aged, ovariectomized rats. Ann Nutr Metab. 1999. 43(1)"52-9.

Ramalakshmi and Raghavan. 1999. Caffeine in coffee: its removal. Why and how? Crit Rev Food Sci Nutr. 39(5):441-56.

Samren EB, van-Duijn CM, Christiaens GC, Hofman A, Lindhout D. Antiepileptic drug regimens and major congenital abnormalities in the offspring. Ann Neurol. 1999. 46(5):739-46.

Simons DH. Caffeine and its effect on persons with mental disorders. Arch Psychiatr Nurs. 1996. 10(2):116-22.

Trevisanato SI, Kim YI. Tea and Health. Nutrition Reviews. 2000. 58(1):1-10.

Wink CS, et al. Effects of caffeine on heart mitochondria in newborn rats. Biol Neonate. 1999. 76(2):114-9.

Yang F, de-Villiers WJ, McClain CJ, Varilek GW. Green Tea Polyphenols Block Endotoxin-Induced Tumor Necrosis Factor-Production and Lethality in a Murine Model. Journal of Nutrition. 1998. 128(12):2334-40.

Turmeric *(Curcuma longa)*

Common name: curcuma

PRESENT DAY KNOWLEDGE

Most of the research that is available on turmeric are *in vitro* experiments and center on curcumin. Curcumin has many effects that have been tested *in vitro* and a few *in vivo*.

Possible cancer prevention is the most heavily researched property of curcumin, and the most promising one. Curcumin is an efficient and powerful antioxidant and anti-inflammatory chemical that also has the ability to cause apoptosis of various types of human cancer cells *in vitro*. Some research has been done showing anticarcinogenic effects in mice or rats as well.

NEGATIVE ASPECTS/SIDE EFFECTS

If consumed in normal dietary amounts turmeric appears to be completely safe. It's not known whether it is an effect of turmeric or of other spice additives, but curry tends to be a very spicy spice, generating some thermal sensations that may vary from mild to extremely hot.

REFERENCES

Bhaumik S, et al. Curcumin mediated apoptosis in AK-5 tumor cells involves the production of reactive oxygen intermediates. FEBS Letters. 1999. 456:311-14.

Deshpande UR, et al. Protective effect of turmeric (Curcuma longa L.) extract on carbon tetra-chloride induced liver damage in rats. Indian Journal of Experimental Biology. 1998. 36:573-7.

Kawamori T, et al. Chemopreventive Effect of Curcumin, a naturally occurring Anti-inflammatory agent, during the Promotion/Progression stages of colon cancer. Cancer Research. 1999. 59(3):597-601.

Kuo ML, Huang TS, Lin JK. Curcumin, an antioxidant and anti-tumor promoter, induces apoptosis in human leukemia cells. Biochemica et Biophysica Acta. 1996. 1317:95-100.

Valerian *(Valeriana officinalis)*

Common names: American valerian, all-heal, capon's tail, common valerian, English valerian, fragrant valerian, garden heliotrope, phu, setewale, stink root, St. George's herb, and vandal root.

PRESENT DAY KNOWLEDGE
Valerian is most commonly used as a sleep-aide or sedative. There are a small handful of studies done on its efficacy. Valerian caused a statistically significant decrease in sleep latency, an increase in sleep quality, and a decrease in night awakenings for irregular sleepers.

NEGATIVE ASPECTS/SIDE EFFECTS
This herb should not be used on a regular basis due to possible cytotoxic effects. There has been evidence that components of valerian may cause liver damage if used for extended durations.

REFERENCES
Balderer G, BorbJly AA. Effect of valerian on human sleep. Psychopharmacology. 1985. 87:406-9.

Chan TY, Tang CH, Critchley JA. Poisoning due to an over-the-counter hypnotic, Sleep-Qik (hyoscine, cyproheptadine, valerian.) Postgrad Med J. 1995. 71(834):227-8.

Duke, James A. and Steven Foster. Peterson Field Guides: Eastern/Central Medicinal Plants and Herbs. Houghton Mifflin Company. 2000. http://www.mus-canet.com/~kschmitt/valerian.html, http://herb.plant.org/valerian.htm, http://herbsforhealth.about.com/health/herbsforhealth/library/weekly/aa091197.htm, http://www.agric.gov.ab.ca/crops/special/medconf/willardi.html

Garges HP, Varia I, Doraiswamy PM. Cardiac complications and delirium associated with valerian root withdrawal. Journal of the American Medical Association. 1998. 280(18):1566-7.

Kirkwood CK. Management of Insomnia. J Am Pharm Assoc Wash. 1999. 39(5):688-96.

Leathwood PD, Chauffard F, Heck E, Munoz-Box R. Aqueous Extract of Valerian Root (Valeriana officinales L.) Improves Sleep Quality in Man. Pharmacology Biochemistry and Behavior. 1982. 17:65-71.

Lindahl O, Lindwall L. Double blind study of a Valerian preparation. 1988. 32:1065-6.

Shepard C. Liver damage warning with insomnia remedy. British Medical Journal. 1993. 306:1477.

Appendix D

Nutrient Tables

Table D.1: Recommended Daily Vitamin Intake (organized by age and gender)

Vitamin	Units	Infants 0-0.5 yr	Infants 0.5-1 yr	Children 1-3	Children 4-6	Children 7-10	Males 11-14	Males 15-18	Males 19-24	Males 25-50	Males 51+	Females 11-14	Females 15-18	Females 19-24	Females 25-50	Females 51+	Pregnant	Lactating
Fat Soluble																		
Vitamin A	RE	375	375	400	500	700	1000	1000	1000	1000	1000	800	800	800	800	800	800	1300
Vitamn D	µg	5	5	5	5	5	5	5	5	5	10	5	5	5	5	10	5	5
Vitamin E	mg	3	4	6	7	7	22	22	22	22	22	15	15	15	15	15	15	18
Vitamin K	µg	5	10	15	20	30	45	65	70	80	80	45	55	60	65	65	65	65
Water Soluble																		
Thiamin	mg	0.3	0.4	0.7	0.9	1	1.3	1.5	1.5	1.5	1.2	1.1	1.1	1.1	1.1	1	1.5	1.6
Folate	µg	25	35	50	75	100	150	200	200	200	200	150	180	180	180	180	400	280
Pyridoxine (B6)	mg	0.3	0.6	1	1.1	1.4	1.7	2	2	2	2	1.4	1.5	1.6	1.6	1.6	2.2	2.1
Riboflavin	mg	0.4	0.5	0.8	1.1	1.2	1.5	1.8	1.7	1.7	1.4	1.3	1.3	1.3	1.3	1.2	1.6	1.8
Niacin	mg	5	6	9	12	13	17	20	19	19	15	15	15	15	15	30	17	20
Biotin (A1)	µg	5	6	8	12	16	20	25	30	30	30	20	25	30	30	30	30	35
Cobalamine	µg	0.3	0.5	0.7	1	1.4	2	2	2	2	2	2	2	2	2	2	2.2	2.6
Pantothenic Acid	mg	1.7	1.8	2	3	3	4	5	5	5	5	4	5	5	5	5	6	7
Vitamin C	mg	30	35	40	45	45	90	90	90	90	90	75	75	75	75	75	75	95

Table D.2: Sources of Water-Soluble Vitamins

foods	biotin	thiamin	panto. acid	riboflavin	folate	niacin	vit. B12	vit. B6	vit. C
asparagus (6 spears, boiled)					131 µg				
bagel (plain, 1)									
banana (1 med)				0.22 mg				0.66 mg	
beans (baked, 1 cup)									
beef (top round, braised, 3 oz)		0.34 mg						0.24 mg	
bread (wheat, fortified, 1 slice)					20 µg				
broccoli (1 cup, boiled)			0.8 µg						116 mg
brown rice (1 cup)						3.0 mg			
cantaloupe (1 cup)									68 mg
cereals (fortified, ready-to-eat)					100–400 µg	5–20 mg	1.5–6 µg		
cheese (cottage / feta, 1/2 cup)				0.21 mg					
chicken (light meat, 3 oz)			0.97 mg			10.6 mg	0.3 µg	0.51 mg	
chickpeas (1/2 cup)					80 µg				
chocolate	32 µg								
clams (canned, 3 oz)				0.36 mg					
cod (cooked, 3 oz)								0.24 mg	
corn (cooked, 1/2 ear)			0.72 mg						
dates (10)			0.65 mg						
egg (whole, cooked)	20 µg			0.25 mg					
fish and shellfish	20 µg						2.1 µg		

Table D.2 continued

water-soluble vitamins / foods	vit. C	vit. B6	vit. B12	niacin	folate	riboflavin	panto. acid	thiamin	biotin
grapefruit juice (8 oz)									
ground turkey (cooked, 3 oz)									
ham (lean, 3.5 oz)									
ice milk (soft serve, 1 cup)						0.36 mg	0.78 mg		16–24 µg
instant milk									
kidney beans (1/2 cup)					62 µg				
kiwi	74 mg								
lentils (1/2 cup, boiled)					179 µg				
malt-o-meal (1 cup)								0.38 mg	
mango (raw, 1)	57 mg								
milk (2% fat, 1 cup)						0.40 mg	0.78 mg		
milk, soy (1 cup)								22–31 µg	
mozzarella cheese (1 oz)			0.2 µg						
mushrooms (raw, 1/2 cup)							0.77 mg		22–31 µg
oatmeal									
orange juice (1 cup)	97 mg				109 µg				
papaya	188 mg						0.33 mg		
papaya juice (1/2 cup)								0.29 mg	
pasta (enriched, 1 cup cooked)				2.3 mg	60 µg				
peanut butter (2 T)				4.0 mg					

Table D.2 continued

water-soluble vitamins / foods	vit. C	vit. B6	vit. B12	niacin	folate	riboflavin	panto. acid	thiamin	biotin
peanuts (roasted)									34 µg
peppers (raw, 1/2 cup)	45 mg								
pork chop (lean, 3.5 oz)				3.5 mg		0.24 mg		0.82 mg	
potato (bake w/ skin, 7 oz)								0.22 mg	
rice (white, 1 cup)								0.26 mg	
roast beef (cooked, 3 oz)			2.20 µg		68 µg				
salmon, Atlantic (3 oz)		0.55 mg							
skim milk (8 oz)			0.90 µg						
spinach (boiled, 1/2 cup)		0.22 mg			131 µg				
strawberries (1 cup raw)	84 mg								
sunflower seeds (shld 1 oz)							0.5 mg	0.59 mg	
top round steak (3 oz)			2.70 µg	3.3 mg					
tuna (canned, 3 oz)			2.54 µg	4.9 mg					
turkey breast (3 oz)			1.70 µg						
vegetable juice (6 oz)		0.24 mg							
walnuts								37–39 µg	
watermelon (1 cup)		0.23 mg							
wheat bran									22.5 µg
wheat germ							0.65 mg	0.55 mg	22–38 µg
whole wheat bread (1 slc)				1.1 mg					
yogurt (fruit flavored, 8 oz)			1 µg			0.37 mg			

Table D.3: Sources for Fat-Soluble Vitamins

foods	fat-soluble vitamins	vitamin A	vitamin D	vitamin E	vitamin K
almonds (roast, 1 oz)			22 IU		
apricots (dried, 5)		253 µg			
broccoli (frozen, 1/2 cup)					63 µg
cabbage (raw, 1/2 cup)					52 µg
canola or corn oil (1 t)			20 IU		
cantaloupe (1 cup)		515 µg			
carrot (1 raw)		2025 µg			
cereals (fortified, 1 cup)				1.6 mg	
chickpeas (1 oz)					74 µg
egg substitute (1/4 cup)				1.4 mg	
egg (large)		84 µg		1.0 mg	
evaporated milk (2 T)				1.2 mg	
flour (whole, 1 cup)					36 µg
Italian salad dressing			24 IU		
liver (3.5 oz, braised)		10602 µg			
lobster (cooked, 3 oz)				1.6 mg	
mango (1 medium)		805 µg			
margarine (1 t)				0.9 mg	
milk (1 cup)		149 µg		1.6 mg	
mozzarella (1 oz)		50 µg			
olive oil (1 t)				5.3 mg	
peanut butter (1 T)			25 IU		
pork (3.5 oz.)					88 µg
salmon (with bones 3 oz)			10 IU	0.6 mg	
soybean oil (1 T)					76 µg
spinach (1/2 cup, boiled)		737 µg			
spinach (frozen, 1/2 cup)					131 µg
strawberries (1 cup)					21 µg
sunflower seeds (2 T)			100 IU		
sweet potato (4 oz)		2487 µg			
tuna (white, 3 oz)				7 mg	
turnip greens (1/2 cup)					82 µg
wheat bran					23 µg
wheat germ (1/4 cup)			40–100 IU		

Table D.4: Vegetable and Fruit Nutrients

Vegetables	calcium (mg)	zinc (mg)	potass. (mg)	phosph. (mg)	niacin (mg)	magnes. (mg)	iron (mg)	folate (µg)	vit E (mg)	vit C (mg)	vit B12 (mg)	vit B6 (mg)	vit A (RE)	fiber (g)	sodium (mg)	fat (g)	protein (g)	carbs (g)	Kcal	serv. size (g)
alfalfa sprouts	5	0.2	13	12	0.1	4	0.2	6	—	1	—	—	3	—	1	—	1	1	5	16.5
asparagus	14	0.3	183	38	0.8	12	0.6	86	1.3	9	—	0.1	39	1	1	—	2	3	15	67
bean sprouts	55	1.4	378	144	0.7	64	0.3	85	—	2	—	—	60	—	167	5	9	6	83	66.7
beets	14	0.3	259	32	0.3	20	0.7	68	0.3	3	—	0.1	3	1	65	—	1	8	37	85
broccoli	21	0.2	143	29	0.3	11	0.4	31	—	41	—	0.1	132	—	12	—	1	2	12	44
brussel sprouts	28	0.3	247	44	0.5	16	0.9	47	0.7	48	—	0.1	56	3	16	—	2	7	30	78
cabbage	33	0.1	172	16	0.2	11	0.4	40	—	36	—	0.1	9	—	13	—	1	4	17	70
carrots	16	0.1	194	26	0.6	9	0.3	8	0.3	6	—	0.1	1688	2	21	—	1	6	26	60
cauliflower	11	0.1	152	22	0.3	8	0.2	29	—	23	—	0.1	1	1	15	—	1	3	13	50
celery	24	0.1	172	15	0.2	7	0.2	17	0.2	4	—	—	8	1	52	—	—	2	10	60
collards	10	—	61	4	0.1	3	0.1	4	0.8	8	—	—	120	1	7	—	1	3	11	36
corn (white)	2	0.3	208	69	1.3	28	0.4	35	0.2	5	—	—	—	2	12	1	2	15	66	77
corn (yellow)	2	0.3	208	69	1.3	28	0.4	35	0.1	5	—	—	22	2	12	1	2	15	66	77
cucumber	7	0.1	75	10	0.1	6	0.1	7	—	3	—	—	11	—	1	—	—	1	7	52
egg plant	3	0.1	89	9	0.2	6	0.1	8	—	1	—	—	3	1	0.1	—	—	2	11	41
leeks	31	0.1	94	18	0.2	15	1.1	33	0.5	6	—	0.1	5	1	10	—	1	7	32	52
lettuce (butterhead)	18	0.1	144	13	0.2	7	0.2	41	0.2	4	—	—	54	1	3	—	1	1	7	56
lettuce (iceberg)	11	0.1	88	11	0.1	5	0.3	31	0.1	2	—	—	18	1	5	—	1	1	7	56
lettuce (looseleaf)	—	38	148	14	0.2	6	0.8	76	0.2	10	—	—	106	1	5	—	1	2	10	56
lettuce (romaine)	20	0.1	162	25	0.3	3	0.6	76	0.2	13	—	—	146	1	4	—	1	1	9	56
mushrooms	2	0.3	130	36	1.4	4	0.4	7	—	1	—	0.1	—	—	4	—	4	2	9	35
okra	41	0.3	152	32	0.5	29	0.4	44	0.3	11	—	0.1	33	1	2	—	1	4	19	50
onion	16	0.2	125	26	0.1	8	0.2	15	0.1	5	—	0.1	—	1	7	—	1	7	30	79.9
parsnip	24	0.4	249	47	0.5	19	0.4	44	0.7	11	—	0.1	—	3	70	—	1	12	50	66.5
peas	19	0.8	1334	72	1.2	23	1.3	47	0.1	8	—	0.1	54	4	1	—	4	10	59	72.5
pepper (green)	7	0.1	131	14	0.4	7	0.3	16	0.5	66	—	0.2	47	1	1	—	1	5	20	74
pepper (red)	7	0.1	131	14	0.4	7	0.3	16	0.5	141	—	0.2	422	2	1	—	1	5	20	74

Table D.4 continued

Vegetables	serv. size (g)	Kcal	carbs (g)	protein (g)	fat (g)	sodium (mg)	fiber (g)	vit A (RE)	vit B6 (mg)	vit B12 (mg)	vit C (mg)	vit E (mg)	folate (µg)	iron (mg)	magnes. (mg)	niacin (mg)	phosph. (mg)	potass. (mg)	zinc (mg)	calcium (mg)
pepper (yellow)	74	20	5	1	–	1	–	18	0.1	–	136	–	19	0.3	9	0.7	18	157	0.1	8
potato	202	220	51	5	–	1	5	–	0.7	–	26	0.1	22	2.7	55	3.3	115	844	0.6	20
radish (oriental)	44	8	2	–	–	9	1	–	–	–	10	–	12	0.2	7	0.1	10	100	0.1	12
spinach	56	12	2	2	–	44	2	376	0.1	–	16	1.1	109	1.5	44	0.4	27	312	0.3	55
squash (summer)	65	13	3	1	–	1	1	13	0.1	–	10	0.1	17	0.3	15	0.4	23	127	0.2	13
squash (winter)	58	21	5	1	–	2	1	235	–	–	7	0.1	13	0.3	12	0.5	19	203	0.1	18
squash (zucchini)	11	2	–	–	–	–	–	5	–	–	4	–	2	0.1	4	0.1	10	50	0.1	2
sweet potato	100	103	24	2	–	10	3	2182	0.2	–	25	4.6	23	0.4	20	0.6	55	348	0.3	28
tomato	132	26	6	1	–	11	1	76	0.1	–	23	0.5	18	0.6	14	0.8	30	273	0.1	6
turnips	65	18	4	1	–	44	1	–	0.1	–	14	–	9	0.2	7	0.3	18	124	0.2	20
yam	68	79	19	1	–	–	3	–	0.2	–	8	3.1	11	0.3	9	0.1	12	71	0.1	8

Nuts	serv. size (g)	Kcal	carbs (g)	protein (g)	fat (g)	sodium (mg)	fiber (g)	vit A (RE)	vit B6 (mg)	vit B12 (mg)	vit C (mg)	vit E (mg)	folate (µg)	iron (mg)	magnes. (mg)	niacin (mg)	phosph. (mg)	potass. (mg)	zinc (mg)	calcium (mg)
almonds	71	418	16	14	36		8	–	0.1	–	–	11.4	45	3.5	216	2	390	549	3.5	201
cashews	68.5	393	22	10	32	438	2	–	0.2	–	–	0.4	47	4.1	178	1	336	387	3.8	31
peanuts	73	414	12	19	35	4	7	–	0.2	–	–	5.3	91	3.3	123	8.8	274	515	2.4	67
pine nuts	10	52	1	2	5	–	–	–	–	–	–	0.4	6	0.9	23	0.4	51	60	0.4	3
sunflower seeds	72	410	14	16	36	2	8	4	0.6	–	1	36.2	164	4.9	255	3.2	508	496	3.6	84
soy beans	86	387	28	34	19	2	7	2	0.2	–	4	1.7	176	3.4	196	0.9	558	1173	4.1	232

Legumes	serv. size (g)	Kcal	carbs (g)	protein (g)	fat (g)	sodium (mg)	fiber (g)	vit A (RE)	vit B6 (mg)	vit B12 (mg)	vit C (mg)	vit E (mg)	folate (µg)	iron (mg)	magnes. (mg)	niacin (mg)	phosph. (mg)	potass. (mg)	zinc (mg)	calcium (mg)
black beans	86	114	20	8	–	204	–	1	0.1	–	–	–	128	1.8	60	0.4	120	305	1	23
green beans	55	17	4	1	–	3	2	37	–	–	9	0.2	20	0.6	14	0.4	21	115	0.1	20
kidney (canned)	128	104	19	7	–	444	–	–	–	–	2	–	63	1.6	40	0.6	134	329	0.7	35
lima	90	95	18	6	–	26	–	15	0.1	–	5	–	14	1.8	50	0.7	101	370	0.5	25
navy (canned)	131	148	27	10	1	587	7	–	0.1	–	1	0.5	82	2.4	62	0.6	176	377	1	62
pinto (canned)	120	94	17	5	–	499	4	–	0.1	–	1	–	72	1.9	32	0.4	110	361	0.8	44

Table D.4 continued

Fruits	serv. size (g)	Kcal	carbs (g)	protein (g)	fat (g)	sodium (mg)	fiber (g)	vit A (RE)	vit B6 (mg)	vit B12 (mg)	vit C (mg)	vit E (mg)	folate (µg)	iron (mg)	magnes. (mg)	niacin (mg)	phosph. (mg)	potass. (mg)	zinc (mg)	calcium (mg)
apple	138	81	21	–	0	–	4	7	0.1	–	8	0.8	4	0.2	7	0.1	10	159	0.1	10
apricot	106	51	12	1	–	1	3	277	0.1	–	11	0.9	9	0.6	8	.6	20	314	.03	15
avocado	201	324	15	4	31	20	12	123	0.6	–	5	2.7	124	2.1	78	3.9	82	1204	.8	22
banana	114	105	27	1	1	1	3	9	0.7	–	10	.3	22	0.4	33	0.6	23	451	0.2	7
blackberry	144	75	18	1	1	–	6	24	0.8	–	30	1.02	49	0.82	29	.58		282	0.39	46
blueberry	72.5	41	10	–	–	4	2	7	–	–	9	0.7	5	0.1	4	0.3	7	65	0.1	4
cantaloupe	267	93	22	2	1	24	2	860	0.31	–	113	0.4	45	0.56	29	1.53		825	0.43	29
cherry	72.5	52	12	1	1	–	2	15	–	–	5	0.1	3	0.3	8	0.3	14	162	–	11
cranberry	47.5	23	6	–	–	–	2	2	–	–	6	–	1	0.1	2	–	4	34	0.1	3
grape	57	40	10	1	1	–	1	4	0.06	–	6	0.4	2	3	3	0.17		105	0.03	6
grapefruit	185.3	72	17	1	–	–	–	82	0.1	–	70	–	19	0.4	22	0.4	28	300	0.1	4
honeydew	129	45	12	1	1	2	1	5	0.08	–	32	0.19	39	0.09	9	0.77		350	0.11	8
kiwifruit	76	46	11	1	–	13	3	14	–	–	74	0.9	–	0.3	23	0.4		252	–	20
lemon	58	17	5	1	–	4	2	2	–	–	31	0.1	6	0.3	5	0.1	30	80	–	2
lime	246	66	1	22	–	1	1	2	0.11	–	72	0.22	20	0.07	15	0.25	9	268	0.15	22
mango	82.5	54	14	–	1	2	1	321	0.1	–	23	0.9	–	0.1	7	0.5		129	–	8
nectarine	136	67	16	1	–	2	1	101	0.03	–	7	1.21	5	0.2	11	1.35	9	288	0.12	7
orange	131	62	15	1	–	–	3	28	0.1	–	70	0.3	40	0.1	13	0.4	18	237	0.1	4
papaya	304	119	30	2	–	9	5	85	0.1	–	6	–	4	0.6	6	0.3	–	58	0.3	19
peach	87	37	10	1	–	–	2	47	–	–	6	0.6	3	0.1	6	0.9	10	171	0.1	4
pear	166	98	25	1	1	–	4	3	–	–	7	0.8	12	0.4	10	0.2	18	208	0.2	18
pineapple	84	41	10	–	–	1	1	2	0.1	–	13	0.1	9	0.3	12	0.4	6	95	0.1	6
plum	66	36	9	1	–	–	1	21	0.1	–	6	0.4	1	0.1	5	0.3	7	114	0.1	3
pomegranate	154	105	27	1	1	–	5	–	0.16	–	9	0.85	–	0.46	5	0.46		399	–	5
raspberry	61.5	30	7	1	–	1	4	8	–	–	15	0.3	16	0.4	11	0.6	7	93	0.3	14
strawberry	74.5	22	5	–	–	1	2	2	–	–	42	0.1	13	0.3	7	0.2	14	124	.1	10
tangerine	84	37	9	1	–	–	2	77	0.1	–	26	0.2	17	0.1	10	0.1	8	132	0.2	12
watermelon	80	26	6	–	–	2	–	30	0.1	–	8	0.1	2	0.1	9	0.2	7	93	0.1	280

Vegetarian and Global Diet Pyramids

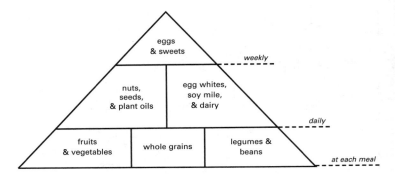

Figure D.1 The Vegetarian Diet Pyramid

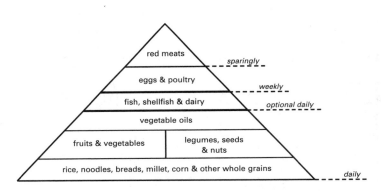

Figure D.2 The Asian Diet Pyramid

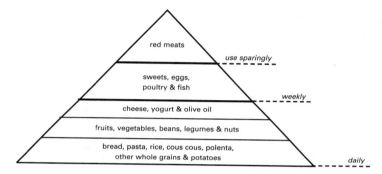

Figure D.3 The Mediterranean Diet Pyramid

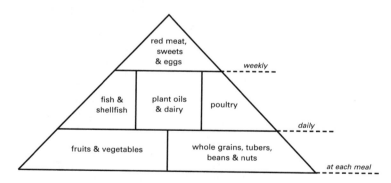

Figure D.4 The Latin Diet Pyramid

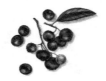

Essential Nutrient Molecular Diagrams

W e have included these chemical structure diagrams for those readers who are interested in understanding the subtle differences in the make-up of the nutrients we need each day. Without these nutrients, our bodies cannot function correctly. Notice the difference that one double bond in place of a single bond can make; notice what one added hydrogen atom can do to the structure of a vital nutrient. Hopefully, this appendix will help you understand visually the danger of toxins and free radicals, which can cause serious damage to these important additions to your diet.

Vitamin C

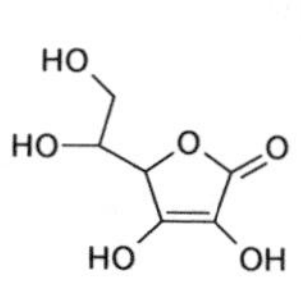

Fig. E.1: (ascorbic acid)

Vitamin D Compounds

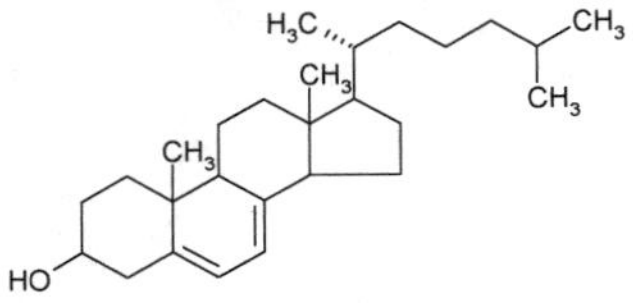

Fig. E.2 (7-dehydrocholesterol)

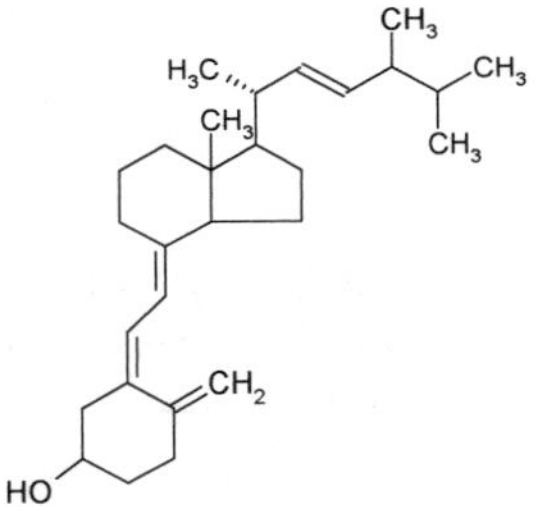

Fig. E.3 (vitamin D2)

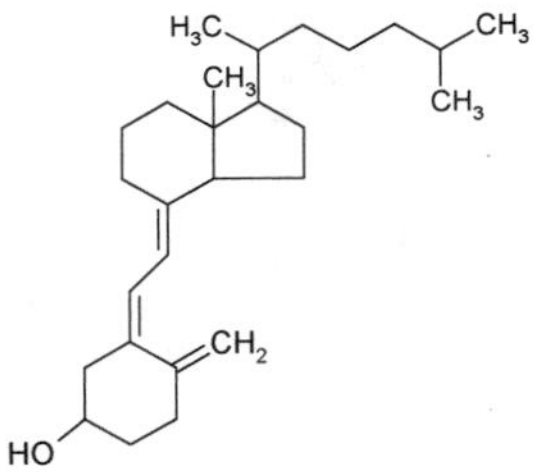

Fig. E.4 (vitamin D3)

Carotenoids

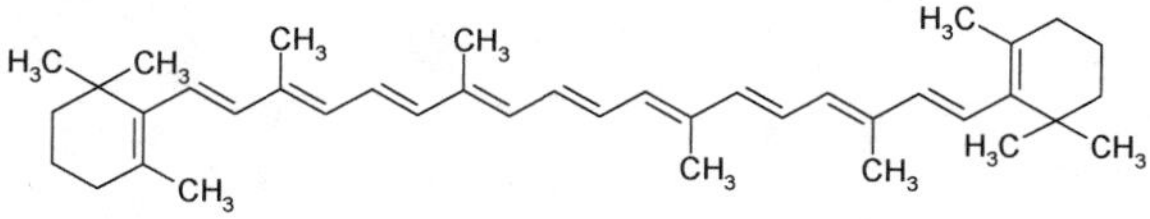

Fig. E.5 (all-trans-beta-carotene)

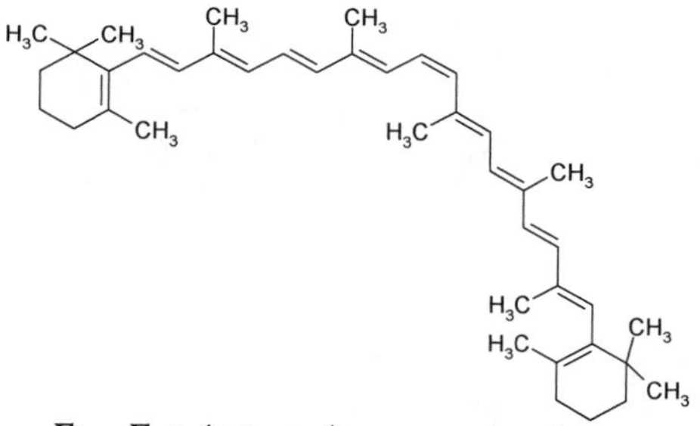

Fig. E.6 (15-cis-beta-carotene)

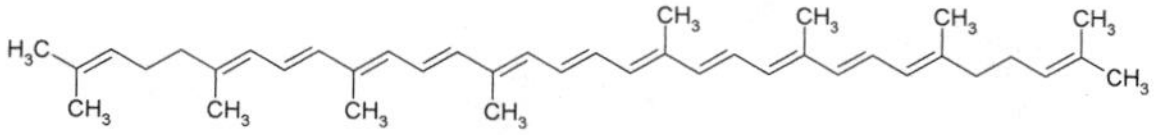

Fig. E.7 (lycopene)

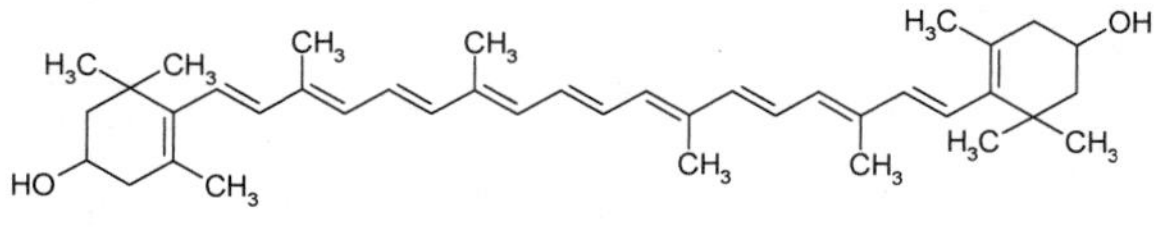

Fig. E.8 (zeaxanthin)

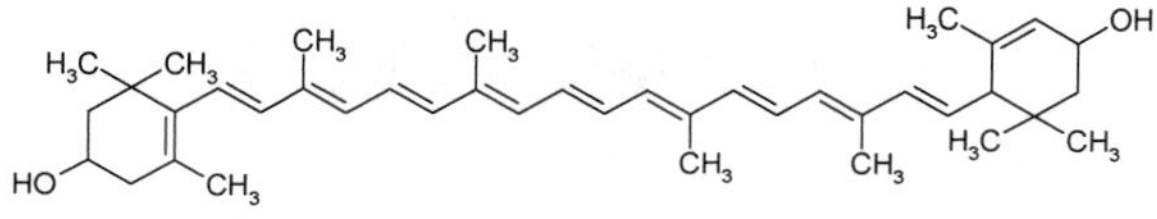

Fig. E.9 (lutein)

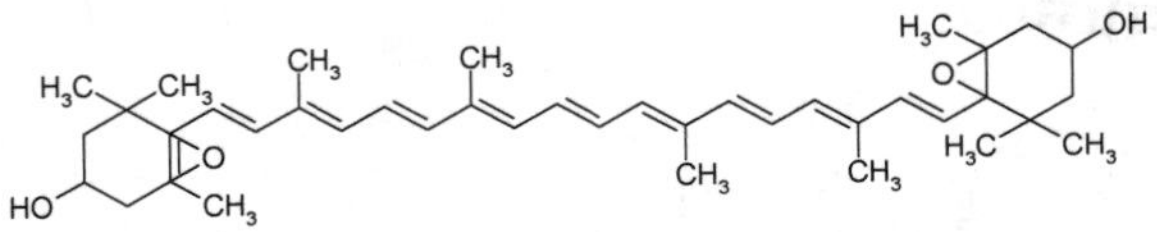

Fig. E.10 (violaxanthin)

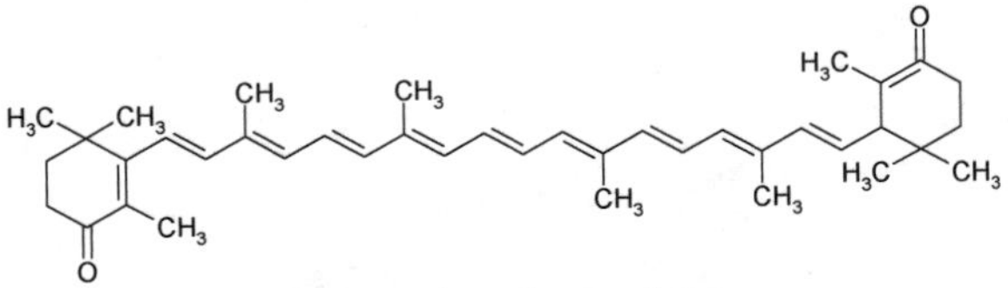

Fig. E.11 (canthaxanthin)

B vitamins

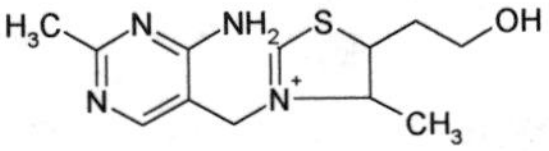

Fig. E.12 (thiamin)

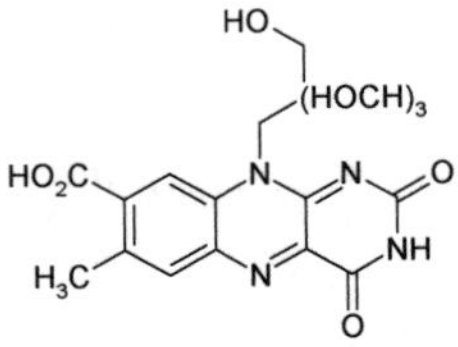

Fig. E.13 (riboflavin)

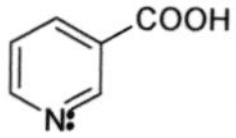

Fig. E.14 (niacin)

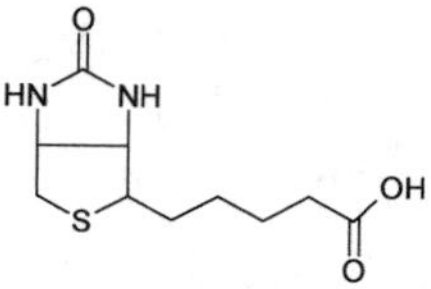

Fig. E.15 (biotin)

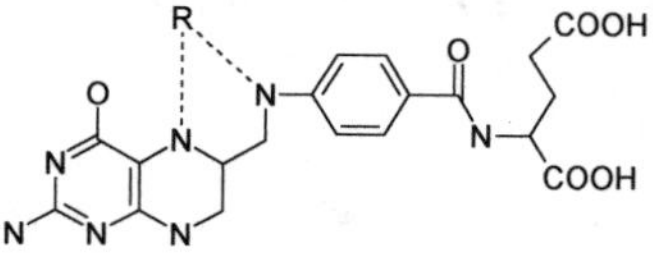

Fig. E.16 (folic acid)

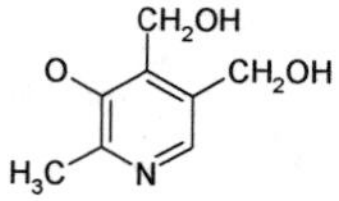

Fig. E.17 pyridoxine)

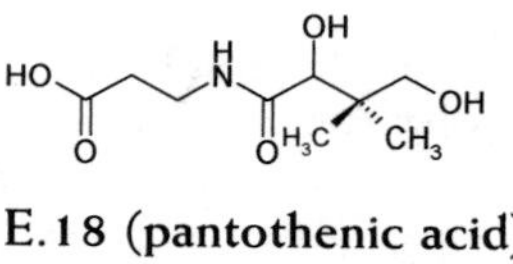

Fig. E.18 (pantothenic acid)

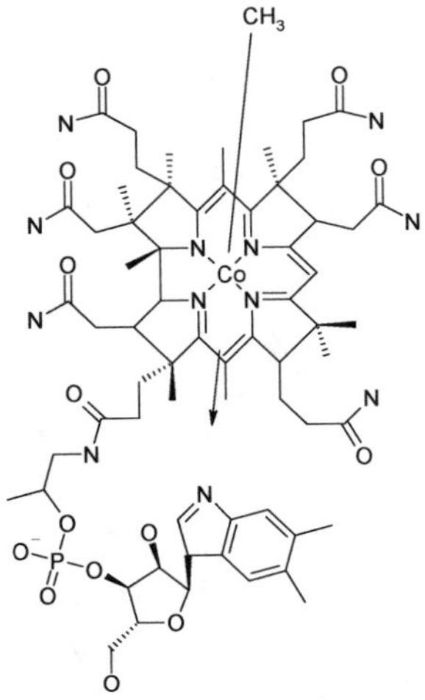

Fig. E.19 (cobalamin B12)

Tocopherols (vitamin E)

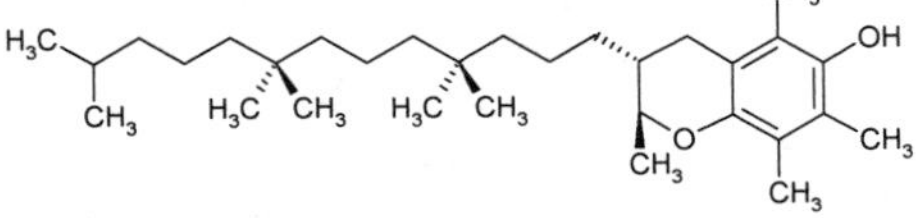

Fig. E.20 (alpha-tocopherol)

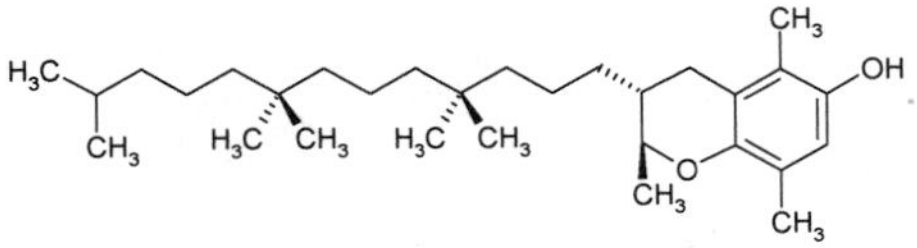

Fig. E.21 (beta-tocopherol)

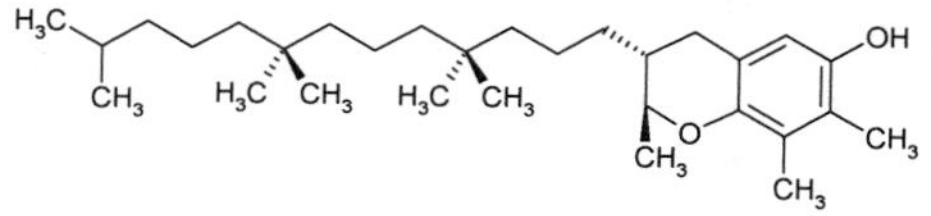

Fig. E.22 (gamma-tocopherol)

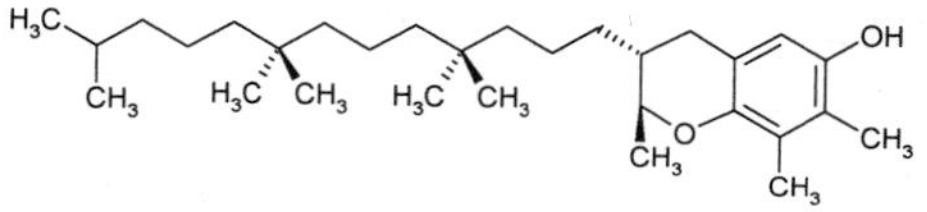

Fig. E.23 (delta-tocopherol)

Tocotrienols (vitamin E)

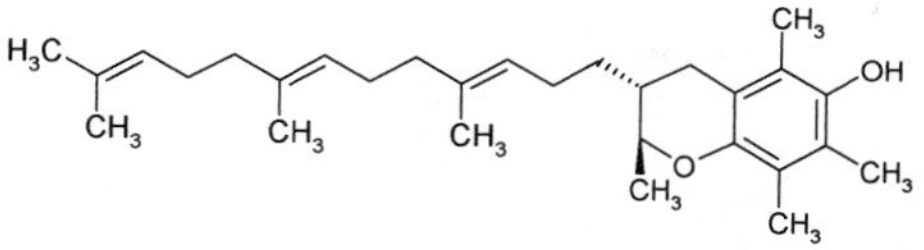

Fig. E.24 (alpha-tocotrienol)

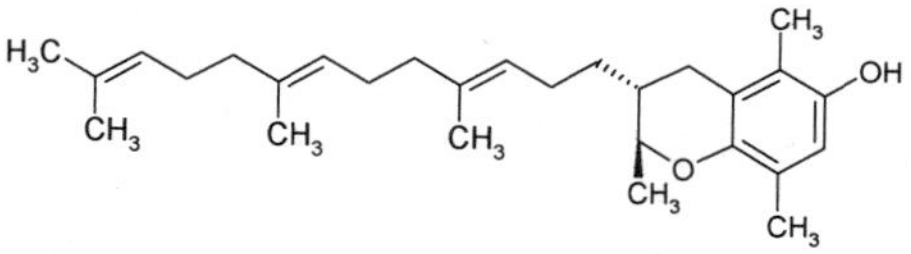

Fig. E.25 (beta-tocotrienol)

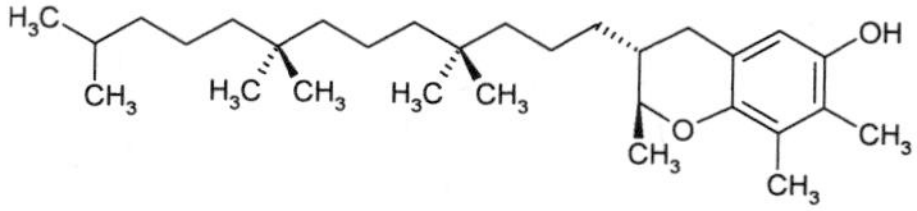

Fig. E.26 (gamma-tocotrienol)

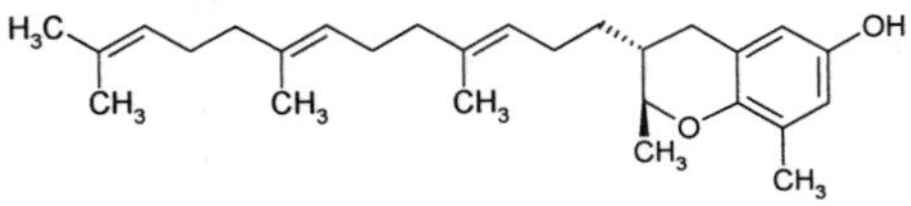

Flg. E.27 (delta-tocotrienol)

Retinoids

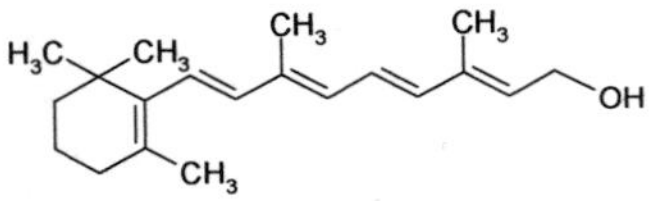

Fig. E.28 (all-trans retinol)

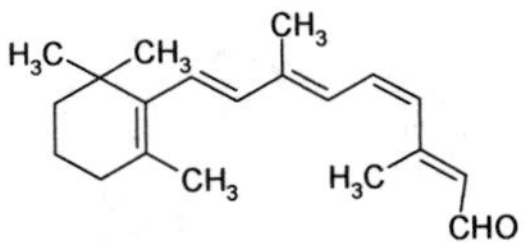

Fig. E.29 (11-cis-retinal)

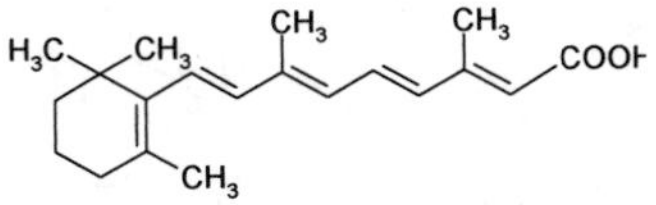

Fig. E.30 (all-trans-retinoic acid)

Terpenes

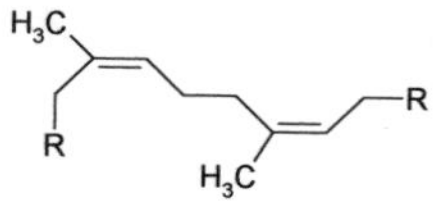

Fig. E.31 (natural rubber)

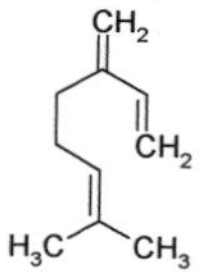

Fig. E.32 (myrcene)

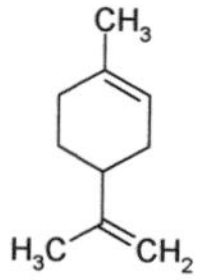

Fig. E.33 (limonene)

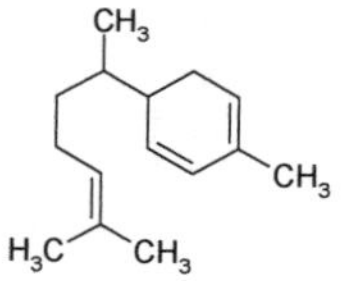

Fig. E.34 (zingiberene)

K vitamins

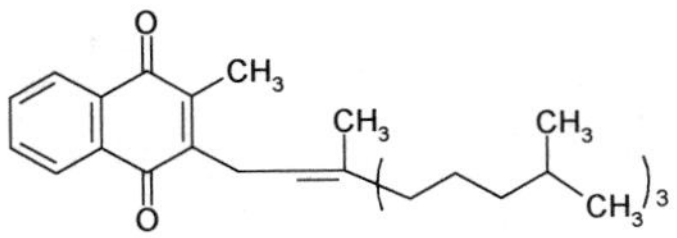

Fig. E. 35 (vitamin K1)

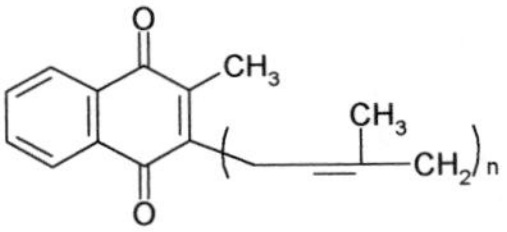

Fig. E.36 (vitamin K2)

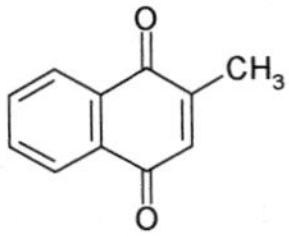

Fig. E.37 (vitamin K3)

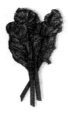

Glossary

ABMC Areal Bone Mineral Content. This is a type of bone density measurement.

active site The part of the enzyme where the reaction occurs. Usually a small pocket in the structure of the enzyme.

active transport The process of transporting certain ions and molecules across a membrane, specifically, active transport requires energy to accomplish the transport.

AI Adequate intake. One of the DRI (Daily Recommended Intake) terms. AI is a term that is used when an RDA is not yet established.

all-rac-alphatocopherol (dl-alphatocopherol) This is vitamin E, made synthetically. Rac is short for racemic, which means that it is a mixture of the active and the inactive form of the molecule.

alpha-linolenic acid This fatty acid is part of the omega-3 family. This essential fatty acid supplies the basic components, or precursors, to other crucial polyunsaturated fatty acids. Alpha linolenic acid helps make another omega-3 polyunsaturated fatty acid, which includes docosahexaenoic acid (important for proper development of the brain and eyes) and eicosapentaenoic acid.

alveoli Tiny air sacs in the lung where gas exchange takes place between the blood and the inhaled air.

Alzheimer's disease A progressive, irreversible disease characterized by degeneration of brain cells and commonly leading to severe dementia. This disease was named after the German physician who first described it.

amino acid An organic acid containing both an amino (-NH2) and an acid (-COOH) group, which serves as the building blocks for protein.

amphipathic The characteristic of having hydrophobic and hydrophilic affinity. Emulsifiers such as bile are amphipathic, and aid in the digestion and absorption of nutrients into the blood.

amylase An enzyme whose specialty is to degrade carbohydrates.

aneurysm A condition where the weakened walls of a blood vessel bulge out.

angina Severe pain in the chest that spreads up the neck, to the shoulders, and sometimes down the arms. Indicative of coronary artery disease.

angiogenesis The process of developing a supply of blood to the tissues. Angiogenesis is necessary for a tumor's progression.

antibiotic A substance that can destroy or inhibit the growth of microorganisms.

antibody A special protein of the immune system that attaches to foreign objects and helps neutralize and expel them from the body.

anticarcinogenic An agent that decreases the likelihood of developing cancer by inactivating cancer-causing substances or agents.

anti-inflammatory An agent that prevents or counteracts the inflammation processes.

antioxidants Substances that prevent oxygen from combining with other substances to cause damage to cells, or cause fat in food to become rancid. Antioxidants are able to donate electrons to electron-seeking compounds, which reduces electron capture and cell damage.

apoptosis "Programmed cell death." It is the death of cells through normal and natural processes, which do not involve inflammatory responses, usually so older cells are replaced with newer ones.

appendicitis Inflammation of the appendix.

arteriosclerosis The hardening of the arteries caused by the deposition of fibrous tissue and calcium minerals in the blood vessel walls.

artery A blood vessel that carries blood away from the heart.

arthritis An inflammatory disease of the joints that results in great pain, loss of movement, and deformation in its most serious cases.

asexual Reproduction without sex, or without union of male and female gametes. Bacteria do this by binary fission, or splitting in half.

aspirin A white crystalline powder, acetylcalicylic acid, used as an anti-inflammatory drug and for reducing fever and relieving headaches.

atherosclerosis The thickening of the arteries caused by the formation of fatty plaques on the arterial walls which leads to blocked blood flow.

atom A basic unit of matter. An atom is composed of a nucleus made of up protons and neutrons. Electrons circle the nucleus in areas called orbitals.

ATP (adenosine triphosphate) The high-energy molecule that provides energy to nearly all of the cell's functions.

augmentation index A measure of arterial stiffness.

autoimmune disease A class of diseases caused by a disorder of the immune system where the immune system recognizes and attacks the body instead of pathogens.

bacteriostatic An agent that inhibits bacterial growth or multiplication of bacteria.

balanced diet A diet providing the recommended intake of all nutrients and containing a wide variety of foods.

base A ringed molecule made up of a carbon, nitrogen, and oxygen atom that is incorporated into the DNA molecule. There are four principle bases used in human DNA: adenine, thymine, guanine, and cytosine.

beriberi Thiamin deficiency disorder characterized by muscle weakness, loss of appetite, nerve degeneration, and sometimes edema.

beta-amyloid Sticky protein that is deposited in the areas of the brain affected by Alzheimer's disease.

bioavailability Describes how readily nutrients are able to be absorbed and used in the body.

biopsy A sample of tissue is removed from a living body in order to determine by closer analysis if a disease and its cause exist in the area.

blood clot A mesh of proteins and platelets that forms when a blood vessel is broken, damaged, or ruptured. The clot serves to stop the escape of blood from the blood vessel.

blood pressure The force that the blood exerts on the walls of the blood vessel. High blood pressure can cause many health problems. A healthy blood pressure will be below 130/85.

blood thinning The process of making the platelets of the blood less likely to stick together resulting in faster flowing, thinner blood and less likelihood for blood clots or poor infiltration.

bond The sharing of electrons between two atoms that results in those atoms being linked together.

bonding orbital The orbital furthest away from the nucleus of an atom. The electrons in this orbital participate in chemical reactions with other atoms.

bone marrow The soft middle portion of the major bones of the body that specializes in the production of white blood cells.

bract A modified leaf, scale, or pouch-like plant part on a flower stalk that is usually at the base of a flower it is protecting. It is usually small and plain but sometimes can be decorative and brightly colored.

caffeine A drug that stimulates the heart and nervous system, constricts the blood vessels, and increases urinary excretion.

calories The amount of heat needed to raise the temperature of one gram of water to one degree celsius.

cancer The condition characterized by uncontrolled growth of abnormal body cells. Cancer can happen in almost every part of the body, from the bladder to the brain.

capillary A tiny blood vessel that specializes in transferring oxygen and nutrients from the blood to the tissues and the absorption of carbon dioxide and cellular wastes from tissues into the blood.

carbohydrate A compound containing carbon, hydrogen, and oxygen atoms; most are known as sugars, starches, and dietary fibers.

carbon A nonmetallic chemical element found in many inorganic compounds and all organic compounds. Diamonds and graphite are pure carbon.

carbon dioxide A colorless and odorless, incombustible gas, CO_2. Is a product of respiration and combustion.

carcinogens Substances that cause cancer.

cardiovascular Anything pertaining to the heart.

cardiovascular disease See heart disease.

carotenoids The red, orange and yellow plant pigments that give fruits and vegetables their vivid colors. A large class of phytochemicals having the general structure described eight isoprene units. In plants, carotenoids function as storage sites for solar energy to support photosynthesis, the process used by plants to make energy. In humans, carotenoids play a key role in immune system support and enhancement. About thirty-four are

found in human syrum, these are associated with certain beneficial antioxidant properties.

cartilage Soft supportive tissue that gives structure to many parts of
the body and functions in the joints to allow for smooth movement.

catalase An enzyme that helps protect the body from oxidation.
Converts hydrogen peroxide to water and oxygen.

catalyze To function so as to speed up a chemical reaction.

cell The most basic unit of life in the human body. Cells form tissues, tissues form organs, organs form systems and systems form
bodies.

cellular membrane A lipid bilayer that bounds the cell and controls what enters and leaves it.

cellulose Straight chained polysaccharide of glucose molecules
that is indigestible; part of insoluble fiber.

chelate To bind a metal in such a way so as to inactivate its free-
radical production capability.

chelator A molecule that chelates metals.

chemokines Chemical messengers that are released from damaged cells as well as cells.

cholesterol A hydrophobic molecule used by the body to stabilize
cellular membranes, synthesize hormones, and absorb fats and
hydrophobic materials from the digestive tract.

circulation The act of moving around in a complete circuit, for
example the movement of blood out of and back to the heart
through the arteries and veins.

coagulation The process of forming blood clots.

coenzyme Molecules that bind to enzymes and enhance or inhibit their activity.

cofactor A small molecule that works in association with an
enzyme to catalyze a specific reaction. Enzymes that require cofactors cannot function without them.

collagen A fibrous protein, known for its strength and resilience,
essential in many tissues. Bone, tendons, ligaments, teeth, and cellular struture are among the tissues that require collagen.

complement proteins Proteins in the blood that attach to foreign
objects and help expel them from the body.

complete proteins Proteins containing all the essential amino
acids in the right balance to meet human needs.

complex carbohydrate Long chains of sugar units arranged to
form starch or fiber; also called polysaccharides.

cone One of the photo sensory cells found in the retina of the eye.

congestive heart failure A chronic condition where the heart is unable to pump enough blood to meet the needs of the body. Characterized by fatigue, swelling of the limbs, and fluid in the lungs.

conjugated bonds Double bonds within a carbon structure that lend themselves to stability.

coronary arteries The blood vessels that supply blood to the heart itself.

coronary artery disease Essentially atherosclerosis of the coronary arteries.

coronary heart disease See coronary artery disease.

cross links Result of oxidative damage to fatty acid chains where chains are connected to one another.

cruciferous vegetables Vegetables belonging to the family *Cruciferae* The family consists of broccoli, cauliflower, brussel sprouts, and cabbage.

cytotoxic A chemical or substance that is capable of producing a toxic effect on healthy, beneficial cells, preventing their reproduction or growth and perhaps even facilitating in their death.

daily values (DV) Set of standard nutrient-intake values developed by the FDA and used as references on food labels showing how much fits into the overall daily diet. Daily values include two types of standards; RDIs (Recommended Daily Intake) and DRVs (Daily Reference Value).

deciduous A plant that sheds its leaves in a certain season then grows them back in another.

deficiency The quality or state of being deficient; absence of something essential; incompleteness.

dehydration To remove water from a compound, substance, or body tissue. To lose water; to become dry.

deoxyribonucleic acid A kind of molecule found in the nucleus of a cell that contains the code for all of our genetic information.

diabetes *(Diabetes mellitus)* A chronic disease where the body mishandles blood glucose levels. Diabetes is caused by the body's inability to produce or respond to the hormone insulin and is characterized by high blood glucose (hyperglycemia), resulting from insufficient insulin action in the body.

diet The usual pattern of food and drink intake by a person.

dietary fiber Collective term for the structural parts of plants that are not digested by humans.

dietary guidelines General goals for nutrient intake and diet composition set by the government agencies USDA (U.S. Department of Agriculture) and DHHS (Department of Health and Human Services.

dietary thermogenesis Energy needed to digest, absorb, transport, and store nutrients in food; also known as specific dynamic action of food, or thermic effect of food.

differentiation, cellular The process of becoming more and more specialized in performing specific functions in the body.

diffusion A natural result of entropy, which causes substances in high consentration to spread out over a larger volume, becoming less concentrated. Diffusion across cellular membranes is one of the most important ways molecules can move. Such molecules diffuse across the membrane.

disaccharide Pairs of single sugars linked together (*di* = two).

diverticulosis The formation of small pockets in the intestines.

DNA See deoxyribonucleic acid.

double blind A testing procedure that is designed to eliminate biased results, in which neither the administrators of the test treatment nor the subjects involved are aware of who is taking the test treatment or the placebo until after the study is completed.

Dowager's hump An abnormal curvature of the upper spine that occurs in people afflicted with osteoporosis. This condition is caused by compression fractures and vertical collapse of the vertebrae.

DRI Daily Recommended Intake. An umbrella term including values such as the RDA, AI, EAR and IU. This system has not been fully developed, and so most values are still listed as RDA.

EAR Estimated Average Requirement. Basically, the EAR is the minimum amount of a nutrient we should eat per day. Typically, we will want to eat much more.

edema The condition of the swelling of the body because of fluid leakage from the blood vessels. This is often seen in protein deficient cases.

EKG or ECG (electrocardiogram) A test that measures the flow of electricity around the heart as it pumps. Erratic measurements can indicate specific heart conditions.

electron affinity The pull that an atom has on electrons.

electron transport chain A series of proteins in the inner mitochondrial membrane that shuttle electrons from high energy electron carriers to oxygen in order to produce energy.

electron A subatomic particle that carries a negative charge. Electrons are found circling the atom's nucleus.

elements A group of atoms that all have the same number of protons in their nuclei. This confers upon them identical chemical properties.

empty calories Foods containing little or no nutritional value compared to the calories they deliver.

emulsification The process of breaking up hydrophobic molecules into small particles that are dissolvable in water.

energy The capacity to do work. The energy in food is chemical energy; it can be converted to mechanical, electrical, heat, or other forms of energy in the body. Food energy is measured in calories.

energy-yielding nutrients Nutrients the body can use for energy. They may also supply building blocks for body structure.

enriched When the vitamins thiamin, niacin, and riboflavin, and the mineral iron are added to grain products to improve nutritional quality.

enzymes A compound that speeds the rate of chemical process but is not altered by the chemical process. Almost all enzymes are proteins.

epidemiology The study of disease patterns, including diet-related disease, in different populations.

essential amino acids Amino acids that are not synthesized efficiently by humans. They therefore must be included in the diet. There are nine essential amino acids.

essential fatty acids Fatty acids that must be present in the diet to maintain health. Linolenic acid and alpha-linolenic acid are the essential fatty acids needed in the body to maintain proper health.

essential nutrients Nutrients that are supplied through foods. Essential literally means, "Needed from outside the body."

fat See lipid.

fat-soluble Describing those compounds that readily dissolve in fats because of their hydrophobic nature.

fat-soluble vitamins Vitamins that dissolve in such substances as ether and benzene, but not readily in water. Fat-soluble vitamins include vitamins A, D, E, and K.

fatty acid A chain of carbon atoms to which hydrogen atoms are linked along its whole length. The body uses fatty acids to store energy. Three fatty acids are connected to a glycerol molecule to form a triglyceride.

ferritin An iron-binding protein in cells that chelates iron to storage.

fiber Collective term for indigestible or partially digestible polysaccharides in food. Containing cellulose, hemicellulose, and pectin.

foam cells White blood cells in atherosclerotic plaques that have engulfed large quantities of fats and cholesterols.

folic acid A crystalline substance $C_{19}H_{19}N_7O_6$, found in green leaves and in certain other plant and animal tissues, exhibiting vitamin B activity.

food Substances taken into the body that maintain life and growth by supplying energy and building and replacing tissue.

food composition The amount of nutrients, chemicals, and ingredients in a food.

food guide pyramid A research-based food guidance system, developed by the USDA, in which foods necessary in large amounts are at the base of the pyramid and foods to be eaten sparingly are at the top.

fortification The addition of nutrients to a food product.

fortified foods Foods with added nutrients, usually vitamins and minerals.

free radicals Short-lived form of compounds that exist with an unpaired electron in the outer electron shell, which make them unstable and highly reactive.

fructose A monosaccharide; sometimes known as fruit sugar.

functional foods Any food with a health benefit.

galactose A monosaccharide; part of the disaccharide lactose (milk sugar).

gall bladder A small organ nestled underneath the liver whose function is to store bile acids needed for digestion.

gas exchange A process that takes place in the alveoli of the lungs where oxygen is absorbed into the blood and carbon dioxide is expelled into the lung to be exhaled.

gene A length of DNA with a specific sequence of nucleotide bases that encodes the information needed to make a protein.

gerontologist A scientist who studies aging.

glucose A single sugar used in both plant and animal tissues for quick energy; known also as dextrose or blood sugar.

glutathione peroxidase An antioxidant enzyme that converts hydrogen peroxide to water though the connection of two glutathione molecules.

glycerol An organic alcohol. When combined with fatty acids it forms a fat.

glycolysis The process by which glucose is broken down into molecules that the mitochondria can use to produce energy.

health Physical and mental well-being; condition of the body and mind.

health food Food considered to be healthful; containing the essential vitamins, minerals, antioxidants, and fiber.

healthy diet A diet that includes a variety of foods from each of the basic food groups.

heart attack An acute, life-threatening condition that occurs when the blood supply to the heart is cut off.

heart disease A disease usually caused by the deposition of fatty material in the blood vessels in the heart. This reduces the blood flow to the heart, which in turn reduces heart function, which can lead to death.

hemicellulose Dietary fiber containing xylose, galactose, glucose and other monosaccharides bonded together.

hemoglobin Protein found in red blood cells that specializes in the transportation of oxygen.

hemorrhage An acute condition where a blood vessel ruptures.

hemorrhoids Pronounced swelling in a large vein, particularly veins found in the anal region.

high density lipoprotein (HDL) The lipoprotein synthesized primarily by the liver and intestines that picks up cholesterol from dying cells and other sources and transfers it to the other lipoproteins in the bloodstream, as well as directly to the liver. A low blood HDL value increases the risk for heart disease.

homocysteine A nonessential amino acid that is believed to contribute to the development of many chronic diseases.

hormones A compound secreted into the bloodstream that acts to control the function of distant target organ cells. Hormones can be either protein like or fat like, example: insulin or estrogen.

hybridize To produce hybrids by crossbreeding and mixture of stocks using parents of different races and varieties.

hydration The addition or absorption of water.

hydrogen A flammable, colorless, odorless, gaseous chemical element. The lightest of all known substances. Needed in the generation of water.

hydrogen peroxide A reactive oxygen species that is involved in the production of many free radicals, but that can also do oxidative damage by itself.

hydrolysis The breaking with water.

hydrophilic Descriptive of a substance that dissolves well in water. The word literally means "water loving."

hydrophilicity (water loving) Able to dissolve readily in water.

hydrophobic Descriptive of a substance that does not dissolve in water. The word literally means "water fearing."

hydrophobicity (water fearing) Does not readily dissolve in water.

hydroxyl radical An extremely reactive free radical composed of an oxygen atom and a hydrogen atom.

hypertension An arterial disease of which chronic abnormally high blood pressure is the primary symptom. May have no apparent cause or can be associated with or caused by other diseases such as heart and kidney diseases, peripheral vascular disease and stroke.

in vitro Outside of the living system. Performed and observed in a simulated state.

in vivo In the living organism. Performed/observed in a living subject.

incomplete protein Proteins lacking, or low in, one or more of the essential amino acids.

inhibition Something that restrains, blocks, interferes, prevents or suppresses a response to a stimulus.

inorganic compounds Minerals do not contain carbon.

insoluble fiber Sometimes called roughage; includes cellulose, lignin, and some hemicelluloses.

insomnia Chronic inability to sleep. Can be total lack of sleep or chronic inadequate sleep.

insulin A hormone produced by the pancreas that induces cells to take up glucose from the blood.

interferon A group of glycoproteins produced by cells as part of the immune response against virus infections. These increase resistance to the infection.

ion An atom or small molecule that has either lost or gained one or more electrons in a chemical reaction. Positive ions have lost electrons while negative ions have gained them.

iron deficiency anemia A blood disorder.

ischemia The blockage of blood flow to a tissue.

ischemia-reperfusion injury Damage done to the heart muscle when blood flow is reintroduced to the areas where it was previously cut off. This damage is likely generated by the production of free radicals.

isoprene Carbon chain units consisting of conjugated bonds, used as precursors to a variety of biochemicals.

keratin Form of structural protein that is fibrous and contributes to the structure of our hair, nails, and skin.

lactose A disaccharide; sometimes known as milk sugars.

latency The time that elapses between a stimulus that should induce a reaction, during which nothing happens, and the eventual response to the stimulus.

LDL Proteins that circulate in blood and transport "bad cholesterol" and other lipid substances to various parts of our bodies.

ligaments Tough, fibrous connective tissue that holds bones together and gives structure to the joints.

limeys A British sailor. Named such because of the lime juice used on British ships to prevent scurvy, a vitamin C deficiency.

linolenic acids Part of the omega-6 family. This essential fatty acid supplies the basic components, or precursors, to other crucial polyunsaturated fatty acids. Linolenic acid is used to make another form of omega-6 fatty acid, arachidonic acid, which is crucial for infant growth.

lipase An enzyme whose specialty is to degrade lipids or fats.

lipid A compound containing much carbon and hydrogen, little oxygen, and sometimes other atoms. Lipids dissolve in ether or benzene and include fats, oils, and cholesterol. It is the primary form of energy storage, acts as a shock absorber for vital organs, maintains skin and hair, stores and transports fat-soluble vitamins, protects cell walls, and keeps our bodies warm.

lipid oxidation The process that makes fat rancid, producing off-odors and off-tastes in food.

lipid peroxidation A kind of damage caused by free radicals that involves the addition of an oxygen molecule to lipid fatty acid. This damages the lipids and contributes to cellular injury and cardiovascular disease.

lipoprotein A compound found in the bloodstream containing a core of lipids with a shell of protein, phospholipid, and cholesterol.

liver An organ whose function is to detoxify the blood and produce bile acids.

low density lipoprotein (LDL) The product of VLDL, containing cholesterol. Elevated LDL is strongly linked to heart disease risk

lymphatic system A system of vessels that collects fluid from the tissues and returns it to the bloodstream.

lymphocyte Any of the nearly colorless cells formed in lymphoid tissue. They function in the development of immunity and include two specific types, B-cells and T-cells.

lyophilic Having a strong affinity for, and stabilized by, the liquid dispersing medium; said of colloidal medium.

macrominerals Minerals recommended in amounts greater than 100 milligrams per day. They are calcium, phosphorus, sodium, potassium, chloride, magnesium, and sulfur.

macronutrients Nutrients that are needed in large amounts. They produce energy (measured in calories) for physical activities. They also assist in the chemical reactions that occur in living cells, and provide material for building the body's tissues and regulating its activities. They consist of carbohydrates, proteins and fats.

macrophage A cell of the immune system that specializes in engulfing foreign objects.

maltose A disaccharide composed of two glucose units; sometimes known as malt sugar.

mammogram An x-ray image of the soft tissues of the breast that is used to detect breast cancers early, before the lumps are large enough to detect by hand.

megadosing The process of taking extremely high concentrations of vitamins or minerals.

melanoma A skin tumor, mostly malignant, derived from cells capable of melanin formation.

memory loss To lose the ability or power of recalling to mind facts previously learned or past experiences.

metabolism A term used to describe all of the chemical processes that go on in the body.

micelles A submicroscopic aggregation of molecules, usually lipids.

microflora The bacteria and other microorganisms that normally inhabit a bodily organ or part: intestinal flora.

microminerals Also called trace elements. Minerals recommended in amounts less than 20 milligrams per day. They include iron, zinc, iodine, selenium, fluoride, and copper.

micronutrients Consist of vitamins, minerals and water.

mild cognitive impairment Less serious mental disorder characterized by progressive memory loss, but without the serious loss of function associated with Alzheimer's disease.

minerals Inorganic elements, some minerals are essential nutrients required in small amounts.

mitochondria Organelle whose specialty is the production of energy molecules (ATP) for the cell's energy needs.

moderated diet A diet that is not in excess or extremes of essential nutrients.

monosaccharides A group name for the simplest form of carbo-hydrates, including glucose, fructose, and galactose. These sugars are not broken down further during digestion. Glucose is the most important monosaccharide. (*Mono*=one, *saccharide*= sugar).

monounsaturated fatty acid Containing one double or triple bond per molecule. Can be found in olive oil and canola oil. Reduces blood cholesterol levels.

muscle strength Suggestive of great physical strength; powerful.

myocardial infarction See heart attack.

natural Of or arising from nature; in accordance with what is found or expected in nature.

natural killer cells A killer cell of the immune system that fights off viral infections and tumors.

neurofibrillary tangles The disrupted remnants of the cellular skeletons of neurons affected by Alzheimer's disease.

neurotransmitter A chemical, usually released as an impulse, reaches the end of a nerve and transmits a chemical message across a synapse, or gap between one nerve to another, that can serve to excite or inhibit the receiving nerve.

neutron A subatomic particle that carries no charge. Neutrons are found in the atom's nucleus.

night blindness A condition caused by vitamin A deficiency that does not allow the eye to adjust rapidly from bright lights to darkness.

nitric oxide A free radical used as a chemical messenger to cause inflammation and induce blood vessels to dilate. Also produced by the immune system to kill invading pathogens.

nonpolar molecule A molecule that has charge evenly distributed over the whole molecule.

nonvitamins Chemicals not meeting all criteria to be called vitamins but marketed as vitamins.

nuclease An enzyme whose specialty is to degrade DNA and other nucleic acids.

nucleotide See base.

nucleus The major organelle in human cells that contains the DNA.

nutrient Chemicals in food that nourish the body by providing energy, allowing growth and repair of tissues, and regulating necessary chemical processes in the body.

nutrition The science of food, the nutrients and other substances therein, their action, interaction, and balance in relation to health and disease, and the processes by which the organism (body) ingests, digests, absorbs, transports, utilizes, and excretes food substances.

obesity A condition characterized by excess body fat often defined as 20 percent above the healthy weight, or body mass index above 27 to 30.

omega-3 fatty acids Being or composed of polyunsaturated fatty acids that have the final double bond in the hydrocarbon chain between the third and fourth carbon atoms from the end of the molecule opposite that of the carboxylic acid group. Found especially in fish, fish oils, vegetable oils, and green leafy vegetables.

opsin A protein of the retina that makes up one of the visual pigments.

orbital The area surrounding an atom's nucleus inhabited by a specific electron or pair of electrons. It can be imagined as the path that the electron follows in its "orbit" around the nucleus.

organelle A membrane-bound compartment of a cell that performs a specialized function. Equivalent to an organ in our bodies.

organic Anything containing carbon atoms bonded to hydrogen atoms in the chemical structure.

osteoblasts Bone cells that deposit bone material.

osteocalcin One of many proteins involved in incorporating calcium into the process of bone formation.

osteoclasts Bone cells that reabsorb bone material.

osteomalacia The softening of the bones, usually in women, caused by a deficiency of vitamin D, calcium or both.

osteoporosis A chronic disease of aging most frequently observed in women involving the slow degeneration of the bones.

overdoses To take in too large of amounts.

oxidation The process of removing an electron from an atom or molecule.

oxidative damage Damage done to the body by free radicals via the oxidation of molecules that make up the body.

oxidative stress A condition where the amount of free radicals in the body overwhelms the oxidative defenses.

oxygen Colorless, odorless, tasteless, gaseous chemical element that occurs freely in the atmosphere.

pancreas An organ whose function is to produce hormones needed for digestion and other processes. The most notable hormone that it produces is insulin, the lack of which causes diabetes.

pathogen A microorganism capable of causing disease.

pectin Dietary fiber containing chains of galaturonic acid and other monosaccharides; characteristically found between plant cell walls.

peptide See protein.

peristalsis The rhythmic squeezing of the intestines that pushes the food through the digestive tract.

peroxynitrite A nitrogen free radical that is highly reactive.

perspiration The act of perspiring a salty moisture (sweat) from the skin.

pH A measure of acidity. Rated on a scale of 0 to 14. Zero is the most acidic while 14 is the least acidic.

photosynthesis The process by which plants harness the energy of the sun and convert water and carbon dioxide into sugar.

phytochemicals Nonnutrient compounds in plant-derived foods having biological activity in the body. Some phytochemicals may contribute to a reduced risk of cancer or heart disease in people who consume them regularly.

placebo A ineffectual substance containing no medication that is given to some of the subjects in an experiment as a comparison to determine the effectiveness of a medicinal substance.

plasma The liquid portion of the blood. Made up mostly of water, this phase carries dissolved proteins, nutrients, and other substances for distribution and transportation around the body.

platelets Tiny disks that circulate in the blood whose function is to clot the blood in the event of damage to the blood vessel.

polar molecule A molecule that has positive and negative charges localized on different poles.

polarity When involved in chemical descriptions, this property describes complete or partial charge orientation on a molecule. For example, water is partially positive on one side of the molecule, while being partially negative on the other side.

polymer A large molecule made up of many repeating subunits.

polypeptide See protein.

polysaccharide Another term for complex carbohydrates, compounds of long strands of glucose units linked together.

polyunsaturated fatty acids Having in each molecule many chemical bonds in which two or three pairs of electrons are shared by two atoms Reduces blood cholesterol. Can be found in vegetable oils, nuts, and high-fat fish.

preformed vitamin These are vitamins that are already in the form that the body needs them when they are absorbed.

protease An enzyme whose specialty is to degrade proteins.

protein A large molecule made up of many amino acids linked together in a chain. The chain of amino acids takes on a specific shape that allows the protein to perform a specific function.

proton A subatomic particle that carries a positive charge. Protons are found in the atom's nucleus.

provitamins These are compounds that are converted into a vitamin (usually associated with vitamin A). Beta-carotene is an A provitamin.

pyruvate A small molecule produced by the process of glycolysis that is used by the mitochondria to produce energy.

quench A type of reaction involving singlet oxygen that results in the energy of that molecule being dissipated so that it returns to its normal state.

randomized The subjects in an experiment are randomly distributed among treatments so as to control bias in the experiment.

RE (retinol equivalent) Equal to 1 mg of retinol.

reactive nitrogen species (RNS) Any compound of nitrogen that reacts readily with other molecules. Includes, but is not limited to, free radicals.

reactive oxygen species (ROS) Any compound of oxygen that reacts readily with other molecules. Includes, but is not limited to, free radicals.

recommended dietary allowance (RDA) The amounts of selected nutrients considered adequate to meet the known nutrient needs of practically all healthy people. RDAs have been set for: energy, protein, vitamins (A, D, E, K, C, thiamin, riboflavin, niacin, B6, folate, and B12), and minerals (calcium, phosphorus, magnesium, iron, zinc, iodine, and selenium).

red blood cells Cells that circulate in the blood that specialize in the transportation of oxygen. They are red because of their high content of hemoglobin.

reduction Process of adding an electron to an atom or molecule.

reperfusion The restoration of blood flow to ischemic tissues.

respiration (1) The process by which we inhale and exhale in order to provide oxygen to our tissues and expel carbon dioxide. The act of breathing.

respiration (2) The process by which cells release the energy contained in our food in order to fuel cellular processes.

retinoid A group of molecules that are related to retinol. These include retinoic acid and retinal.

rhizome A horizontal plant stem, also called the rootstalk or rootstock, that is usually underground and sends shoots of the plant upwards and roots downwards. They may serve as an asexual reproductive structure.

rhodopsin A pigment in the retinal rods of the eyes, consisting of opsin and retinene.

rod Rod-shaped cells in the retina that respond to dim light.

satiety State in which there is no longer a desire to eat; a feeling of satisfaction.

saturated fats Raises blood cholesterol more than any other form of fat. Saturated fats come from meats, milk, and milk products. They have all the hydrogen atoms they can hold. They are appropriately named because they are saturated with hydrogen. They are thus highly efficient for storing energy because they utilize more bonds. Diets high in saturated fats are linked with higher risks of heart disease, certain cancers, and stroke. Saturated fats are straight chains. The structure of saturated fats lends itself more easily to accumulation and compression at body temperature.

saturated fatty acid A fatty acid without any double bonds and thus has the maximum amount of hydrogen atoms possible linked to its carbon chain.

scavenge Action of antioxidants whereby they intercept and neutralize free-radicals.

scurvy The deficiency disease resulting after a few weeks of consuming a diet that lacks vitamin C.

selenium A transition metal that is found in the active sites of many antioxidant enzymes.

serrated The edges are serrate, like a saw, having tooth-like projections lined up along the margin.

simple carbohydrates Sugar, including both single sugar units and linked pairs of sugar units. The basic sugar unit is a molecule containing six carbon atoms, together with oxygen and hydrogen atoms.

singlet oxygen A reactive oxygen species that is composed essentially of an oxygen molecule that has been energize by the reception of light energy.

smoking One of the most damaging things to the health of an individual. Smoking introduces massive quantities of free radicals into the body where they cause extensive destruction and lead to diseases such as cancer and heart disease.

soluble fiber Consists of pectins, gums, mucilages, and hemicelluloses; makes about one-third of the total fiber in typical diets.

spleen An organ whose function is to clean the blood of aging red blood cells.

starch A plant polysaccharide composed of glucose; highly digestible by human beings. Also known as complex carbohydrates.

sterioisomer Set of isomers whose molecules have the same atoms bonded to each other but differ in the way these atoms are arranged in space.

stroke An acute, life-threatening condition where blood is cut off parts of the brain.

structural proteins Include ligaments, bone and teeth cores, scars, filaments of hair, materials of toenails and fingernails, and more.

sucrose A disaccharide composed of glucose and fructose; sometimes known as table, beet, or cane sugar.

sugars Relatively small compounds of carbon, hydrogen, and oxygen that form the basic source of fuel for our bodies.

superoxide dismutase An enzyme that neutralizes free radicals by converting superoxide to hydrogen peroxide.

superoxide ion A free radical composed of an oxygen molecule that has acquired an extra electron.

supplementation Sources of nutrients separate from food products either synthesized artificially or extracted from natural sources.

synovial fluid Lubricating fluid found within the synovium. It also acts as a shock absorber.

synovium A membrane bound sac that encloses all joints.

terpenoids Any of various unsaturated hydrocarbons, $C_{10}H_{16}$, found in essential oils.

toxicants Chemicals that harm people, animals, or plants.

toxicity The extent, quality, or degree of being poisonous.

transferrin A protein that binds iron in the intestines and successfully chelates it for safe transportation in the body.

transition metals Metals located in the middle of the periodic table that participate readily in the formation of free radicals because of their ability to shuttle electrons.

triglycerides The major form of lipid in the body and in food. It is composed of three fatty acids bonded to glycerol, an alcohol.

UL (Tolerable Upper Intake Level) ULs represent the maximum amount of a given nutrient that we can eat without experiencing any of the toxic side effects from having too much of that nutrient.

unsaturated fats Unsaturated fats do not have all of the hydrogen atoms they are capable of holding. Unsaturated fats are thus not as efficient for storing energy as saturated fats. They have have important functions in the body. They are found in vegetable oils (olive, canola, peanut, safflower, sunflower, and soybean), nuts and in fatty fish. Some research suggests that unsaturated fatty acids may help prevent heart disease, reduce blood clotting, lower blood pressure and possibly aid in preventing irregular heart beats.

unsaturated fatty acid A fatty acid that has one or more double bonds thus decreasing the amount of hydrogen atoms linked to the carbon chain. Usually has a bent shape due to the double bond(s).

USDA United States Department of Agriculture.

vegetarian A person who avoids eating animal products to a varying degree, ranging from consuming no animal products to simply not consuming animals.

vein A blood vessel that carries blood to the heart.

vertigo The sensation of dizziness, confusion or disorientation, in which stationary objects appear to move and the person finds it difficult to remain standing and may feel like they are falling.

vitamers A group of compounds having related structures, and called under the same vitamin family name. For example, vitamin E has at least eight different vitamers.

vitamins Essential organic nutrients required in small amounts by the body for health.

water of metabolism The water produced in the mitochondria by the reduction of oxygen at the end of the electron transport chain.

water-soluble vitamins Vitamins that dissolve in water, which consists of the B vitamins and vitamin C.

white blood cells Any of a number of various kinds of cells that pertain to the immune system. They guard the body against unwanted visitors.

working proteins These proteins include enzymes, antibodies, transport vehicles, hormones, cellular "pumps," and oxygen carriers. In essence, these proteins perform all the hard chemical labor that keeps us alive.

xerophthalmia A condition during a deficiency of vitamin A, the front of the eye, which is moist and protected in normal individuals, becomes dry and susceptible to infection.

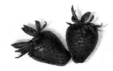

General References

Ambau. 1997. The Importance of Good Nutrition, Herbs and Phytochemicals. For your Health, Good Looks and Longevity. Falcon Press International.

Barberán and Robins.1997. Phytochemistry of Fruit and Vegetables. Oxford Science Publications, Claredon Press.

Baskin and Salem. 1997. Oxidants, Antioxidants and Free Radicals. Taylor and Francis Publishers.

Beling. 1997. Power Foods. Harper Perennial. Harper Collins Publishing.

Berning and Steen. 1998. Nutrition for Sport and Exercise 2nd Edition. An Aspen Publication.

Bidlack, Omaye, Meskin and Topham. 2000. Phytochemicals as Bioactive Agents. Technomic Publishing Co., Inc. Lancaster, Basel.

Boulos. 1983. Medicinal Plants of North Africa. Reference Publications, Inc.

Burke and Berning. 1996. Training Nutrition. Cooper Publishing Group.

Byung Pal Yu. 1993. Free Radicals and Aging. CRC Press.

Cadenas and Packer. 1996. Handbook of Antioxidants. Marcel Dekker, Inc.

Carper. 1996. Stop Aging Now! Harper Perennial. HarperCollins Publishers.

Carper. 1997. Miracle Cures. Harper Perennial. HarperCollins Publishers.

Carper. 2000. The Miracle Heart. Harper Paperbacks. HarperCollins Publishers.

Cerutti, Fridovich and McCord. 1988. Oxy-Radicals in Molecular Biology and Pathology. Alan R. Liss, Inc. New York.

Chow. 1988. Cellular Antoxidant Defense Mechansims Volume I–III. CRC Press.

Cremlyn. 1996. An Introduction to Organosulfur Chemistry. John Wiley and Sons.

Driskell. 2000. Sports Nutrition. CRC Press.

Duke. 1986. Handbook of Northeastern Indian Medicinal Plants. Quarterman Publications Inc., Lincoln, Mass.

Duke. 1999. Dr. Duke's Essential Herbs. Rodale Reach. An Imprint of Rodale Books.

Eastwood. 1997. Principles of Human Nutrition. Chapman and Hall.

Firshein. 1998. The Nutraceutical Revolution. Riverhead Books, New York.

Frei. 1994. Natural Antioxidants in Human Health and Disease. Academic Press.

Gabriel. 1975. Herb Identifier and Handbook. Sterling Publishing Co., Inc. New York Oak Tree Press Co. Ltd. London and Sydney.

Garewal. 1997. Antioxidants and Disease Prevention. CRC Press.

Goodwin. 1976. Chemistry and Biochemistry of Plant Pigments Volume 1 and 2. Academic Press. Harcourt Brace Jovanovich, Publishers.

Graci. 1999. The Power of Superfoods. Prentice Hall Canada Inc. Scarborough, Ontario.

Griggs. 1986. The Food Factor. Viking.

Groff and Gropper. 2000. Advanced Nutrition and Human Metabolism 3rd Edition. Wadsworth Thompson Learning.

Halliwell and Gutteridge. 1999. Free Radicals in Biology and Medicine 3rd Edition. Oxford University Press.

Haslam 1989. Plant Polyphenols: Vegetable Tannins Revisited. Cambridge University Press.

Haslam. 1998. Practical Polyphenolics. Cambridge University Press.

Hegarty. 1995. Nutrition: Food and the Environment. Eagan Press.

Heinerman. 1998. Dr. Heinerman's Encyclopedia of Nature's Vitamins and Minerals. Prentice Hall Press.

Hodges. 1980. Nutrition in Medical Practice. W.B. Saunders Company.

Hostettmann and Marston. 1995. Saponins. Cambridge University Press.

Hutchens. Indian Herbalogy of North America. 1973. MERCO.

Jacobs. 1994. Diet and Cancer: Markers, Prevention, and Treatment. Plenum Press.

Joossens, Hill and Gegoers. 1986. Diet and Human Carcinogenesis. Elsevier Science Publishing Company, Inc.

Kellog Company. 1985. A Citizen's Petition: The Relationship Between Diet and Health. Kellog Company. Battle Creek, Michigan.

Kretchmer and Robertson. 1978. Human Nurtition. Scientific America, Inc.

Kreutler. 1980. Nutrition in Perspective. Prentice Hall, Inc. Englewood Cliffs, New Jersey.

Kritchevsky and Bonfield. 1997. Dietary Fiber in Health and Disease: Advances in Experimental Medicine and Biology Volume 427. Plenum Press. New York and London.

Kwiterovich. 1998. The Johns Hopkins Complete Guide to Preventing and Reversing Heart Disease. Prima Health. Prima Publishing.

Larson. 1997. Naturally Occurring Antioxidants. Lewis Publishers.

Lehninger, Nelson and Cox. 1993. Principles of Biochemistry with an Extended Discussion of Oxygen-Binding Proteins 2nd Edition. Worth Publishers

Lin and Lonsdale. 1993. Free Radicals and Disease Prevention. Keats Publishing, Inc. New Canaan, Conn.

Linskens and Jackson. 1994. Alkaloids. Springer-Verlag.

Lloyd, McDonald, and Crampton. 1959. Fundamentals of Nutrition. WH Freeman and Company.

Mahan and Escott-Stump. 2000. Krause's Food, Nutrition, and Diet Therapy 10th Edition. W.B. Saunders Company. A division of Harcourt and Brace Company.

Manthey and Buslig. 1998. Flavonoids in the Living System: Advances in Experimental Medicine and Biology Volume 439. Plenum Press. New York and London.

Mark and Mark. 1999. Reversing Memory Loss. Houghton Mifflin Company.

Matkovics and Kal<sz. 1990. Radicals, Ions and Tissue Damage. Akadémiai Kiadó, Budapest.

Mazza and Miniati. 1993. Anthocyanins in Fruits, Vegetables, and Grains. CRC Press.

McCaleb, Leigh and Morien. 2000. The Encyclopedia of Popular Herbs. Prima Health. Prima Publishing.

McCully. 1997. The Homocysteine Revolution. Keats Publishing, Inc. New Canaan, Conn.

Mettlin and Aoki. 1990. Recent Progress in Research on Nutrition and Cancer. Wiley-Liss.

Meyskens. 1989. Nutrients and Cancer Prevention. The Humana Press, Inc.

Miquel, Quintanilha, and Weber. 1989. Handbook of Free Radicals and Antioxidnats in Biomedicine Volume I–III. CRC Press.

Mitchell. 1996. Biological Interactions of Sulfur Compounds. Taylor and Francis.

Mitchell and Bernard. 1955. Food in Health and Disease. F.A. Davis Company. Philadelphia.

Moerman. 1986. Medicinal Plants of Native America Volume I. Ann Arbor.

Montagnier, Olivier, and Pasquier. 1998. Oxidative Stress in Cancer, AIDS, and Neurodegenerative Diseases. Marcel Dekker, Inc.

Moslen and Smith. 1992. Free Radical Mechanisms of Tissue Injury. CRC Press.

Null. 1999. Gary Null's Ultimate Anti-Aging Program. Broadway Books. New York.

Packer and Colman. 1999. The Antioxidant Miracle. John Wiley and Sons, Inc.

Packer, Hiramatsu, and Yoshikawa.1999. Antioxidant Food Supplements in Human Health. Academic Press.

Papas. 1999. Antioxidant Status, Diet, Nutritionm and Health. CRC Press.

Passwater. 1975. Supernutrition. The Dial Press. New York.

Pizzorno and Murray. 1999. Textbook of Natural Medicine Vol. I and II 2nd Edition. Churchill Livingstone. Harcourt Publisher's Limited.

Raffauf. 1996. Plant Alkaloids: A Guide to Their Discovery and Distribution. Food Products Press, The Haworth Press, Inc.

Raven and Johnson. 1995. Biology 3rd Edition. Wm. C. Brown Communications, Inc.

Rice-Evans and Packer. 1998. Flavonoids in Health and Disease. Marcel Dekker, Inc.

Roberts. 1998. Cornucopia: The Lore of Fruits and Vegetables. Saraband Inc.

Roberts and Wink. 1998. Alkaloids. Biochemistry, Ecology, and Medicinal Applications. Plenum Press. NY.

Rosen, Huang, Osawa and Ho. 1994. Food Phytochemicals for Cancer Prevention I and II. Series 546, 547. American Chemical Society. Washington D.C.

Salunkhe and Kadam. 1995. Handbook of Fruits Science and Technology: Production, Composition, Storage, and Processing. Marcel Dekker, Inc.

Salunkhe and Kadam. 1998. Handbook of Vegetable Science and Technology. Marcel Dekker, Inc.

Sen, Packer, and Hänninen. 1994. Exercise and Oxygen Toxicity. Elsevier.

Shahidi. 1997. Natural Antioxidants. AOCS Press. Champaign, Illinois.

Shibamoto, Terao and Osawa. 1998. Functional Foods for Disease Prevention. Medicinal plants and other foods. American Chemical Society. Oxford University Press.

Shibamoto, Terao and Osawa. 1998. Functional Foods for Disease Prevention I. Fruits, Vegetables and Teas. American Chemical Society. Oxford University Press.

Shils, Olson, Shike and Ross. 1999. Modern Nutrition in Health and Disease 9th Edition. Williams and Wilkins, a Waverly Company.

Sizer and Whitney. 1997. Nutrition: Concepts and Controversies. West/ Wadsworth.

Smolin and Grosvenor. 2000. Nutrition: Science and Applications 3rd Edition. Saunders College Publishing. Harcourt College Publishers.

Smythies. 1998. Every Person's Guide to Antioxidants. Rutgers University Press.

Spatz and Bloom. 1992. Biological Consequences of Oxadative Stress: Implications for Cardiovascular Disease and Carcinogenesis. Oxford University Press.

Stafford. 1990. Flavonoid Metabolism. CRC Press, Inc.

Stryer. 1988. Biochemistry 3rd Edition. W.H. Freeman and Company. New York.

Stryer. 1995. Biochemistry 4th Edition. W.H. Freeman and Company. New York.

Sundberg. 1996. Indoles. Academic Press. Harcourt Brace and Company, Publishers.

Tamarin. 1996. Principles of Genetics 5th Edition. WCB Publishers.

The American Institute for Cancer Research. 2000. Stopping Cancer Before It

Starts. St. Martin's Griffin, New York.

Turner and Szczawinski. 1991. Common Poisonous Plants and Mushrooms of North America. Timber Press, Inc.

Voet and Voet. 1990. Biochemistry. John Wiley and Sons.

Voet, Voet and Pratt. 1999. Fundamentals of Biochemistry. John Wiley and Sons.

Waller and Yamasaki. 1996. Saponins Used in Food and Agriculture. Plenum Press.

Waller and Yamasaki.1996. Saponins Used in Traditional and Modern Medicine. Plenum Press.

Wardlaw. 1997. Contemporary Nutrition. Issues and Insights 3rd Edition. Brown and Benchmark Publishers.

Watson, Ronald R. 2000. Vegetables, Fruits, and Herbs in Health Promotion. CRC Press

Weil. 1998. Natural Health, Natural Medicine. Houghton Mifflin Company.

Weil. 2000. Eating Well for Optimum Health. Alfred A. Knopf. New York. Borzoi Book.

White and Selvey. 1974. Nutritional Qualities of Fresh Fruit and Vegetables. Futura Publishing Company.

Wilson and Gillespie. 1997. Rooted in America: Foodlore of Popular Fruits and Vegetables. The University of Tennessee Press.

Wolinsky. 1998. Nutrition in Exercise and Sport 3rd Edition. CRC Press.

Yang and Tanaka. 1999. Advances in Plant Glycosides, Chemistry and Biology. Elsevier Science B.V.

Zappia, Salvatore, and Ragione. 1993. Advances in Nutrition and Cancer. Plenum Press.

Zappia, Ragione, Barbarisi, Russo and Dello Iacovo. 1999. Advances in Nutrition and Cancer 2. Kluwer Academic/Plemun Publishers.

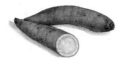

Index

About the Authors

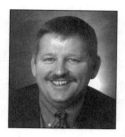

KIM O'NEILL, PH.D., is a professor in Microbiology at Brigham Young University and serves as Associate Director of the Brigham Young University Cancer Research Center. He received his Doctorate in Biomedical Sciences from the University of Ulster in Northern Ireland. His impressive credentials include over 75 published scientific papers in cancer research and over 100 professional presentations. Dr. O'Neill invented the TK1 Monoclonal Immunoassay, an inexpensive, highly accurate cancer-detection instrument. He belongs to a number of societies, including the American Association for Cancer Research, the American Society for Microbiology, the American Society for Cell Biology, and the Environment Mutagen Society.

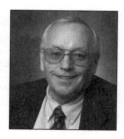

BYRON MURRAY, PH.D., served as the Director of the Brigham Young University Cancer Research Center and continues to serve on the Board of Directors. He received his Doctorate in Microbiology from Brigham Young University and has over 30 years' experience in medical research. Dr. Murray's research includes studies of infectious disease prevention by medicinal plant compounds, cancer prevention by vitamins in fruits and vegetables, and the biochemistry of nutritional phytochemicals, from which there are numerous peer reviewed papers and presentations at national and international scientific meetings. He belongs to a number of societies. including the American Association for Cancer Research, the American Society for Microbiology, and the American Association for the Advancement of Science.